Supportive Care in Radiotherapy

For my parents, my husband and my daughters
MW

For David and William for their laughter and perspective
SF

*And for every person who has to go through radiotherapy treatment,
in the hope that the care they receive is supportive in its widest sense*

MW and SF

For Churchill Livingstone:

Senior Commissioning Editor: Ninette Premdas
Project Development Manager: Dinah Thom
Project Manager: Samantha Ross
Design Direction: Judith Wright

Supportive Care in Radiotherapy

Edited by

Sara Faithfull BSc(Hons) MSc PhD RGN Onc Cert ILTM
Senior Lecturer (Clinical) in Advanced Practice, European Institute of Health and
Medical Sciences, University of Surrey, Guildford, UK

Mary Wells BSc(Hons) MSc RGN Onc Cert
Lecturer and Clinical Research Fellow in Cancer Nursing,
School of Nursing and Midwifery, University of Dundee,
Ninewells Hospital and Medical School, Dundee, UK

Foreword by

Jessica Corner BSc PhD
Professor in Cancer and Palliative Care, School of Nursing and Midwifery,
University of Southampton, Southampton, UK

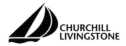
CHURCHILL
LIVINGSTONE

EDINBURGH LONDON NEW YORK OXFORD PHILADELPHIA ST LOUIS SYDNEY TORONTO 2003

Dawson Books   unv. C862324
22/03/04   €18.95

CHURCHILL LIVINGSTONE
An imprint of Elsevier Science Limited

First published 2003

ISBN 0 443 06486 5

British Library Cataloguing in Publication Data
A catalogue record for this book is available from the British Library.

Library of Congress Cataloging in Publication Data
A catalog record for this book is available from
the Library of Congress.

Notice
Medical knowledge is constantly changing. Standard safety
precautions must be followed, but as new research and clinical
experience broaden our knowledge, changes in treatment and drug
therapy may become necessary or appropriate. Readers are advised to
check the most current product information provided by the
manufacturer of each drug to be administered to verify the
recommended dose, the method and duration of administration, and
contraindications. It is the responsibility of the practitioner, relying on
experience and knowledge of the patient, to determine dosages and
the best treatment for each individual patient. Neither the Publisher
nor the authors assume any liability for any injury and/or damage to
persons or property arising from this publication.

The Publisher

The URLs quoted were correct at the time of going to press,
however, information on the internet, including URLs,
are subject to constant change.

your source for books,
journals and multimedia
in the health sciences
www.elsevierhealth.com

The
publisher's
policy is to use
paper manufactured
from sustainable forests

II

Printed in China by RDC Group Limited

Contents

Contributors

Douglas Adamson MD MRCP(UK) FRCR
Consultant Clinical Oncologist, Tayside Institute for Cancer Care, Ninewells Hospital and Medical School, Dundee, UK

Hazel Colyer BA(Hons) MA TDCR(T) SRR
Principal Lecturer and Programme Director, MSc Interprofessional Health and Social Care, Faculty of Health, Canterbury Christ Church University College, Canterbury, UK

Helen Dryden BSc(Hons) RGN RM MN(CancerNursing) CeLTHE
Macmillan Clinical Nurse Specialist Palliative Care, Macmillan Hospital Palliative Care Team, Ninewells Hospital and Medical School,
Dundee, UK

Sara Faithfull BSc(Hons) MSc PhD RN Onc Cert ILTM
Senior Lecturer (Clinical) in Advanced Practice, European Institute of Health and Medical Sciences, University of Surrey, Guildford, UK

Jill Ireland BA(Hons) MSc RGN PgDip (Cancer Care)
Consultant Nurse & Lead Clinician Cancer Care, The Whittington Hospital NHS Trust, London, UK

Vincent Khoo MBBS MD(Lon) FRACR
Senior Lecturer and Honorary Consultant in Radiation Oncology, Academic Department of Radiation Oncology, Christie Hospital, Manchester, UK

Sheila MacBride BSc(Nursing) RGN MN NDN Onc Cert
Macmillan Senior Clinical Nurse Facilitator, Western General Hospital, Edinburgh, UK

Alastair J Munro BSc(Hons) FRCR FRCP (E)
Professor of Radiation Oncology, Department of Surgical and Molecular Oncology, University of Dundee, Ninewells Hospital and Medical School, Dundee, UK

Caroline Nicholson BSc(Hons) MSc RGN HV DN
Lecturer in Palliative Care, Centre for Cancer and Palliative Care Studies, Institute of Cancer Research/Royal Marsden Hospital, London, UK

Mary Wells BSc(Hons) MSc RGN Onc Cert
Lecturer and Clinical Research Fellow in Cancer Nursing, School of Nursing and Midwifery, University of Dundee, Ninewells Hospital and Medical School, Dundee, UK

Isabel White BEd(NursingEd) MSc(Nursing) DipLScNursing RGN RSCN RNT Onc Cert
Lecturer Practitioner in Cancer Care, St Bartholomew's School of Nursing and Midwifery, City University, Barts and the London NHS Trust, London, UK

Angela E Williams BSc(Hons) RGN DipDN
Health Outcomes Manager, Health Outcomes Research Group, GlaxoSmithKline UK Ltd, Hatfield, UK

Foreword

Daily there are news headlines about cancer and cancer treatment. We are showered with media stories of scientific discoveries and new treatments, heralding a new age when cancer will no longer be the scourge it is now portrayed to be. The counterpoint to these discovery stories are those of inadequate cancer services: delayed and mistaken diagnoses, unacceptably long waiting times for treatment, damaging and disfiguring treatments, insensitive communication, insufficient information. It seems that cancer is a huge industry, and at the same time an isolating experience of personal tragedy made worse by scientific aspiration and healthcare's failure to address what is personal and everyday about having cancer.

If cancer is an industry, then, like any other, it has its glossy showrooms or front of house areas as well as its dusty cupboards and back corridors, cancer biology, genetics and drug discovery being the former; vast industrial processes, brilliant minds, Nobel prizes, and occasionally progress so that lives are saved. Radiotherapy treatment and care, on the other hand, might be better represented metaphorically as one of a number of dusty cupboards. Beyond the huge machines needed to deliver treatment, it cannot be commodified in the ways in which chemotherapy agents are and therefore it is of little interest to the pharmaceutical or other health-related industries. For some reason it has not entered the popular, nor indeed the professional imagination as life-saving treatment in the way that chemotherapy has. Yet radiotherapy plays a central role in the treatment of cancer and around half of people with cancer have radiotherapy at some time during their illness.

Radiotherapy, it seems, has been rather neglected and there is a lack of detailed research into the experience of treatment. Little work has been undertaken into the various physical, social and emotional effects of treatment or into the kinds of support people undergoing radiotherapy or living with the short- and long-term effects of treatment need. There has been an emphasis on getting the job of radiotherapy treatment done, on ways of working out the right dose of therapy, and on measuring the ways in which radiotherapy is toxic. There has unfortunately been a lack of serious scholarship into aspects of care and into understanding what it is like to be treated with radiotherapy.

Sarah Cutler (1996) in *A Survivor's Tale* describes her experience of her husband's radiotherapy treatment.

To reach the radiation laboratory [Mike] journeys by wheelchair, later by trolley, down several floors and through a building complex to the basement of another. There he waits his turn among other miserable human beings in various stages of debilitation. Some speak in hushed tones with relatives whose faces are creased with worry... Others, more dead than alive, lie mute and hollow eyed on trolleys... 'Halloween' masks moulded to the features of those receiving brain irradiation are stacked on the floor against the concrete walls ... Each symbolises a family's tragedy, a grim reminder, should one be needed, that ours is shared suffering.

Stopping treatment was no less difficult. Sarah Cutler describes her meeting with the doctor who broke the news to her that treatment should stop because it wasn't doing any good, as *'bearing all the marks of a hit and run accident'*. While this account tells you little about the physical effects of radiotherapy treatment, it highlights how traumatic it can be, and how as health professionals we may be unaware of the wider experience of treatment or its effect on family members and carers. If this kind of experience is typical, then something must be seriously amiss with the territory that might be called 'supportive care in radiotherapy'.

As the title suggests, this book seeks to redress the lack of attention to the experience of radiotherapy, particularly, although not exclusively, from the point of view of those undergoing radiotherapy treatment, and from the point of view of those trying to organise radiotherapy services. One conclusion that could be drawn from reading this book is that there may be value in founding a new area of work into supportive care in radiotherapy.

As with other forms of cancer treatment, radiotherapy is difficult and demanding. Treatment frequently requires daily trips to hospital, may cause an array of short- and long-term side effects, and finishing treatment, although a relief, also entails a loss of close contact with the cancer treatment team. Despite the demanding nature of treatment, little information exists about what to expect of radiotherapy treatment or how to manage physical and other problems that arise. There has been relatively little discussion about how to establish and maintain effective multidisciplinary teams that can offer supportive care to people undergoing treatment or about how best to structure services to optimise treatment within a highly supportive environment.

This book may represent the first serious attempt to collate into a single volume such evidence that exists so that it is made available to treatment teams. One hopes that it will provide a springboard for wider activity and interest as well as being a useful resource for those studying radiotherapy treatment and care. If it succeeds in this ambitious task, then an important step forward will have been achieved.

Jessica Corner

REFERENCES

Cutler S 1996 A Survivor's Tale. The Pharos, Spring 37–40

Preface

Most radiotherapy textbooks concentrate on the principles of treatment and the technical aspects of planning and treatment delivery. In contrast, this book addresses the supportive care of patients undergoing this high-tech treatment. By considering the experience and impact of treatment on the individual alongside the assessment and management of radiation toxicity, it aims to place the experience of radiotherapy in context. Issues relating to the technical, scientific and organisational aspects of radiotherapy care are brought together with those related to the physical and psychosocial side effects of treatment.

The first six chapters of the book address the challenges of radiotherapy care today, highlighting organisational and psychosocial issues at different stages of the treatment trajectory, and clarifying the radiobiological basis of side effects and the importance of assessment. Chapters 7–13 deal with the general and site-specific acute effects of radiotherapy, using evidence from research and clinical experience to provide strategies and suggestions for the assessment and management of individual symptoms. The underlying problems facing patients with cancer are considered in tandem with the additional issues arising as a result of radiotherapy. Finally, Chapters 14–19 summarise the potential late effects of radiotherapy treatment, illustrating the fact that the impact of radiotherapy can be felt long after treatment is ended. Throughout the book we have highlighted areas for further research, and key clinical points for practice.

This book is aimed primarily at nurses and therapy radiographers caring for patients having radiotherapy, but it will also be relevant to hospital and community doctors and nurses who encounter patients before, during and after radiotherapy. We hope that it will inform both undergraduate and postgraduate teaching so that this important but neglected area of oncology practice has a more central place in the education of future cancer care practitioners. Finally, we hope that the book will stimulate further research and discussion into the development of supportive care in radiotherapy.

Mary Wells
Sara Faithfull

Dundee and London 2003

Acknowledgements

This book stems from a joint conviction that patients' needs for supportive care during radiotherapy are not fully addressed. Many people have influenced the development of the book's philosophy and we are indebted to them. We particularly want to acknowledge all the patients who have shared their experiences with us and have been so honest about what it really feels like to have radiotherapy. We also want to thank the nurses, oncologists and therapy radiographers we have worked with over the last 15 years, many of whom have contributed to our vision of what supportive care should be. Our experiences at Barts, the Royal Marsden, Oxford and Dundee have shaped the way in which we have approached this book. There are a number of specific individuals who deserve particular mention: Louise Becker, Nancy Hallett, Sally Dickinson, the nursing and medical staff of Heath Harrison Ward in the early 1990s, Jessica Corner, Anne Lanceley, Chris Alcock, Rebecca Davis, David Dearnaley, Sarah Helyer, Bridget Suter and, of course, our families, who have put up with our involvement in this all-consuming project. We would also like to acknowledge the support and forbearance of colleagues at our respective workplaces: the School of Nursing and Midwifery and Ninewells Hospital, Dundee and the Centre for Cancer and Palliative Care Studies, Institute of Cancer Research. We hope that this book gives them some return on their investment.

Abbreviations

5-HT	5-hydroxytryptamine
ACE	angiotensin-converting enzyme
ALARM	activity, libido, arousal, resolution, medical history
AUA	American Urological Association
BACUP	British Association of Cancer United Patients
BCG	bacillus Calmette-Guérin
BDS	beam directional shell
BED	biologically effective dose
BMI	body mass index
BS	British Standard
BTE	basic treatment equivalent
CHART	continuous hyperfractionated accelerated radiotherapy
CHI	Centre for Health Improvement
CNS	central nervous system
CoR	College of Radiographers
CPD	continuing professional development
CSB	Clinical Standards Board Scotland
CT	computerised tomography
CTC	common toxicity criteria
CTV	clinical target volume
CTZ	chemoreceptor trigger zone
DNA	deoxyribonucleic acid
DoH	Department of Health
DXT	deep X-ray therapy
EBM	evidence-based medicine
ECOG	Eastern Cooperative Oncology Group
EORTC	European Organisation for Research and Treatment of Cancer
EU	European Union
FACT	Functional Assessment of Cancer Therapy
FBC	full blood count
FLIC	Functional Living Index – Cancer
FSH	follicle-stimulating hormone
G-CSF	granulocyte colony-stimulating factor
GM-CSF	granulocyte-macrophage colony-stimulating factor
GM%	gram percentage
GP	general practitioner

GTV	gross tumour volume
Gy	gray
HAD	Hospital Anxiety and Depression scale
HBO	hyperbaric oxygen
HDR	high-dose-rate
HRQOL	health-related quality of life
HTBS	Health Technology Board for Scotland
IASP	International Association for the Study of Pain
ICSI	intracytoplasmic sperm injection
IGRT	image-guided radiation therapy
Il-1	interleukin-1
IM	interal margin
IMRT	intensity-modulated radiotherapy
IPSS	International Prostate Symptom Score
ISL	International Society of Lymphology
LA	linear accelerator
LDR	low-dose-rate
LENTSOMA	Late Effects Normal Tissues/Subjective/Objective/Management/Analytic
LET	linear energy transfer
LH	luteinising hormone
MDR	medium-dose-rate
MIBG	metaiodobenzylguanidine
MLC	multileaf collimation
MLD	manual lymphatic drainage
MPA	medroxyprogesterone acetate
MRC	Medical Research Council
MRI	magnetic resonance imaging
MST	malnutrition screening tool
MV	megavolts
NCRI	National Cancer Research Institutes
NHP-1	Nottingham Health Profile Part 1
NHS	National Health Service
NICE	National Institute for Clinical Effectiveness
NMC	Nursing and Midwifery Council
NSAID	non-steroidal anti-inflammatory drug
OECD	Organisation for Economic Cooperation and Development
PAIS	Psychological Adjustment to Illness Scale
PEG	percutaneous endoscopic gastrostomy
PET	positron emission tomography
PGI	patient-generated index of quality of life
PNS	peripheral nervous system
PTV	planning target volume
PUC	probability of uncomplicated cure
QLQ	quality-of-life questionnaire
RAGE	Radiation Action Group Exposure
RBE	relative biological effectiveness
RCN	Royal College of Nursing

RCR	Royal College of Radiologists
RCT	randomised controlled trial
RISRAS	Radiation-Induced Skin Reaction Assessment Scale
RNA	ribonucleic acid
RP	radiation pneumonitis
RSCL	Rotterdam Symptom Checklist
RTOG	Radiation Therapy Oncology Group
SCCAC	Scottish Cancer Co-ordinating and Advisory Committee
SEIQoL	schedule for the evaluation of individual quality of life
SGA	subjective global assessment
SIGN	Scottish Intercollegiate Guidelines Network
SM	set-up margin
SoDoH	Scottish Office Department of Health
START	Standardisation of Breast Radiotherapy Trial
TBI	total body irradiation
TCP	tumour control probability
TENS	transcutaneous electrical nerve stimulation
TGF-α	transforming growth factor-alpha
TGF-β	transforming growth factor-beta
THC	terazosin hydrochloride
TNF	tumour necrosis factor
TPN	total parenteral nutrition
TURP	transurethral resection of the prostate
U&E	urea and electrolytes
UKCC	UK Central Council
WHO	World Health Organization

1

The context of radiotherapy care

Hazel Colyer

INTRODUCTION: THE ORGANISATION AND STRUCTURE OF RADIOTHERAPY IN THE UK

There are currently 64 centres in the UK in which radiotherapy treatment is delivered; most are discrete units with dedicated professional, technical support and administrative staff. People with cancer who may require a course of radiotherapy are referred to the treatment centre for assessment and, where appropriate, a treatment regime is planned and delivered. This regime may be curative or palliative in intent and is frequently given in conjunction with surgery and cytotoxic chemotherapy. Supportive care is an integral part of the process of treatment and must take account of the combined effects of these other therapies as well as the effects of the radiotherapy. The quality of care given within and across the different elements of the cancer care system depends on a thorough understanding of the structures and relationships that support each one. The purpose of this chapter is to provide an insight into the complex organisational and unique interprofessional context of radiotherapy care.

Since the implementation of the Report of the expert advisory group on cancer to the chief medical officers of England and Wales (DoH 1995), and the corresponding Scottish Cancer Co-ordinating and Advisory Committee (SCCAC) report (1996), radiotherapy departments are all almost entirely located in designated cancer centres. The Calman–Hine Report, as the English report is better known, is founded on the principle of networking expertise to promote collaborative care pathways, advocating a 'hub-and-spoke' approach, with the cancer centre at the hub, and the majority of care being delivered within the primary sector. Common cancers are assessed and managed in designated cancer units by clinical teams with sufficient expertise, and rare cancers are referred to cancer centres, where expertise is most concentrated. Each cancer network has developed as a 'virtual service organisation' with its own management board. Its purpose is to ensure that patients follow a seamless pathway of care, which is appropriate to them as individuals, but is also managed systematically to promote consistency and improve patient outcomes (DoH 2000a).

1

The hallmarks of a cancer centre are specialist expertise and comprehensive care provision. The Calman–Hine report suggests that radiotherapy should normally be confined to centres, although it recognises that, when geographical access is difficult due to distance, a cancer unit may continue to provide a limited radio-therapy service. The report became the blueprint for the subsequent government initiatives to develop national service frameworks (DoH 1998) – specific managed-care groups, based on sound evidence, whose purpose is to ensure that patients receive consistent, optimal standards of seamless care through interprofessional team working.

Like the majority of health services, radiotherapy departments developed through the twentieth century on an ad hoc basis, triggered by scientific discover-ies and increasing clinical experience. Departments grew out of diagnostic radiog-raphy units with the discovery that X-rays could not only be used to image bone and other body structures, but were also useful in the treatment of cancerous tumours. Deep X-ray therapy (DXT) departments emerged in the 1930s, usually with one or two superficial and deep X-ray machines. Gradually, departments evolved into today's sophisticated centres of clinical oncology, as they are now widely known. The change in terminology from radiotherapy to clinical oncology reflects the enormous increase in the number and range of cancer therapies avail-able in most departments, often including access to complementary therapies, which have been shown to improve symptoms and coping in patients with cancer (White 1998).

Initially concentrated in urban areas and teaching hospitals, radiotherapy departments in other areas of the UK developed to meet the needs of rural popula-tions. The high capital and revenue costs of maintaining and investing in services led to a rationalisation in the latter part of the twentieth century, with many small departments closing and a smaller number of large ones opening. Unfortunately, this pattern of service development inevitably created inequity of access. It remains the case that London is well provided for, having 11 departments to serve six million people, while a single centre such as Glasgow serves a population of almost 3 million in the west of Scotland and central belt (Royal College of Radiologists 2000a).

Cancer centres generally cater for populations of between one and two million people. The effective management of several thousand courses of radiotherapy treatment annually poses a significant challenge for each centre, compounded in less densely populated areas where public transport is limited and geographical access difficult. Survival of some small departments existing at the time of the implementation of the Calman–Hine report has been achieved through the estab-lishment of close links with the nearest cancer centre. However, it must be acknowledged that current government policy is predicated on the philosophy that excellence accrues with experience and, therefore, big is beautiful. This has proved a difficult concept for the general public who want local, accessible services. Indeed, the small improvements in overall 5-year survival which may be achieved in centres of excellence for the fewer number of radiocurable cancers have to be set against the inconveniences caused to many patients requiring palliative care, for whom travel difficulties or separation from carers during treatment impacts on both their perception of a quality service and their quality of life.

INFRASTRUCTURE – EQUIPMENT AND STAFF

External beam (teletherapy) equipment producing photons (X-rays) or electrons delivers the majority of radiotherapy treatment. Depending on its energy, the radiation beam deposits a dose of ionising radiation at a specific depth in tissue, measured in Gray (Gy) or centiGray (cGy). The standard treatment unit is the linear accelerator (LA), which operates at a range of specified energies, usually between 6 and 25 megavolts (MV), for both photons and electrons. LAs have sophisticated computerised treatment delivery systems and can deliver tumoricidal doses of radiation to customised treatment volumes in any anatomical site. They generally also have 'record and verify' information systems to assist in patient set-up and information management, and portal imaging systems, which monitor the beam position during treatment delivery and permit field placement errors to be rectified. Using current parameters, it is recommended that departments require four LAs per million population, together with appropriate supporting technology for tumour localisation and planning (Royal College of Radiologists 1991, 1996a). Ideally, machines should be networked together so that patients can easily be transferred to a different machine at times of machine service or breakdown. Many of the UK's existing LAs have outlived their useful lifespan, resulting in a need for major capital investment, much of which is being channelled through the New Opportunities fund. The English NHS *Cancer Plan* (DoH 2000a) suggests that the target for machine replacement and commissioning will be met by 2003, but the Scottish plan (Scottish Executive Health Department 2001) is less specific.

In addition to its LAs, a department will also house a variable energy superficial X-ray machine for the treatment of skin cancers and other superficial lesions. Occasionally, cobalt-60 external beam therapy machines can still be found. These contain a large radioactive source which, when exposed, delivers gamma radiation of skin-sparing energy, comparable to the lower range of an LA. Smaller radioactive sources such as caesium-137 and iridium-192, which emit beta and gamma radiation, are also used for intracavitary or interstitial (brachy)therapy. When a radioactive source is placed in or in proximity to tissue, the dose delivered remains more localised, thus protecting surrounding normal tissues. This enables higher radiation doses to be delivered to the target volume. Unsealed radioactive sources, e.g. iodine-131 and metaiodobenzyl-guanadine (MIBG), may also be used in the management of some conditions such as thyroid disorders and carcinoid syndrome. Responsibility for their dispensing and administration usually rests with the nuclear medicine department. The use of both sealed and unsealed radioactive sources raises significant radiation protection issues due to the continuous emission of radiation and the requirement for safe disposal of unsealed source waste.

Ionising radiations do not distinguish between cancerous and normal tissues per se; therefore successful radiotherapy treatment depends on optimising the dose to the tumour and minimising damage to normal tissue, a delicate balance called the therapeutic ratio (Neal & Hoskin 1997). This requires accurate localisation of the clinical target volume (CTV) and delineation of a planning target volume (PTV), which accounts for any potential subclinical spread of the tumour and avoids sensitive normal structures (Fig. 1.1).

This process is accomplished through simulation of the intended treatment area and localisation of the proposed volume using either diagnostic X-rays, or,

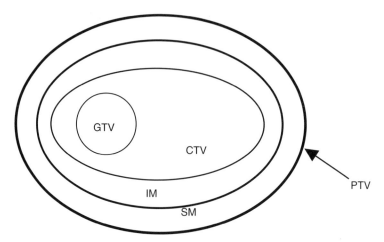

Figure 1.1 Delineation of the planning target volume (PTV). GTV, gross tumour volume (area of tumour itself). CTV, clinical target volume (GTV + an added margin to contain subclinical disease). IM, internal margin (CTV + a margin to compensate for changes in the position, size and shape of the CTV relative to a fixed anatomical point, e.g. vertebra. These changes may occur as a result of breathing, blood flow, peristalsis, patient movement, bladder and bowel filling, tumour shrinkage or weight loss). SM, set-up margin (added to account for uncertainties in day-to-day set-up and variations in beam position and alignment). PTV, planning target volume (CTV with added margins to ensure that the prescribed dose is actually delivered to the CTV). Courtesy of Prof. AJ Munro.

increasingly, computed tomography (CT) and magnetic resonance imaging (MRI). Following localisation, computerised treatment planning systems are used to create a treatment plan which gives a homogeneous dose of radiation to the PTV while reducing normal tissue doses to acceptable levels.

If people with cancer are to receive quality care during their cancer journey, i.e. the right modality at the right time with the right level of information and support, then such a complex undertaking demands multiprofessional input and good interprofessional teamwork both within and without the clinical oncology department. Increasingly, this is facilitated by computerised information management systems, which both enable the flow of patient information and help to support communication and liaison between staff groups.

A referral for radiotherapy is made to a clinical oncologist who has overall clinical responsibility for the patient and the radiotherapy prescription. Clinical oncologists generally have site-specific expertise; they see new patients, identify CTVs and PTVs, confirm acceptability of the treatment plan and prescribe the dose/fractionation schedule. They may review patients during treatment, although radiographers and nurses are increasingly assuming this role.

The largest professional group in clinical oncology is made up of therapeutic radiographers, with an estimated 1480 whole-time-equivalent posts in the UK (Abraham et al 1999). Radiographers have a dual role: the safe, accurate, effective use of radiation technology and the provision of continuous, treatment-specific care, support and information to individual patients. This role extends across the continuum of radiotherapy treatment delivery from localisation, target delineation, planning and dosimetry to management and verification of the treatment and follow-up. Because of the complexity of this continuum, radiographers tend to specialise and there is a broad division between 'pre-treatment' (simulation and planning) and 'treatment' specialist roles, with further differentiation into site-specific groups. Many departments also have specialist information and support radiographers (Colyer & Hlahla 1999), often funded by charitable bodies such as the Macmillan Cancer Relief Fund.

Scientific and technical support is given by medical physicists who provide a specialist physics service to the clinical oncology department, comprising both hands-on and quality management expertise related to brachytherapy, external beam treatment planning, radiation protection, computing, dosimetry, commissioning of radiotherapy equipment and development.

Specialist and outpatient nurses also play a vital role in radiotherapy departments, providing clinical and supportive care to patients on treatment. Wells (1998) highlights some of the historical factors which have delayed the development of specialist nursing roles in radiotherapy, and argues that nurses have a unique contribution to make, complementary to that of their radiographer colleagues. The Calman–Hine report (DoH 1995) stated that nursing care in cancer centres should be led by nurses with at least a postregistration cancer qualification and suggested that the nursing service should be structured so as to enable patients access to specialist nurses; for example, those in breast care and lymphoedema management. The Royal College of Radiologists (RCR) has also endorsed the role of nurses within radiotherapy departments, recognising their potential to contribute to supportive care (RCR, College of Radiographers (CoR) and Royal College of Nursing (RCN) 1999).

It is generally accepted that there are major staff shortages in clinical oncology which are impeding service quality. An RCR report (RCR 2000b) stated that 70% of radiotherapy departments are not meeting the standards for radiographer staffing in the UK. Although the government has proposed measures to increase staffing establishments in England, no specific recommendations for training, recruitment or retention are made in the Scottish cancer plan. The English *NHS Cancer Plan* proposes a 49% increase in clinical oncologists by the year 2005–2006, from 305 to 453, with smaller increases for therapists and medical physicists (DoH 2000a). A number of national initiatives are under way to support these ambitious targets, including government-sponsored projects within the modernising education and training agenda (DoH 2000b).

However, it is also accepted that the proper care of patients is dependent not only on numbers, but also on good interprofessional collaboration and teamwork, particularly where the roles and responsibilities of team members may be blurred rather than professionally demarcated (RCR and CoR 1999). Wengstrom & Haggmark (1998) identified that lack of communication, lack of knowledge of their work and competence, and lack of comprehension of each other's professions were significant problems for nurses working in radiotherapy. It could be argued that these problems are magnified for therapeutic radiographers, without whom radiotherapy treatment could not take place, but whose needs and development were given little attention in strategic documents until recently (DoH 2000a, Scottish Executive Health Department 2001). However, the joint publications by the professional bodies highlighted above have endorsed the development of new ways of working, which are improving the quality of patient care within existing staffing levels. These are discussed in more detail below.

CURRENT PRACTICES IN RADIOTHERAPY

Radiotherapy continues to play a crucial role in the curative and palliative treatment of cancer. Many common cancers have poor overall 5-year survival rates – less than 10% for lung cancer and less than 40% for cancer of the colon (DoH 2000a). For radiocurable tumours, suitability for treatment by radiotherapy depends on the possibility of exploiting the therapeutic ratio. However, the often narrow differential between the dose required to produce lethal damage to the tumour and that which causes irreversible damage in normal tissues makes it difficult to achieve a radical, tumoricidal dose without causing considerable, sometimes unacceptable, radiation morbidity. In order to preserve normal tissue, treatment may inevitably be suboptimal. Current technological developments hold out the promise that real improvements may occur in both the process of treatment and also in the proportion of patients achieving complete local control of their disease.

A technically successful course of radical radiotherapy is dependent on a number of factors:

- accurate localisation and assessment of the clinical target volume
- effective patient immobilisation to ensure reproducibility of position both for planning and on each occasion of treatment
- correct delineation of the PTV
- production of a treatment plan which delivers a uniformly high dose of radiation to the PTV whilst sparing radiosensitive critical structures and normal tissues
- selection of the optimal dose/fractionation schedule
- accurate, consistent setting-up and execution of the treatment prescription.

Each step in this process involves cooperation, liaison and mutual respect between the different staff groups if the patient's progress is to be as seamless as possible.

Following referral and consultation, accurate localisation and staging of tumours using an X-ray simulator, CT or MRI scanner is the first crucial pre-treatment stage. It includes consideration of patient immobilisation and, in the case of people with head and neck tumours, the production of a close-fitting perspex shell to be worn during treatment. A further appointment may be necessary to fit the shell and for outlines to be taken of the patient's contour at various levels throughout the proposed treatment volume. Sometimes these outlines are taken directly from the CT or MRI scans and the data entered into the treatment planning system. The clinical oncologist delineates the CTV and PTV, together with any critical structures, and a treatment plan is computed. This normally comprises a complex, multiple-field arrangement.

In the past, treatment machines could only produce beams (fields) which were square or rectangular, and any change in shape was achieved by placing lead blocks between the machine and the patient. Variations in beam intensity across the field could only be achieved by the use of simple wedges or tissue compensators, similarly positioned. Recent equipment developments, involving multileaf collimators and three-dimensional inverse treatment-planning systems, permit irregularly shaped treatment fields which can be more closely conformed to the CTV and produce complex variations in beam intensity across the field. This technology is called intensity modulated radiotherapy or IMRT. These advances hold out the possibility of decreasing treatment margins and enabling dose escalation across PTVs, with a concomitant increase in tumour control probability (TCP). The effect of introducing such complex technology is an increase in the number of fields per patient and a greater workload.

Recommended good practice is for radical radiotherapy to begin within 2 weeks of referral (RCR 1996a). The proposed radiotherapy treatment plan must be verified, either on the simulator or using a portal imaging system, before the first treatment can be given. This can be a difficult period for patients at a time of immense uncertainty in their lives. Patients may feel that, having been diagnosed with cancer, treatment should begin immediately, hence they may find the pre-treatment period difficult to accept or understand. The importance of this preparation period cannot, however, be overstated; there is only one chance to get radical radiotherapy right.

Following localisation and planning, radical radiotherapy frequently extends over a 5 or 6 week period, and patients require support and encouragement to persevere, not least because of the side effects associated with treatment. On average, a multiple-field treatment takes 10 min to complete. The patient is immobilised in the treatment position and the machine is positioned accurately using the parameters on the treatment plan. While the radiographers set and deliver the precise radiation dose for each treatment field, the patient remains alone in the treatment room.

Brachytherapy may be administered using high-dose rate (HDR), medium-dose rate (MDR) or, rarely, low-dose rate (LDR) equipment. Radioactive sources are stored in protected containers and moved by remote control to prepositioned applicators, either in body cavities or directly into tissues – a technique called afterloading. When MDR is used to treat gynaecological cancers, for example, treatment may take between 24 and 48 h to complete. Such equipment is usually sited in specially designated wards in the hospital. Patients are anaesthetised for the positioning of the applicators and, after their position has been checked, they are loaded with the radioactive sources in the ward. Sources can be withdrawn for short periods to enable nursing staff to give care without being unnecessarily exposed to radiation. Interstitial afterloading therapy can be used to treat cancers of the tongue, breast, anus and prostate, but these sources cannot generally be removed during treatment.

HDR brachytherapy equipment, used mainly for the treatment of bronchial, oesophageal and gynaecological cancers, is generally sited in the clinical oncology department. After applicators have been positioned and checked for accuracy, the patient receives a single fraction of treatment lasting only a few minutes, normally as a day case, although a second fraction may be given 1 or 2 weeks later, depending on the dose/fractionation schedule. Brachytherapy is not available in every UK centre, as its use often depends on the existence of a clinician with specialist interest and expertise in the modality.

THE DELIVERY OF TREATMENT

It is estimated by Blyth et al (2001) that approximately 50% of patients attending a clinical oncology department are receiving palliative treatment, the aim of which is to relieve symptoms without adding to the burden of illness. Whilst care must be taken to ensure that target volumes are localised accurately, there is less need to apply the rigorous standards of radical treatment delivery. Generally, palliative techniques are simple, the number of treatments is kept to a minimum and treatment takes place as soon as possible after referral, often on the same day. The comfort of the patient is a more effective predictor of immobilisation than a technical device and the appropriate dose should be determined by the degree to which symptom control, such as pain relief or haemostasis, is achieved. Nevertheless, it is most important to ensure that doses are biologically effective.

The biological radiation dose has three components: number of fractions, overall treatment time and total dose. Fractionating the dose permits a larger overall total dose to be given to the tumour, while small fractions minimise normal tissue effects. The aim of treatment is to optimise the tumour dose whilst permitting recovery of normal tissues. Clinical oncology departments use a great variety of dose/fractionation schedules, the rationale for which is often historical. These differences may or may not be biologically significant. Comparisons can be made between the practices of different departments by calculating the biologically effective dose (BED) for a particular treatment regime (Jones et al 2001). Such calculations also demonstrate when treatment regimes are suboptimal. Current clinical research studies, such as the Standardisation of Breast Radiotherapy Trial (START) trial for breast cancer treatment, are seeking to optimise and standardise dose/fractionation schedules nationwide.

Historically, many centres adopted the 'gold standard' course of radical radiotherapy treatment; 60 Gy in 30 daily fractions, given Monday to Friday, over 6 weeks. Biologically equivalent variations of this regime exist, incorporating permutations of larger fractions, fewer fractions and reduced overall treatment times. Most clinical oncology departments, however, employ a variety of schedules. Although increasing numbers of protocols exist to guide the radiotherapy management of specific tumour sites, individual clinicians still exercise their clinical freedom to prescribe whatever dose/fractionation schedule they believe is in the patient's best interest.

The weekend break was, and still is, seen as recovery time for patients (and staff). However, following mounting evidence about the detrimental effect on tumour control of unplanned extensions of overall treatment time caused by machine breakdown or patients being unfit for treatment, guidelines for the management of treatment gaps were published (RCR 1996b). These identify patients at risk and advocate the development of local protocols to ensure that overall treatment times are maintained, by transferring patients to other machines in the event of equipment failure and treating patients during public holidays to minimise the effect of long breaks. However, as James (1997) pointed out, the implications of these guidelines for such a complex, labour-intensive service, depending as it does on major technical and clinical support, are considerable.

Similarly, there is strong evidence for the effectiveness of accelerated treatments such as continuous hyperfractionated accelerated radiotherapy (CHART) in the local control of lung and head and neck tumours (Saunders et al 1988). The CHART regime comprises three fractions per day given daily for 12 days – a total dose of 54 Gy in 36 fractions over 12 days. Despite the length of time that has elapsed since the work was published, the subsequent modification of overall time to include a weekend break and confirmation of benefit, this regime has not been adopted widely. Again, the implications it has for service delivery are far-reaching, including the need for patients to be hospitalised during treatment, and the requirement for radiographic, physics and medical staff to provide extended day cover 7 days a week.

Overall, the work of a clinical oncology department is complex, often unpredictable and very diverse in its nature and scope. Each patient with cancer is unique and requires an individualised treatment plan whose execution depends for its success on a range of professional and other personnel who can work together to deliver treatments using sophisticated and potentially dangerous technologies. Patients frequently find this experience difficult and disempowering at a time when many of them are coming to terms with a life-threatening cancer diagnosis.

THE RADIOTHERAPY EXPERIENCE

Of the 200 000 people who are diagnosed with cancer each year, it is estimated that 60% will have contact with secondary or tertiary services. Estimates of the percentage of cancer patients who access radiotherapy services are variable, and inequity of access is likely. It is difficult to find the evidence on which reported rates are based, but the RCR (2000b) has suggested that service planning initiatives should presume that around 45% of cancer patients will require radiotherapy treatment. However, actual workloads are reported by service managers to be increasing by between 7% and 15% per year due to population growth, increasing incidence of cancer and expanding indications for radiotherapy and greater treatment complexity. This is leading to waiting lists that are well in excess of the recommended 2 weeks (RCR 1996a).

What can be said unequivocally is that many people with cancer will have contact with radiotherapy services, either as part of the radical management of their disease or for palliative treatment, with some patients returning several times. Radiotherapy plays a significant role in the management of the most common cancers; breast, lung, colorectal, head and neck, oesophageal, gynaecological, bladder and prostate. It also makes a valuable contribution to the palliation of metastases, particularly those in the bone and brain.

However, a course of radiotherapy is only one part of the cancer journey. Nearly all patients will undergo some kind of surgical procedure to confirm their diagnosis, and many will also require surgical resections prior to or after their radiotherapy treatment. Some may return for further radiotherapy following recurrence or metastasis, and others may require concomitant or adjuvant chemotherapy.

The additional toxicity associated with combined modalities can place an increased burden of side effects on patients.

Typically, the majority of patients attending a clinical oncology department are adult outpatients. During the past 30 years, the management of most childhood cancers has been transformed by the advent of combination chemotherapy, so that radiotherapy treatment in children is now rarely a treatment of choice, except where irradiation of the central nervous system is required. However, both the incidence and prevalence of cancer in adults is increasing, with many more cases in younger adults and many people with cancer surviving for extended periods of time.

Senior staff in the treatment team manage individual machine caseloads. A large number of patients will be having fractionated courses of treatment, requiring multiple attendances on different days of the week. In general, patients are encouraged to make their own way to the department if possible, although a carer will accompany many. Exceptionally, ambulance transport is required, which adds a degree of unpredictability to the treatment schedule. Emergencies also have to be accommodated occasionally, and there are generally a number of inpatients to be fitted into schedules, all of which may cause difficulties for the organisation of workload. This can be particularly complicated where combined chemo/radiotherapy is prescribed. Radiography staff may only be able to treat patients at a specific time, but ward staff first have to ensure that patients are admitted, cannulated, premedicated, comfortable and connected to their chemotherapy infusion, which has to be ordered and obtained from pharmacy.

Greater mutual understanding of the pressures on both ward and machine staff, as well as efficient communication systems, can significantly enhance this process. However, the logistics of planning and organising the work of a clinical oncology department are formidable. A centre serving a population of one million will see approximately 2000 new referrals annually. The national average number of exposures per LA in 1997 was 20 000 (RCR 1998a) and most centres are working extended days, with staff doing shifts to accommodate this. With an LA treating on average between 45 and 55 patients per day, most having an individually planned multiple-field technique, there is enormous pressure on resources. The high throughput of patients inevitably diminishes the quality of care given, with staff having to concentrate on vital technical details, leaving less time to support patients through the experience.

It is difficult to prioritise patients for treatment since all are urgent. With a few exceptions, such as the treatment of someone with spinal cord compression or superior vena cava obstruction, emergencies are rare. In the main, patients are added to waiting lists for treatment according to clinical need, creating further pressure for both patients and staff as these lists build up. *A National Audit of Waiting Times for Radiotherapy* (RCR 1998b) concluded that 28% of patients fell outside their maximum waiting time for treatment to begin and there is evidence that this figure is worsening, despite the government's published targets for referral to treatment times (DoH 2000a). There is also now some evidence that delays in starting treatment may be leading to outcomes being compromised (O'Rourke & Edwards 2000).

All patients receiving radical doses of radiation will experience acute side effects from treatment. These are broadly categorised as systemic and local effects, with many patients experiencing fatigue, anorexia and some degree of nausea. Local effects occur at the site of treatment delivery, and are generally dose- and tissue-dependent. The response of tissues and organs to radiation varies; those with active stem cell and differentiating populations tend to be more radiosensitive, thus the skin, mucous membranes and bone marrow are likely to be most affected by local irradiation. Reactions generally arise within the first 2 weeks of treatment and increase in severity, reaching a peak some 10 days after completion and gradually subsiding within 6 weeks to 6 months. These physical reactions are managed by the staff in the department through a combination of advice, support and medication; radiographers assess patients at each visit and patients are also reviewed more specifically at weekly intervals, increasingly by radiographers or nurses rather than doctors (Campbell et al 2000, Collins 2001, Colyer & Hlahla 1999, Sardell et al 2000).

Chronic effects are those which occur between 6 months and 2 years after treatment has been completed and are usually caused by a decrease in blood supply to the tissue irradiated, leading to fibrosis, stenosis or, in extreme cases, necrosis. Examples of this are restricted shoulder movement, lung fibrosis and increased risk of myocardial infarct in women treated for breast cancer. Treatment is usually restricted to supportive or rehabilitative measures, including, for example, colostomy in the extreme situation where a patient develops a rectovaginal fistula following treatment for cervical cancer. The literature puts the occurrence of long-term side effects at about 5% and it is suggested that optimum tumour control is 'inseparable from acceptance of a long-term complication rate' (RCR 1995, p. 3). More details of late effects can be found in Chapters 14, 18 and 19.

The persistence of radiation side effects and the ever-present risk of tumour recurrence require patients to be followed up regularly by staff from the clinical oncology department. Follow-up clinics are held both at radiotherapy treatment centres and at peripheral hospitals or primary care health centres. Initially patients are seen monthly and this usually extends until the patient is discharged around 5 years later. The value of conventional follow-up clinics is increasingly being questioned; evidence suggests that disease recurrence is not detected at routine clinic visits and that alternative models of supportive follow-up may be more appropriate (Brada 1995, GIVIO Investigations 1994, Moore et al 1999). Current government initiatives are actively encouraging supportive care in the community as the norm, generating the need for closer liaison between primary and secondary services and a sharing of expertise among professional groups.

THE QUALITY OF THE RADIOTHERAPY EXPERIENCE

The picture painted above is of a service under considerable pressure from all directions – increasing incidence of cancer, government directives, more complex equipment and patients living longer than ever before with their disease. The quality of the service provided depends on many factors related to service structure, treatment processes and outcomes measured both in overall survival times and expressed quality of life. The government's modernisation agenda and increased levels of funding may address some of the structural issues around staffing and technology in the longer term, but new trainees in therapeutic radiography, physics and radiation oncology still have to be recruited and educated.

Additionally, there is much to do in relation to the process and outcomes of cancer care and treatment. Giving the right treatment at the right time with the right amount of information and support should therefore be the aim of all staff in clinical oncology departments.

Giving the right treatment at the right time depends crucially on ensuring that the equipment used is functioning optimally and that systems exist to monitor and improve its performance and ensure its effective utilisation. Following two major radiation dose accidents in the late 1980s, a government-sponsored working party under the chairmanship of Professor Bleehan produced a report about quality assurance in radiotherapy (DoH 1991). The report took the form of a quality standard and proposed a system of total quality management for radiotherapy services, using the British Standard (BS) 5750, which had been written for manufacturing practice. The working party decided not to be prescriptive but to recommend its implementation to all clinical oncology departments in England, Wales and Northern Ireland.

Two departments were selected and funded for a comparative study of the feasibility of applying BS5750 to their practice (Scholl-Evans 1992). In one department, the scope was limited to aspects of the work which directly affected the delivery of radiation according to the direction of the prescribing clinicians, while the second took a wider stance, including all activities which contributed to the overall care and treatment of patients having radiotherapy. Positive features identified from the study included enhanced communication between staff groups and departments, clarification of responsibilities and opportunities for review and improvement of working practices. The labour intensive nature of developing quality assurance systems and the subsequent bureaucratisation were noted as the major negative features (DoH 1994). It is interesting that the contentious issue of the quality of clinicians' dose/fractionation prescriptions was excluded from one of the pilot studies.

In 1994, the DoH released an advisory document, *Quality Assurance in Radiotherapy*, containing advice and sample documentation to encourage departments to develop their own systems and seek accreditation from the British Standards Institute when they were ready. By this time, BS5750 had been revised and an international equivalent, BS EN ISO 9000, was published in 1994. This internationally agreed set of standards for the design and implementation of quality management systems has now been adopted throughout the UK. It comprises a series of documents of differing scope, enabling departments of clinical oncology to utilise the most appropriate for their needs.

The introduction of systematic programmes to assure the quality of radiotherapy treatment given to cancer patients seems to have come somewhat late in the day. Departments have always carried out quality control checks of equipment when commissioning and using treatment machines, with responsibility being divided between the radiographers and the physicists. However, the systematic setting and monitoring of technical and care standards to promote improvements in service delivery across the board through the implementation of quality assurance is both recent and optional, rather than mandatory.

During the 1990s, robust data from the Eurocare study (Beerino et al 1995) finally confirmed what many had believed for some time – that people with cancer are more likely to die when treated in the UK than in most European countries. The Calman–Hine report (DoH 1995) can be seen as a recognition of and response to this grim reality; however, the introduction of the clinical governance framework (DoH 1999) into the National Health Service (NHS) has injected a new urgency into the situation.

Clinical governance imposes a duty of quality on service provider organisations with a named person being held responsible (Buetow & Martin 1999). It is a framework for managing and monitoring NHS performance in the context of a nationally coordinated programme of clinical guideline development and service standards. In England and Wales, this takes place under the aegis of the National Institute for Clinical Excellence (NICE) and Commission for Health Improvement (CHI). In Scotland, the Clinical Standards Board (CSBS), Scottish Intercollegiate Guidelines Network (SIGN) and Health Technology Board for Scotland (HTBS) fulfil these roles. Clinical governance is, above all, about changing the culture of healthcare practice to enable excellence to flourish and poor practice to be addressed (DoH 1998). Among others, it is intended to encourage openness, accountability, the sharing of good practice and collaborative working and to dispel secrecy and the 'blame' culture. Its implementation is currently exerting a major influence on the generation and dissemination of outcome data and the development of quality management systems with a focus on the patient's perspective.

Within cancer services in England and Wales, this national service framework is well advanced, with the publication of core standards and performance indicators (NHS Executive 2000) against which organisations are required to produce a self assessment report and are accredited through peer review site visits. Simultaneously, patient pathways and experiences are being reviewed by the CHI. A similar process exists in Scotland, through the publication of standards and minimum data sets by the CSBS and SIGN, which are then monitored through external peer-review visits and reports.

An important aspect of the quality process is the demonstration of clinical competence. The clinical governance framework addresses this through professional self-regulation, rather than the imposition of an external system to monitor professional performance. Underpinning self-regulation is the concept of continuing professional development (CPD) to ensure the maintenance and development of professional knowledge and skills. Individual performance is usually monitored through the staff appraisal system and will shortly be linked to a performance management system of pay and rewards, while registration bodies such as the Health Professions' Council (for radiographers and physicists), NMC (Nursing and Midwifery Council) (for nurses) and General Medical Council (for doctors) are expected to ensure that their members demonstrate appropriate CPD to comply with the criteria for professional registration.

CONCLUSION: A SEAMLESS APPROACH TO CARE AND TREATMENT

It will be apparent from the description of the service given above that the potential exists for fragmentation and lack of coordination of care through poor teamwork and poor communication. Thus, one of the keys to improving the patient's experience of radiotherapy is to develop a genuine interprofessional approach to teamwork, and foster new ways of working. Historically, there has been considerable rigidity in terms of role definition, social status and hierarchy between groups of healthcare professionals. Throughout the latter half of the twentieth century, however, non-medical groups of staff involved in healthcare delivery have embarked on a drive for greater professional recognition; developing a unique knowledge base, seeking autonomy over their practice, controlling entry and regulating membership and conduct of their professions. This professionalisation of health work has resulted in a clearer professional identity for specific groups such as nurses and radiographers, defined in relation to the knowledge and skills of other professions. Although this has been largely positive, in that it has given nurses and allied health professionals a more confident voice, it has also, to some extent, created boundaries between professional groups, sometimes expressed through rivalry and lack of acknowledgement of each other's contribution. These boundaries are now becoming more fluid, and it is imperative that we take the opportunity to reconsider the roles and responsibilities of individual staff groups and to enhance the relationships between them (Colyer 1999).

Research into the effectiveness of teams has been mainly undertaken in the primary care sector. Poulton & West (1999) demonstrated that team processes were the best predictors of overall effectiveness, suggesting that 'teams which are more participative and collaborative are more likely to achieve a patient-centred service, (p. 16). To improve the quality of team working in radiotherapy, what is needed is further realignment of professional relationships and a relinquishing of power (though not necessarily of leadership) by the dominant medical profession. At the heart of this realignment is respect for the core skills and professionalism of others, which will not only improve efficiency, but will also enable genuine interprofessional teamwork to become a reality. Leadership development programmes may provide impetus to this process, introducing new styles of transformational leadership, which develop teamwork through sharing and devolving responsibility, in contrast to the traditional, top-down approaches of the past.

Recent white papers such as *Designed to Care* (DOH 1997) and *The NHS Plan* (DoH 2000b) commit us to finding collaborative and innovative ways of improving the quality of care given to patients. They make it clear that patients, not professionals, are at the centre of services and that there should be an emphasis on competence rather than professional tribalism when it comes to judging who should be responsible for particular aspects of patient care. Medical staff shortages are creating opportunities for nurses and radiographers in particular to develop their knowledge and skills to advanced and consultant practitioner levels. Communication and liaison skills are fundamental to these developments, and staff in these developed roles must be able to work with others across both professional boundaries and care sectors to give patients the support to which they are entitled.

Clinical oncology services have developed beyond recognition since the early days of the twentieth century. There is no sign of any slowing down; rather, at a time of increasingly sophisticated technology, high expectations and demographic change, the opposite is the case. This chapter has tried to show that, although all patients are vulnerable to misinformation, cancer patients are especially so because of the complexity of clinical oncology services and the potential for fault lines between different aspects of the service and the multiplicity of professions involved in the delivery of care. Although much has been achieved in terms of improvements in the treatment and care of patients with cancer, greater understanding and recognition of the context in which care takes place are required from those of us whose responsibility it is to support patients through their treatment.

REFERENCES

Abraham M, Jackson M, Johnson J 1999 Shortage of therapy radiographers: local problem or UK crisis. Journal of Radiotherapy in Practice 1:45–49
Beerino F, Sant M, Verdecchia A et al 1995 Survival of cancer patients in Europe: the Eurocare study. Larc Scientific Publications, Lyon
Blyth C M, Anderson J, Hughson W et al. 2001 An innovative approach to palliative care within a radiotherapy department. Journal of Radiotherapy in Practice 2:85–90
Brada M 1995 Is there a need to follow up cancer patients? European Journal of Cancer Part A General Topics 31(5):655–657
Buetow S, Martin R 1999 Clinical governance: bridging the gap between managerial and clinical approaches to quality of care. Quality in Healthcare 8:184–190
Campbell JL, German L, Lane C et al. 2000 Radiotherapy outpatient review: a nurse-led clinic. Clinical Oncology (Royal College of Radiologists) 12:104-107
Collins D 2001 Telephone follow-up clinics. Macmillan Voice 17:11–12
Colyer H 1999 Interprofessional teams in cancer care. Radiography 5:187–189
Colyer H, Hlahla T 1999 Information and support radiographers: a critical review of the role and its significance for the provision of cancer services. Journal of Radiotherapy in Practice 1:117–124
Department of Health 1991 Report of the working party standing scientific committee on cancer of the standing medical advisory committee. Quality assurance in radiotherapy. Department of Health, London
Department of Health 1994 Quality assurance in radiotherapy. HMSO, London.
Department of Health 1995 A policy framework for commissioning cancer services: a report by the expert advisory group on cancer to the chief medical officers of England and Wales. Available:www.doh.gov.uk/cancer/calmanhine.htm 2 Aug 2001
Department of Health 1997 Designed to care: reviewing the National Health Service in Scotland. HMSO, London
Department of Health. 1998 A first class service: quality in the NHS. HMSO, London
Department of Health 1999 Clinical governance: quality in the NHS. HMSO, London
Department of Health 2000a The NHS cancer plan. HMSO, London
Department of Health 2000b The NHS plan. HMSO, London
GIVIO investigations 1994 Impact of follow-up testing on survival and health related quality of life in breast cancer patients. Journal of the American Medical Association 271:1587–1592
James S 1997 Changing clinical practice. Synergy April:14,15
Jones B, Dale R G, Deehan C et al 2001 The role of biologically effective dose in clinical oncology. Clinical Oncology (Royal College of Radiologists) 13:71–81
Moore S, Corner J, Fuller F 1999 Development of nurse-led follow-up in the management of patients with lung cancer. Nursing Times Research 4 (6):432–445
Neal A J, Hoskin P J 1997 Clinical oncology, 2nd edn. Arnold, London
NHS Executive 2000 Improving the quality of cancer services. HSC/021. NHS Executive, London
O'Rourke N, Edwards R 2000 Lung cancer treatment, waiting times and tumour growth. Clinical Oncology (Royal College of Radiologists) 12:141–144
Poulton B, West M 1999 The determinants of effectiveness in primary health care teams. Journal of Interprofessional Care 13:7–18
Royal College of Radiologists 1991 Cancer care and treatment services: advice for purchasers and providers. Royal College of Radiologists, London
Royal College of Radiologists 1995 Risk management in clinical oncology. BFCO(95)1. Royal College of Radiologists, London

Royal College of Radiologists 1996a Guidance on the structure and function of cancer centres. BFCO(96)1. Royal College of Radiologists, London

Royal College of Radiologists 1996b Guidelines for the management of the unscheduled interruption or prolongation of a radical course of radiotherapy. BFCO(96)4. Royal College of Radiologists, London

Royal College of Radiologists 1998a Equipment, workload and staffing in the UK, 1992–1997. BFCO(98)2. Royal College of Radiologists, London

Royal College of Radiologists 1998b A national audit of waiting times for radiotherapy. BFCO(98)3. Royal College of Radiologists, London

Royal College of Radiologists, College of Radiographers and Royal College of Nursing 1999. Skills mix in clinical oncology. BFCO(99)2. Royal College of Radiologists, London

Royal College of Radiologists and the College of Radiographers 1999 Interprofessional roles and responsibilities in a clinical oncology service. BFCO(99)0. Royal College of Radiologists, London

Royal College of Radiologists 2000a Equipment, workload and staffing for radiotherapy in Scotland 1992–1997. BFCO(00)1. Royal College of Radiologists, London

Royal College of Radiologists 2000b The provision and replacement of radiotherapy equipment. BFCO(00)2. Royal College of Radiologists, London

Sardell S, Sharpe G, Ashely S et al 2000 Evaluation of a nurse-led telephone clinic in the follow-up of patients with malignant glioma. Clinical Oncology (Royal College of Radiologists) 12(1):36–41

Saunders M, Dische S, Fowler J et al 1988 Radiotherapy with three fractions per day for twelve consecutive days for tumours of the thorax and head and neck. Frontiers of Radiation Therapy and Oncology 22:99–104

Scholl-Evans B 1992 Developing quality assurance in a radiotherapy department. Radiography Today November: 42,43

Scottish Cancer Co-ordinating and Advisory Committee 1996 Commissioning cancer services in Scotland (SCCAC report) Scottish Office Department of Health, Edinburgh

Scottish Executive Health Department 2001 Cancer in Scotland: action for change. Scottish Executive Health Department, Edinburgh

Wells M 1998 What's so special about radiotherapy nursing? European Journal of Oncology Nursing 2(3):162–168

Wengstrom Y, Haggmark C 1998 Assessing problems of importance for the development of nursing care in a radiation therapy department. Cancer Nursing 21(1):50–56

White P 1998 Complementary medicine treatment of cancer: a survey of provision. Complementary Therapies in Medicine 6(1):10–13

2

Challenges to radiotherapy today

Alastair J Munro

INTRODUCTION

This chapter has been written from a perspective that is almost entirely British. The challenges that radiation oncology faces in the UK are, however, little different from those that face the speciality elsewhere in the developed world. The issue of supply and demand is both critical and universal. The lack of investment in, and planning for, cancer services in the UK between 1975 and 1995 means that, in the UK, we have already had to confront many of the issues that are starting to arise elsewhere.

Inadequate resources and a lack of strategic planning have meant that cancer services in the UK are attempting to cope with a gross imbalance between supply and demand. There are lessons for everyone here. Third-party payers, whether within a system of socialised medicine or a privately funded system, are increasingly influencing clinical decision-making. This influence is not necessarily harmful – there is nothing wrong with being both efficient and effective. Nevertheless, as a discipline, we need to be able to make our case persuasively. We need to identify that which is best about current practice, and defend it. We also need to have the courage to abandon those practices that the evidence shows to be ineffective, inefficient, or both. These are the issues with which we are grappling in the UK. From our mistakes, others might learn.

At times of environmental change, the rule is adapt or fade away. The main challenge to radiation oncology is to adapt to a rapidly changing environment. Box 2.1 summarises the changes that are occurring in the milieu within which cancer care in general and radiation therapy in particular is delivered.

Box 2.1

- Increasing knowledge concerning the basic biology of cancer and advances in our understanding of the biological effects of radiation
- Technological advances in the delivery of radiation therapy
- Organisational changes in the structures and systems for managing cancer
- An absolute and relative increase in workload superimposed upon a total lack of strategic planning either for equipment or for workforce
- Changes in working practice, in particular multidisciplinary team working
- Changes in public perceptions and expectations concerning cancer and its treatment
- The increasing need to justify interventions within an evidence-based framework, i.e. the need to build the evidence base and then to translate that knowledge into practice
- The challenge of effective palliation and the avoidance of double jeopardy (risk or harm without benefit)
- An exponential increase in the volume of information available coupled with the obligation, when making decisions concerning the management of an individual patient, to include all relevant, but no irrelevant, information in the decision-making process
- The general public, and members of other health-related professions, are insufficiently amazed by what radiation therapy can do, how comparatively cheap it is, and just how sophisticated and safe modern equipment is

---

The challenges listed in Box 2.1 are not separate, they are interrelated, and it is perhaps the need to recognise the interconnectedness of things that poses one of the greatest challenges to our speciality. As human beings we find it both convenient and comfortable to compartmentalise our existence. Categorisation is one way in which we try to make sense of the world, but the categories we construct are no more than artefacts – they have no independent existence as entities in their own right. The natural world is seamless and our attempts to parse it are no more than convenient fictions.

Those of us who look after people with cancer are dealing with individuals. We are not treating tumours, or disordered body parts, we are caring for people. Again the principle of integration is crucial; individual human beings are far more than a collection of components bolted together in a predictable and categorical fashion. We are each more than the sum of our parts. If there is one major challenge to radiation oncology it is to be able to recognise and accommodate this whilst still ensuring that the management of all those individuals who come to us for care is firmly placed on a rational and equitable base. We must do our best for each individual and yet make sure that, by so doing, we have not put any other individual at a disadvantage.

CANCER CELL BIOLOGY AND THE BIOLOGICAL BASIS OF RADIATION THERAPY

Up until 15 years ago we thought that radiation was an effective treatment for cancer solely because, through physicochemical interactions with the DNA within the nucleus of the cell, it produced genetic damage that prevented cells from

---

Box 2.2

- Free radicals cause damage to base pairs of DNA molecule so that, at next mitosis, the cell is unable to divide properly (the classical explanation for the biological effects of radiation)
- Radiation triggers immediate programmed cell death (apoptosis)
- Radiation influences genes controlling the cell cycle, e.g. RB gene, p53, A-T gene.
- Radiation can affect the expression of over 100 separate genes. Early-response genes, such as jun and EGR1, are directly switched on by radiation. Intermediate or later-response genes are usually induced indirectly: radiation causes damage to DNA and it is the DNA damage that, in turn, influences gene expression (Munro 2001a, pp. 204–205)
- Radiation damages cell membranes. This causes signals to be transmitted to the nucleus and these signals influence cell behaviour

---

subsequently dividing. We were wrong. We now appreciate that radiation was doing all sorts of other things as well. Our current understanding of radiation effects on cells is summarised in Box 2.2.

We are only now, after 100 years, learning how to use radiation properly. Radiation therapy has evolved as an empirical art, not an exact science. Fractionation (Ch. 5) was introduced not because of an appreciation of the nuances of radiobiology, but because the vacuum pumps available to French tube manufacturers in the early years of the twentieth century were inferior to those produced by the Germans. This affected the reliability of the X-ray tubes and so French radiotherapists had to use multiple short exposures, in contrast to their German counterparts who were able to employ single fraction treatments (therapia magna sterilans). The clinical results were better with the French approach and the past 90 years have been spent trying to understand the biological basis for this crucial clinical observation.

The challenge for the future will be to incorporate the recent discoveries in the biological basis of cancer and of radiation therapy into the design and testing of new approaches to treatment. The question of selective toxicity is critical. There is little to be gained if an innovative approach increases normal tissue damage to the same extent as it improves local control of the tumour. There is no net therapeutic gain from such an approach. The much-vaunted 'success' of chemoradiation in head and neck cancer is somewhat vitiated by the fact that the rate of severe mucositis is increased with combined treatment, and to an extent that is almost identical to the improvement in local control. An observation which begs the question: might not the same improvement have been achieved simply by increasing radiation dose (Munro 2001b)? A converse argument applies to radioprotectors: it is essential to demonstrate that the tumour and normal tissues are not protected equally. If this were the case then, once again, there would be no therapeutic gain.

The major challenge to radiobiology in the twenty-first century is to provide the tools that will enable us to put radiotherapy on a rational basis for each individual. We all differ in the way our normal tissues respond to radiation. Tumours, even when histologically identical, differ in their response to radiation. The result is that, when groups of patients are considered, the dose–response curves for tumour control and for normal tissue damage are flattened (Fig. 2.1A). This makes it difficult to choose an optimal dose or schedule suitable for the group as a whole. The 'optimal' regimen will be a statistical compromise in which individuals are disadvantaged. Some are treated with a dose that is above the tolerance of their normal tissues; others are treated with doses that fail to control their tumours, even though their particular normal tissues could have tolerated a higher dose (Fig. 2.1B). The development of clinically feasible predictive assays for the radiosensitivity of tumours and of normal tissues will allow disagreggation of the composite, flattened, dose–response curves and a return to the steep individual curves (Fig. 2.1C). This would give us the ability to define a regimen for each individual patient that would give the maximum probability of uncomplicated cure.

ADVANCES IN THE TECHNOLOGY OF RADIATION THERAPY

Radiation therapy equipment and techniques have evolved rapidly over the past decade or so. Some innovations may save time; some may add to the time taken to deliver each fraction. The main technological advances that are likely to affect the clinical practice of radiotherapy within the next decade are summarised in Box 2.3.

It is difficult to estimate the impact of these advances upon the workload of clinical departments. If the past is any guide, these innovations will be introduced in an ad hoc, unplanned fashion, funded from soft money with no provision made for revenue costs or for the implications in terms of the workforce. Such is the excitement associated with novelty that the problems of opportunity cost are overlooked. As we invest money, time and effort in introducing new techniques, we often take resources away from other areas of clinical activity. The overall result is that we do the new things badly, because we are learning how to do them, and what we used to do well we now do badly, because we have diverted the resources into the new technique. Everyone – in the short term at least – loses.

Managing technological evolution within finite resources is a major challenge to the technical development of radiation therapy. Were there but world enough, and time, we would be able to innovate and maintain standards: but there isn't, and we can't, unless new developments attract increased resources.

We need to reflect on potential developments, to place them within the context of real patients in the real world and make rational judgements as to whether the money and effort expended will be worth the gains experienced by those who really matter – the patients. Conformal therapy is a case in point: many techniques have been developed and published based on work with tissue-equivalent phantoms, rather than patients. But we treat people, not ghosts. The tangible benefits from conformal treatment have, so far, been fairly minimal. The extra time taken per patient is not insignificant. Data from Addenbrooke's Hospital (Burnet et al 2001) suggest that conformal therapy, as part of the Medical Research Council RT01 prostate trial, will double the machine time taken to treat each patient. Unless capacity is increased, the consequence would be that every patient randomised to conformal therapy would mean adding another patient to the waiting list for radiation treatment.

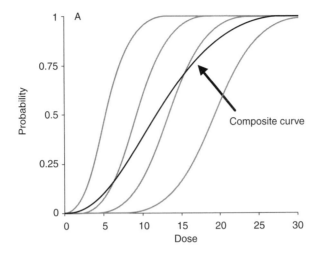

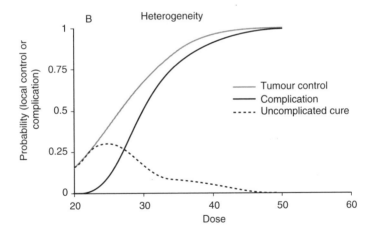

Figure 2.1   This series of dose–response curves shows that, when disparate individual dose–response curves are combined, the overall composite curve is, relative to each of the component curves, flattened (A). The composite curve (shown in black) is the result of plotting the averaged-out data from the four individual curves (shown in grey). In other words, when pooling data from a mixed group of subjects, the dose–response curve will be flatter, rather than steeper. This causes problems when, using the concept of therapeutic ratio, we try to define the optimal dose for treating patients. We wish to use that dose which gives us the best compromise between controlling the tumour and causing damage to normal tissues. This dose can, using the formalism of dose–response curves for tumour control and normal tissue damage, be defined as the probability of uncomplicated cure (PUC). Heterogeneity, as in (B), smears the PUC curve so that there is, at best in this example, only a 30% chance of achieving an uncomplicated cure.

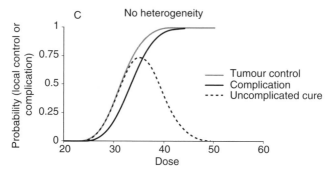

Figure 2.1 (Continued) If we could disaggregate the composite curve, and get back to the data from individual patients, or highly homogeneous groups of patients, then the PUC curve is narrower and taller (C). It is now possible to choose a dose that would achieve an uncomplicated cure rate of nearly 75%.

Box 2.3

- Portal imaging
- Intensity-modulated therapy (IMRT)
- Image-guided radiation therapy (IGRT)
- Conformal therapy
- Multileaf collimation
- Stereotactic radiotherapy
- Gated treatment (pulsed according to the phase of the respiratory cycle)
- Therapy with portable photon sources, e.g. intraoperative
- Intraoperative external beam therapy
- Prostate brachytherapy
- Intraoperative brachytherapy using Flab (flexible tissue-equivalent material)

The basic treatment equivalent (BTE) concept (Delaney et al 1997a,b) provides an extremely useful tool for assessing the impact of technological innovation upon machine utilisation. By modelling the effect of innovation using the BTE it should be possible to anticipate, and mitigate, any adverse consequences arising from the introduction of the new technology. One of the advantages of the BTE formula is that it contains a factor, based on Eastern Cooperative Oncology Group (ECOG) performance status, that indicates a patient's general fitness. It explicitly incorporates the common-sense observation that, regardless of treatment technique, it takes longer to treat sicker patients.

Multileaf collimation (MLC) offers a potential method for increasing the throughput of linear accelerators. It will also save the backs of many radiographers. Lifting and positioning shielding blocks takes time and, for a three-field treatment, with shielding, MLC will save about 10–20% of machine time each fraction. For a typical case-mix on a linear accelerator this would be equivalent to an extra three or four patients each day. This benefit may, however, be offset by an increase in the number of fields treated with shielding. The seductive ease with which individually shaped shielding can be obtained with MLC may prove hard to resist. Work expands to exploit the available technology – a variant of Parkinson's law.

Portal imaging devices providing data in real time will increase the accuracy of alignment of each field used for radiation treatment. Eventually, given the confidence thus provided, we may be able to reduce field sizes without compromising the dose delivered to the tumour. This should, by decreasing treatment-related morbidity, improve the therapeutic ratio. It will take time to achieve the confidence to reduce field size and so, after the introduction of portal imaging, there will be an interim period during which machine throughput is decreased by the time spent on portal imaging but without there being any demonstrable benefit to patients.

Image-guided radiation therapy (IGRT) is an extension of portal imaging in which motion, of patients or their internal organs, is monitored during treatment and, if such motion is beyond specified parameters, then the linear accelerator will switch itself off: just as my electric hedge clippers do when I try to use them to cut through tree trunks. This is another technique which might permit a decrease in the volume of the planning target volume (PTV) relative to that of the clinical target volume (CTV) but, once again, the benefits are hypothetical rather than proven. What is, however, totally certain is that such technology will decrease the number of patients that can be treated per linear accelerator per day. This is definitely good news for the manufacturers of linear accelerators.

Absolute safety is a desirable ideal, but safety always comes at a price. Modern radiotherapy equipment has sophisticated interlocks to prevent treatment being given unless the whole system is functioning perfectly. These precautions are necessary but, as they become more rigorous, will through false alarms and other malfunctions again tend to decrease the number of patients that can be treated per day. It is absolutely right that we concentrate on safety but, in so doing, we should be aware that, when crude productivity is the metric, new machines may not be as efficient as those machines they replace. There is an interesting ancillary point here. Most day-to-day difficulties with linear accelerators involve problems with safety interlocks rather than machine failure per se. And yet we talk, amongst ourselves and to patients, of 'machine breakdowns'. We know what we mean, but the patients are likely to take a quite different meaning: imagining the machine to be a smouldering mass of melted metal and plastic emitting the occasional spark. Pilots are well aware of the psychology here. Why aren't we? As the plane aborts take-off during a thunderstorm the pilot doesn't come on the intercom to say 'Sorry about that, but the plane broke down as we were trying to take off, we'll just take a few minutes to fix it and then try again'. He says something along the lines of 'Well, we have a little problem with a warning indicator, the light seems to have jammed on, we'll take a few moments to check it out and then we should be on our way'.

ORGANISATIONAL CHANGES IN THE STRUCTURES AND SYSTEMS FOR MANAGING CANCER

The organisation of cancer services in the UK is rapidly changi ng as a result of several separate but interrelated developments (reviewed in Ch. 1). There were two main spurs to this reorganisation. One was the demonstration that there were geographic and social inequalities in the delivery of cancer care within the UK, and that these disparities might be associated with an effect upon survival. In the South Thames region, for women diagnosed with breast cancer between 1980 and 1989, there was a 7.4% difference in 5-year survival between the most and the least deprived (Schrijvers et al 1995).

Survival is only a proxy measure of the care people receive. Under a National Health Service (NHS) your income should not influence the care you or your family receive. This applies not just to how quickly you obtain access to specialist care, but also to the treatment you receive and to the information and support you are given. The literature on psychosocial oncology is heavily biased towards the care of breast cancer. The very nature of this research is such that the articulate and the middle classes tend to be overrepresented. We should not disenfranchise people who are less articulate, or less well off, or who have tumours that, because of their association with tobacco and alcohol, are judged to be self-inflicted.

The other stimulus to change was the appreciation that survival rates for British patients with cancer were poor compared with those for patients in the rest of western Europe. Five-year survival rates for colon cancer in England and Wales are around 40%, compared with an average in the European Union (EU) of 48%. The corresponding figures for lung cancer are 5% (England and Wales) and 11% (EU). Put simply, if you have lung cancer you are, on average, twice as likely to survive if you live in an EU country other than England or Wales. These findings should have come as no surprise. The political history of the UK between 1979 and 1995 was that of a nation in which the biblical prescription 'Unto every one that hath shall be given, and he shall have abundance; but from him that hath not shall be taken away even that which he hath' (Holy Bible 1611) was adopted as government policy. The result was overall underinvestment in public services, including health, and an increasingly steep socioeconomic gradient between the haves and the have-nots. The epithet 'postcode prescribing' only scratches the surface of the latter problem: it is not just about having access to new drugs, it is about access to the healthcare system as a whole; it is about poverty and hopelessness, about wilful neglect. The farce that was the internal market only compounded the difficulties.

The Calman–Hine report (DoH 1995), the various cancer plans (Department of Health 2000, Scottish Executive 2001a), as well as the NHS plan (Department of Health 1998) represent attempts by government to improve matters. The centralisation of cancer services (cancer centres) has advantages, in terms of concentrating expertise, but disadvantages, in terms of increased time spent travelling – for both patients and staff. We immediately encounter the centralisation paradox: all individuals wish to be treated by an expert but all individuals want their treatment to be available at once, and within a few minutes of home. There is no easy solution here, and the arrangements that are being put into place are no more than compromises. The challenge for radiation oncology will be to harness new technology, particularly information technology and data transfer, to resolve the paradox. One example might be to link several simulators, at different sites, to a central planning system at a different site. This could help to make sophisticated planning techniques available to a greater number of patients without increasing the distances for either patients or staff to travel.

The new structures and systems make considerable demands on staff at a time when there are too few of us. We are charged with providing more information: informing patients of choices; gathering and analysing statistics on referrals and outcomes. The resources to do this are only gradually becoming available, but the demands to deliver are immediate. Once again, improved information technology might come to our aid. The challenge is to make it work: the problem is that the NHS has a dismal record when it comes to managing information.

The bizarre emphasis on waiting times as a metric for health service performance also causes difficulty. Should admissions of new patients, waiting for investigation and treatment of cancer, be cancelled so that beds can be freed in order to achieve waiting-list targets for hernia repair or hip replacement? The challenge here is to put our patients' case firmly and clearly, otherwise they might be put at a disadvantage as hospital managers pursue a politically imposed agenda.

INCREASING WORKLOAD AND INADEQUATE RESOURCES

Radiotherapy services in the UK have suffered from a lack of strategic planning over the past 25 years. The net result has been that, in England and Wales, the government's own figures suggested that, in the year 2000, 56 new linear accelerators would be immediately required: 14 extra machines and 42 to replace linear accelerators which were more than 11 years old. These machines are to be purchased using money from the National Lottery. The money is welcome, but the sudden need to find over £50 million simply to keep up with demand illustrates just how parlous the position had been allowed to become.

Providing machines is, of course, relatively straightforward: a simple matter of capital investment. Running the machines effectively is a much more difficult problem. Staff are required to run and maintain the machines and this requires long-term training and funding. The numbers of trained staff are currently, and for the immediate future, inadequate. It takes 7 years to train a medical physicist, 3 years to train a radiographer and about 12 years to train a clinical oncologist. *The NHS Cancer Plan* for England and Wales estimates that, by 2005, an extra 214 therapy radiographers and 65 medical physicists will be required (DoH 2000). These are increases of, in proportional terms, 16% for radiographers and 12% for medical physicists. It is not immediately obvious where these highly skilled individuals will come from. The challenge will be to continue to provide a high standard of clinical service whilst trying to recruit, train and retain personnel in these key areas. The number of currently unfilled posts, and the high drop-out rate from radiography training, indicate that the problem is here now. Unless we can rise to the challenge, departments will have expensive new machines lying idle through lack of staff to service and operate them.

The Cottier report (Forbes & Cottier 1999) clearly demonstrated that resources for radiotherapy in England and Wales were unevenly distributed and that, in addition, utilisation was equally heterogeneous. Such anomalies can, potentially at least, exacerbate inequalities in the standard of care. Figure 2.2 shows that, when adjusted for population on a pro rata basis, there is an approximately threefold variation (best to worst) for three main parameters: machines, radiographers and

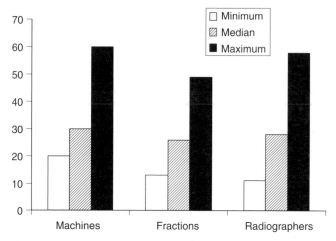

Figure 2.2   Uneven allocation and consumption of resources for radiotherapy in England and Wales. Data adapted from Forbes and Cottier (1999). The figures are for machines per 10 million population served, fractions per 1000 population, and radiographers per million population. When values are explicitly related to population served there is a consistent threefold difference between the lowest and highest figures. The data also suggest that those centres with relatively more machines use a relatively higher number of fractions: work expanding to fit the space available?

fractions of treatment per head of population. The Organisation for Economic Cooperation and Development (OECD) average for the developed world is 48 megavoltage machines per 10 million population: the figure for England is 38, for Scotland, 30.

The data on fractionation are disconcerting, but unsurprising. The Royal College of Radiologists' fractionation survey (Priestman et al 1989) showed that different centres had very different policies for managing common clinical problems. Three centres in Forbes & Cottier's (1999) survey used more than 45 fractions per 1000 population; all three were south of Watford and two of them were in greater London. A similar survey of the nine cancer centres in Ontario, Canada (Dixon & Mackillop 2001) showed that mean number of fractions per course varied from centre to centre, ranging from 10.9 to 16.0. There were 64 megavoltage machines in use in the province during the study period. If all centres had used the policies that were employed at the centre that used the fewest number of treatments, then this would liberate capacity equivalent to 14 machines, or over one-fifth of the total capacity.

Waiting times for treatment are an inevitable consequence of inadequate or patchy resources, or of the inefficient use of those resources. There is some evidence, and for obvious ethical reasons the amount of such evidence is limited, that delay in starting radiotherapy might compromise cure (Mackillop et al 1995, O'Rourke & Edwards 2000). There is also the psychological impact upon patients forced to wait for essential treatment. A study from Ontario in the 1990s, at a time of some difficulty with the provision of radiotherapy services, showed the balance that patients were prepared to strike. Patients with early breast cancer who required postsurgical adjuvant radiotherapy were prepared to wait up to 7 weeks if that was the price to pay for having their treatment locally (Palda et al 1997). If they had to wait any longer than this then they were prepared to travel several hundred miles and spend 6 weeks away from home having treatment at a distant centre. The waiting time for treatment at the local centre at the time this study was performed was 13 weeks.

We not only have to ensure that resources are adequately distributed to deal with current workload but also have to anticipate future requirements. The incidence of cancer rises with age (Fig. 2.3). As individual life expectancy increases, then, so the proportion of older people in the general population will rise. Currently around 15% of the British population are aged 65 or over. Recent Scottish estimates suggest that, largely because of the anticipated changes in the age distribution of the population, the number of new cases of cancer per annum in Scotland (population around five million) will rise from the current level of 26 000 to 33 000 by the year 2014 – an increase of 27% over 15 years, nearly 2% per annum (Scottish Executive 2001b). Even if only half of this anticipated increase were translated into increased workload for radiotherapy departments, this would still produce an annual increase in workload of 1%, year on year. This absolute increase in the number of patients with cancer is, however, only part of the story.

Radiotherapy plays an increasing role in the management of cancer: a decade ago about 40% of all patients with cancer were treated with radiotherapy at one time or another during their illness. Nowadays the figure is nearer 50%. Thus, even if the absolute number of new patients developing cancer each year were to

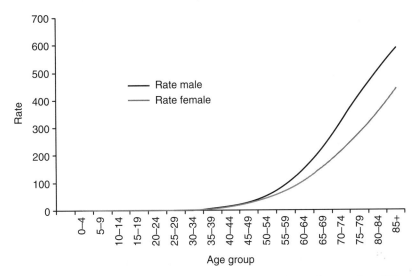

Figure 2.3 The risk of cancer rises with age: data on colorectal cancer from ISD Scotland. Age-specific incidence rate (per 100 000 person-years at risk) in Scotland 1986 to 1995.

remain constant, we could still anticipate an increase in referrals for treatment. Recent changes in the management of rectal cancer provide a practical illustration of this point.

In 1993 only three patients with rectal cancer were treated with adjuvant radiotherapy in Tayside. By 1999, the figure was 20: a sevenfold increase. The increase arose, not through some caprice or statistical quirk, but because evidence-based guidelines published in 1997 (Scottish Intercollegiate Guidelines Network 1997) recommended that adjuvant radiotherapy be considered for patients with operable rectal cancer. If this local experience were in any way typical then, by extrapolation, this would suggest that referrals for adjuvant radiotherapy for rectal cancer might have increased by 1500 per annum in the UK over the past 7 years. This corresponds to an increase in workload equivalent to one linear accelerator. Similar shifts in emphasis are occurring in other cancers – prostate cancer, breast cancer and oesophageal cancer.

THE NEED TO DEVELOP EFFECTIVE WORKING PRACTICES, IN PARTICULAR MULTIDISCIPLINARY TEAM WORKING

The wide variations in radiotherapy prescribing practice were alluded to in the previous section (Fig. 2.2). These have arisen mainly because, historically, consultants have been all-powerful figures within radiotherapy departments. Teamwork is the fundamental principle underlying modern cancer care and the domineering, by their very nature, cannot work in teams. The challenge for the future is to build effective multidisciplinary teams with flexible working practices and mutual respect between team members. Given that, for many, this represents a new way of working, there is a pressing educational challenge: how to train the team members? The challenge is made more difficult because, as has been pointed out (Finch 2000), there is a certain lack of clarity amongst policy-makers as to what exactly is meant by 'interdisciplinary working'. The possible educational goals include (adapted from Finch 2000):

- understanding what exactly it is that other professional groups do (do nurses really know what radiographers get up to, and vice versa?)
- learning how to work with each other (it takes a degree of professional self-confidence both to relinquish territory and to take advice, particularly if you have a medical degree)
- enabling staff to take on roles normally associated with other professional groups (can, or should, radiographers take blood, or administer chemotherapy?)
- allowing individuals to change careers easily (should there be core training for cancer nurses, oncologists and therapy radiographers which could provide academic credit for any subsequent move between disciplines?)

Whatever the difficulties, these challenges must be met. It is difficult to work effectively in a team if the lead decision-maker in that team is making decisions based on the beliefs and habits of 20 years ago rather than upon the best of contemporary evidence. It is soul-destroying to have to obey stale orders whilst realising that there are better and more effective ways of doing things. Quaint practices, such as the use of 10 fractions to treat bone metastases, are often indulged despite a wealth of evidence demonstrating that such regimens are no more effective than properly administered single fractions. The reasons for adhering to such practices are complex; sometimes it seems to have more to do with the doctor's desire to be in control than with the patient's best interests. There are two far more important issues here. One is the needless time that patients, whose life expectancy may be short, spend attending for treatment. When you have only 20 weeks to live, then a fortnight is 10% of your remaining lifespan – the equivalent of 5 years to a healthy 30-year-old. The other issue is that squandering scarce resources means that other patients suffer. Each patient treated with 10 fractions gratuitously consumes machine time that could have been used, without detriment to anyone, to treat nine other patients. Quaint is both unaffordable and unjust.

Consistency in decision-making poses a major challenge in contemporary oncology. Guidelines and departmental protocols represent attempts to introduce a degree of consistency but there is a difficult balance to be struck between clinical freedom, to make decisions in the best interests of individual patients, and corporate accountability and responsibility, to formulate policies and procedures that ensure the greatest possible good for the greatest possible number. On the one hand, an approach that is too dictatorial will produce disgruntlement and disdain. On the other hand, failure to agree on how to manage common problems will lead to confusion, anarchy and, more often than not, profligate consumption of resources. A properly functioning team, with access to the relevant information, offers the best solution to the dilemma. The important proviso being that the individual patient should never be excluded from the team.

Recognising that teamwork is essential is relatively easy. Putting the concept into practice is far more difficult. Useful practical guidance on the composition of the multidisciplinary team in radiation oncology can be found in the document produced jointly by the Board of Faculty of Clinical Oncology, Royal College of Radiologists, the College of Radiographers and the Royal College of Nursing (1999a). The potential pitfalls of changes in working practice are succinctly summarised: inadequately defined lines of responsibility; compromised training; interprofessional rivalry; fragmentation of care. When the approach works, it is very very good. When it doesn't, it is horrid. A complementary document (Board of Faculty of Clinical Oncology, the Royal College of Radiologists and the College of Radiographers 1999b) deals with the issues of delegation and responsibility primarily from a medical perspective. It is based on the advice given by the General Medical Council and emphasises such crucial issues as competence, written agreed protocols, audit of both process and outcome and clearly defined responsibility. It emphasises that, no matter to whom a task or procedure may be delegated, the medical responsibility remains with the doctor.

CHANGES IN PUBLIC PERCEPTIONS AND EXPECTATIONS CONCERNING CANCER AND ITS TREATMENT

Fifty years ago, doctors only rarely told patients with cancer their diagnosis. In a remarkable change during the middle decades of the last century, there was a shift from opacity and prevarication to full disclosure; by the 1970s nearly all patients with cancer had been told their diagnosis. This openness has diffused into society as a whole and, by and large, the message has been one of optimism. Newspapers and magazines feature celebrities who have 'beaten' cancer. The major cancer charities collude in this optimism: press conferences hail minor advances as major breakthroughs and a cure is always just about to be found. The truth is that, for common tumours, there have been no major discoveries that have had a major impact on cure rates. The improvements that have occurred have arisen as the result of incremental progress, not major leaps: as a result of more effective application of existing knowledge rather than because of spectacular new insights. True, we know far more of the biology of cancer than we did 10 years ago, but it will be another decade or so before any new therapies based on recent advances find widespread, affordable, clinical application. And so we have, on the one hand, a climate of raised hopes and expectations and, on the other hand, a reality that demonstrates only limited advances. This creates a challenging tension for those responsible for the clinical care of patients and their families. How do we maintain patients' hopes without pandering to unreal expectations? How do we deal with the son-in-law who has looked up every latest treatment on the internet?

Patients also have, quite rightly, higher expectations of the clinical environment than they did 20 years ago. They are unwilling to wait quietly. They see immediate attention as a right, not a privilege. They see information and emotional support as essentials, not optional extras. They expect the architectural environment to be civilised and, in its own way, therapeutic. They do not expect to be undressed and left lying terrified in a shabby cubicle before being subjected to a brusque assessment by a consultant with the communication skills of a regimental sergeant major. They expect to be involved in decisions about their care; they expect their preeminent role in the process to be both acknowledged and honoured. All of these expectations are totally and absolutely justified. The challenge is to make sure that for each and every patient, and without favouring some over others, these expectations are completely fulfilled.

EVIDENCE-BASED ONCOLOGY

The term evidence-based medicine (EBM) is relatively new, but the concept is not: 'an old field with a new name' (Sackett 2000). The best medicine has always been evidence-based. The main achievement of the EBM movement has been to indicate clearly that clinical decisions should not be based on the ex cathedra pronouncements of experts but should be based on a systematic and objective appraisal of the relevant facts. A concise definition has been proposed by its original proponent: 'the conscientious, explicit and judicious use of current best evidence in making decisions about the care of individual patients' (Sackett et al 1996). The authoritarian, but poorly substantiated, pronouncements of the past are to be replaced by a more scientific and intellectually rigorous approach. There is certainly evidence to demonstrate that experts do not always give the best advice. A classic paper showed that, even when the cumulative evidence from randomised trials showed the effectiveness of immediate thrombolytic therapy in patients with acute myocardial infarction, expert opinion still considered such treatment experimental or even dangerous (Antman et al 1992). There was a time lag of about 10 years between knowledge becoming available and its incorporation into standard medical texts or review articles.

Appropriately, and unsurprisingly, EBM has spawned evidence-based oncology (Bentzen 1998). The concept is easy to criticise, on both practical and intellectual grounds, but the challenges raised will not go away simply because, like the poor, we find them embarrassing and a little inconvenient. One very practical objection is that, if the appropriate evidence is unavailable, how can you possibly make an evidence-based decision? To which the reply would be: well, at least formulating the problem in this way has defined what is lacking, always remembering that absence of evidence is not evidence of absence. A simple catechism summarises the problem of evidence:

The evidence we have is not the evidence we want
The evidence we want is not the evidence we need
The evidence we need is not the evidence we can obtain
The evidence we can obtain costs more than we can afford
The evidence we can afford may be imperfect

(adapted from Bernstein 1996).

Perhaps one major argument in favour of evidence-based oncology is to consider it in terms of its negation, 'oncology that is not based on evidence' – scarcely an attractive prospect in either scientific or ethical terms. A variety of other approaches can be defined.

- Desperation-based oncology: action because inaction would be unacceptable, the 'do something' imperative, a variant of which is:
- Pascal-based oncology: when a treatment offers even an infinitesimal probability of success then, provided there are no adverse consequences, it is logical to treat rather than to withhold treatment
- Nervousness-based oncology: when management is modified because of fear of litigation or other punishment. An example would be overcautious interpretation of the limited clinical data on the radiation tolerance of the spinal cord (Fowler et al 2000)
- Empire-based oncology: when decisions are based on a desire to build a personal or institutional reputation, or to corner the market in a particular intervention
- Technology-based oncology: a variant of Parkinson's law: we have a new technique, so let's find some patients to fit it
- Habit-based oncology: probably the most widely practised style of oncology, and not necessarily always the worst, but not the easiest proposition to defend intellectually

(adapted from Isaacs & Fitzgerald 1999).

The challenge for the future is to retain the best of the past – the art of oncology as it were – and to integrate it with a more rigorous approach to obtaining, weighing, interpreting and deploying evidence. The ultimate quandary will, however, always remain: evidence based on statistics will apply to populations; we can calculate average probabilities and risks. Patients, however, come to us as individuals and statistics do not really help us here: death and recurrence are, like pregnancy, all-or-none phenomena. There is no such thing as 0.25 of a recurrence, or 75% of a death. Our ultimate responsibility is to individuals – the challenge is to interpret the statistics of populations in order to provide each individual patient with the management that is appropriate to their particular predicament.

EFFECTIVE PALLIATION AND THE PROBLEM OF DOUBLE JEOPARDY

Over 40% of all courses of radiotherapy treatment in the UK are prescribed with palliative intent. They are given in order to relieve symptoms in patients for whom cure is no longer considered a possibility. It is a fundamental tenet of palliative treatment that the treatment should not itself produce problems that are greater or worse than those produced by the cancer. In a perfect world, palliative treatment would relieve all symptoms, in all patients, without itself causing any disruption or discomfort. Our world is far from perfect and we will only rarely provide ideal palliation. We can, nevertheless, make sensible attempts to achieve that goal. If however, the purpose of fractionation in palliative treatment is to make doctors feel important, rather than to make patients feel better, then there is an immediate confusion of aims. Fractionated treatment is disruptive and patients who are attending hospital for 2 or 3 weeks of palliative treatment are unable to do other things: they cannot take holidays, go off for a day at the races or spend time doing absolutely nothing. They are imprisoned by the schedule set by the hospital and a major part of the opportunity cost of unnecessarily protracted treatment is paid by the patients (Munro & Sebag-Montefiore 1992). This is not merely a theoretical argument. There is abundant evidence from randomised clinical trials that single fractions of radiotherapy are as effective as multiple fractions in relieving pain in patients with bone metastases (Hoskin et al 2000). There is, equally, an impressive volume of evidence demonstrating that clinicians are reluctant to use single fractions of radiotherapy in the palliative treatment of such patients (Bentzen et al 2000, Booth et al 1993, Maher 1991). A small minority of radiotherapists, even when the evidence is explicitly drawn to their attention, will still persist in prescribing multiple fractions (Booth et al 1993). Added disruption without demonstrable additional benefit flouts the basic principles of palliative treatment.

A patient who experiences the disruption, and possible toxicity, of palliative treatment and who does not obtain significant relief of symptoms has been placed in double jeopardy: pain plus pain, no gain. A major challenge for palliative radiotherapy is not simply to devise the simplest and most effective schedules and techniques but also to develop tools for predicting which patients will benefit from such interventions and, more importantly, which patients will not. Although the use of predictive assays in radiation oncology has, classically, been investigated in patients being treated for cure, these assays may be equally relevant for patients being treated palliatively. Decisions concerning palliative treatment are much more difficult than those concerning radical treatment: a difficulty which is inversely reflected in the funding for research and in the published literature. There are many more trials of radical therapies, many more publications on curative treatment. The fact that palliative treatment is more emotionally and intellectually challenging than radical treatment is no excuse for evading the issues involved.

INFORMATION: AN EXPONENTIAL EXPANSION OF BOTH SUPPLY AND DEMAND

The problems with evidence, outlined above, highlight issues to do with the quality of information: relevance, accuracy and availability. There is, however, another problem – that of quantity. Sources of information can be split into those that are generally accessible to patients and staff alike and those that are designed for a more restricted distribution.

Generally accessible

- Television and videos
- Radio
- Newspapers, magazines and books
- Specific guides (e.g. British Association of Cancer United Patients (BACUP) booklets, guides to complementary or alternative therapies)
- Worldwide web.

Restricted distribution or access

- Specialist journals and books
- Specialist websites
- Company representatives (drugs, radiotherapy equipment)
- Professional organisations (colleges, institutes, etc.)
- Mailshots (advertisements, meeting announcements)
- Guidelines
- Government reports and circulars
- Correspondence: letters from consultants, general practitioners
- E-mail
- Laboratory reports: imaging, haematology, biochemistry.

'Information overload' is one definition of senility. We are all being driven prematurely senile by the sheer volume of information we are asked to process. A major challenge for clinical oncology is to develop systems based on information technology that store and transmit information electronically, have filters built in so that important information is flagged up immediately and enable team members at different locations to communicate in real time. How much time do radiographers and nurses spend trying to track down a doctor to deal with a relatively simple query?

We are also asked to provide information. As radiation oncology services become increasingly managed, the demands for information increase. Each department is expected to collect, store and, when asked, pass on vast amounts of data concerning workload, resource utilisation and outcomes. The system in the UK has, for far too long, relied on individual consultants or other groups keeping and maintaining their own data sets. The result is fragmentation with many isolated pockets, each containing data relevant to one aspect of a problem, each on a separate computer system and each unable to communicate with any other because of software incompatibility or disputes over ownership of the data.

There needs to be a far more integrated approach to the recording and retrieval of data on cancer and its treatment.

Audit is an essential prerequisite for progress and, without data of high quality that is immediately available, much audit activity is, at best, deeply frustrating and, at worst, a totally meaningless waste of time. If we don't really know what we have been doing, how can we possibly define how we might make things better?

Patients with cancer, particularly those who are about to undergo a complex and potentially frightening course of treatment, have an absolute right to be fully informed of the options open to them and to have the advantages and disadvantages of each explained to them in terms that they can understand and which have relevance for them as individuals. Again, there is a huge amount of information out there and the challenge is to bring to all individuals that which they need and want to know, no more and no less. Too much information may be as bad as too little (Dunn et al 1993). Simply to thrust a fistful of booklets and information sheets at the hapless victim and smugly tick the box marked 'patient fully informed of risks and benefits associated with proposed treatment' is a totally inadequate approach to the problem. All individuals live in a world that is personal to them; their illness (and its management) have a meaning that is equally personal. There are no class solutions to the problem of adequately informing each individual patient. Once again, it may be possible to harness the power of computer-based technology to address the issue. Menu-driven information systems, using touch-sensitive screens, offer an effective means of ensuring that patients are able to titrate the information they acquire against the information they need (Jones et al 1999).

This approach also provides the option for automatically auditing the process of informed consent. This is a contentious issue and a challenge which, as a profession, we have not yet met. Although the official advice is that all patients undergoing a course of radiation treatment should sign a written consent form, there is no agreement on what information this form should actually contain. The legal position is also opaque. Signed written consent is no legal guarantee that informed consent has been obtained: the medicolegal value of these forms is therefore limited. Most consent forms are like Sam Goldwyn's verbal contracts – not worth the paper they are printed on. They may be regarded as being better than nothing; the absence of such forms could be viewed unfavourably by a court, but not as being very much better than nothing. A court could still rule that patients had failed to give adequate informed consent, even though they had signed a consent form. The problem, and the challenge, here hinges on the question of disclosing risk. What should be the probability threshold for disclosing the existence of a potentially adverse consequence of treatment? Should this threshold be influenced by the severity of the adverse event? All individuals vary in their approach to risk: some are risk-seeking and others risk-averse (Kahneman & Tversky 1984). How might this human attribute be incorporated into the process of informed consent? Some individuals would not want to know much about trivial side effects, for example, mild nausea, no matter how common. They might, however, insist on knowing about catastrophic potential complications, such as radiation myelopathy and paresis, no matter how rare. Others might take the view that they did not wish to be gratuitously frightened by being told about very rare, but very serious, complications. They would, in contrast, like to know everything about the things they might reasonably expect during a course of treatment, no matter how apparently trivial. These questions lie at the very root of how we choose to live our lives. Informed consent is not about protecting ourselves from litigation; it is about protecting the right of all individuals to make their own choices and to have the information that is for them both adequate and accurate. The challenge is, human variety and fallibility notwithstanding, to make this right a reality.

Information technology, with data acquisition, processing and transfer carried out by a nationally networked system of PCs, is no panacea, but it would be an interesting start. The challenge is to take the best from information technology and fuse it with the best of old-fashioned caring and nurturing and produce a solution that ensures that all individual patients, and their families, receive the appropriate level of information and support.

THE GENERAL PUBLIC, AND MEMBERS OF OTHER HEALTH-RELATED PROFESSIONS, ARE INSUFFICIENTLY AMAZED

Modern radiation therapy, if it is nothing else, is a triumph of precision engineering. The gantry of a linear accelerator weighs 3 tons, the couch 1.5 tons. The gantry can be rotated through 360° and positioned with an accuracy of one-tenth of a degree. Working together, the 4.5 tons of couch and gantry, weighing as much as three family cars, can be moved so that the isocentre can be located within a sphere of 2 mm diameter. Scaling down to the size of a dartboard: we are able to place an object, weighing 750 kg, so that it will lie within 0.05 mm of any desired position on the periphery of the dartboard. Every time we treat a patient we take this technological miracle for granted, and this is before we have even started to consider such complexities as safety interlocks, MLC and the ability to shape isodoses in three dimensions. Given this astonishing complexity and accuracy, the sheer reliability of the equipment is more surprising than the occasional problem, frustrating though those problems can be.

In public, we tend to make light of all of this. We are motivated, I suspect, by a desire not to intimidate patients. In this we are most unlike colleagues in other specialities who are often more loquacious about the technical wizardry or mystique associated with their disciplines. We are simply too modest. This has led to a vocabulary of denigration within the wider world of oncology: 'just pop them into the toaster'; 'give them a little heat treatment'; 'zap them in the microwave'. One challenge for our profession is, without boasting or intimidating, gently to point out that day in and day out, and with minimal fuss, we deliver effective treatment of the utmost sophistication and complexity. Like the best magicians and athletes, we make the barely possible seem ordinary.

We have another problem. Radiotherapy is often perceived by both colleagues and the public as an unsuccessful treatment of last resort: 'well, after the tumour came back they gave him the ray treatment, but he still died'. There is no doubt that radiotherapy can cure even fairly advanced cancers: it is still a source of wonder to me that, after radical radiotherapy, up to 40% of bladder cancers which have invaded deeply into muscle (T3) will disappear, never to return. There are no external scars, any side effects are usually temporary and self-limiting and, at follow-up, the bladder lining looks normal. The tumour appears to have dissolved and, although we can invoke apoptosis, genetic damage, necrosis and many other biological mechanisms to explain what has happened, there is still something magical about an invisible treatment that can produce such impressive results. One major challenge to radiation oncology is to combine the science with the art of radiation oncology so that each individual enjoys this type of therapeutic success. The poor reputation that we have as a speciality stems from the fact that, too often, we get it wrong. We doubly jeopardise our patients – they suffer from the treatment and they suffer from the failure of the treatment. We need to fuse basic science with clinical experience so that all individuals receive the treatment that is appropriate both for them and for their tumour. This goes far beyond our current horizons, investigating the value of predictive assays for radiosensitivity on tumour cells and on normal tissues. It demands that we incorporate into the decision-making process patients' informed choices. These choices reflect each individual's attitudes to benefit, to harm, to risk, to regret, and to the balance between certain disruption in the short term and the – less certain – longer-term gain.

Supportive care for the patient undergoing radical radiotherapy is important, not simply because it relieves distress but because, both directly and indirectly, it can improve the probability of eradicating the tumour. The direct effect is easy to define: by allowing a patient to complete a course of treatment that, in the absence of such support, might have been intolerable, supportive care has ensured the best possible chance of cure for that patient. The less obvious aspect is this. Given adequate supportive care, we can assume that a greater proportion of patients will be suitable for a radical, as opposed to a palliative, approach to treatment; we may also be able, cautiously, to increase the dose of radiation used in radical treatment. Thus we could increase not only the chances of cure for those individual patients whom we treat radically but also, at the population level, increase the proportion of patients who are selected for radical therapy.

We are too modest about the effectiveness of radiotherapy for the relief of symptoms in patients with advanced cancer. Again, we are often the option of last resort. Patients with painful bone metastases may spend weeks in hospital or at home, constipated and drowsy on opiates, before they are referred for palliation of bone pain, a single simple outpatient procedure costing about £150. We have, to some extent, only ourselves to blame for this. For too long we have preoccupied ourselves with curative treatment, to the exclusion of thinking rationally, or writing clearly, about palliative treatment. We have pretended to be that which we are not – a specialty solely concerned with curing cancer – and to offer that which we cannot – cure for the majority of patients we treat. One challenge is to be more honest with ourselves, with our colleagues and, most importantly, with our patients. We need to accept that, nowadays, 40–50% of the patients we treat with radiation are treated palliatively. We need to invest resources in the clinical and scientific investigation of palliative treatment. We need to draw more attention to the importance of the palliative role of radiotherapy. A recently completed book chapter on the management of head and neck cancer, a chapter of which I confess to being the principal author, was 43 000 words long. The word palliative, or a derivative thereof, was used only 20 times. There were 929 words (2% of the total) on the subject of palliative treatment. Overall, only about 55% of patients with head and neck cancer are cured, 45% are not: 2% of a chapter was allocated to problems that could affect 45% of the patients.

CONCLUSION

The challenge facing radiation oncology can be viewed as the need to bridge a series of deficits – deficits between that which is required and that which is available. These deficits are encountered across the whole of that broad spectrum of clinical activity that is radiation oncology. The solution is, wherever possible, to match supply to demand. Where resources are not present, be they machines, people or knowledge, then seek out what is missing. When demand seems excessive, then ask why and, if there is no good reason for such excess, seek to reduce it.

Ultimately, however we try to parse and analyse the problems, we inevitably return to the same point: the individual patient. We need to use all that we know, and all that we have available, to ensure that individual patients receive the care they require and deserve. That is the real challenge, and it is the timeless challenge that clinical medicine and its related disciplines have always faced. It will never fully be met, but that is no excuse for not trying.

REFERENCES

Antman E M, Lau J, Kupelnick B et al 1992 A comparison of results of metaanalyses of randomized control trials and recommendations of clinical experts. Treatments for myocardial infarction. Journal of the American Medical Association 268:240–248
Bentzen S M 1998 Towards evidence based radiation oncology: improving the design, analysis, and reporting of clinical outcome studies in radiotherapy. Radiotherapy Oncology 46:5–18
Bentzen S M, Hoskin P, Roos D et al 2000 Fractionated radiotherapy for metastatic bone pain: evidence-based medicine or…? International Journal of Radiation Oncology, Biology, Physics 46:681–683
Bernstein P L 1996 Against the Gods: the remarkable story of risk. John Wiley, New York
Board of Faculty of Clinical Oncology, Royal College of Radiologists, the College of Radiographers and the Royal College of Nursing 1999a Skills mix in clinical oncology. Royal College of Radiologists, London
Board of Faculty of Clinical Oncology, the Royal College of Radiologists and the College of Radiographers 1999b Inter-professional roles and responsibilities in a clinical oncology service. Royal College of Radiologists, London
Booth M, Summers J, Williams M V 1993 Audit reduces the reluctance to use single fractions for painful bone metastases. Clinical Oncology (Royal College of Radiologists) 5:15–18
Burnet N G, Routsis D S, Murrell P et al 2001 A tool to measure radiotherapy complexity and workload: derivation from the basic treatment equivalent (BTE) concept. Clinical Oncology (Royal College of Radiologists) 13:14–23
Delaney G P, Gebski V, Lunn A D et al 1997a Basic treatment equivalent (BTE): a new measure of linear accelerator workload. Clinical Oncology (Royal College of Radiologists) 9:234–239
Delaney G P, Gebski V, Lunn A D et al 1997b An assessment of the basic treatment equivalent (BTE) model as measure of radiotherapy workload. Clinical Oncology (Royal College of Radiologists) 9:240–244
Department of Health 1995 A policy framework for commissioning cancer services: a report by the expert advisory group on cancer to the chief medical officers of England and Wales. Available:www.doh.gov.uk/cancer/calmanhine.htm 2 Aug 2001

Department of Health 1998 Our healthier nation: a contract for health. Stationery Office, London

Department of Health 2000 The NHS cancer plan: a plan for investment, a plan for reform. Available:www.doh.gov.uk/cancer/cancerplan.htm 2 Aug 2001

Dixon P, Mackillop W 2001 Could changes in clinical practice reduce waiting lists for radiotherapy? Journal of Health Services Research and Policy 6:70–77

Dunn S M, Butow P N, Tattersall M H et al 1993 General information tapes inhibit recall of the cancer consultation. Journal of Clinical Oncology 11:2279–2285

Finch J 2000 Interprofessional education and teamworking: a view from the education providers. British Medical Journal 321:1138–1140

Forbes H, Cottier B 1999 A survey of radiotherapy services in England (1999). Department of Health, London, p 1–46

Fowler J F, Bentzen S M, Bond S J et al 2000 Clinical radiation doses for spinal cord: the 1998 international questionnaire. Radiotherapy Oncology 55:295–300

Holy Bible 1611 Gospel according to St Matthew (authorised version). Ch. 25, verse 29

Hoskin P J, Yarnold J R, Roos D R et al 2000 Radiotherapy for bone metastases. Clinical Oncology (Royal College of Radiologists) 13:88–90

Isaacs D, Fitzgerald D 1999 Seven alternatives to evidence based medicine. British Medical Journal 319:1618

Jones R, Pearson J, McGregor S et al 1999 Randomised trial of personalised computer based information for cancer patients. British Medical Journal 319:1241–1247

Kahneman D, Tversky A 1984 Choices, values and frames. American Psychologist 39:342–347

Mackillop W J, Bates J H T, O'Sullivan B, Withers H R 1995 The effect of delay in treatment on local control by radiotherapy. International Journal of Radiation Oncology, Biology, Physics 34:243–250

Maher E J 1991 The influence of national attitudes on the use of radiotherapy in advanced and metastatic cancer with particular reference to differences between the United Kingdom and the United States of America: implications for future studies. International Journal of Radiation Oncology, Biology, Physics 20:1369–1373

Munro A J 2001a Modern oncology: an A–Z of key topics. Greenwich Medical Media, London

Munro A J 2001b Anticipating the future role of radiotherapy and chemotherapy in the management of head and neck cancer: a lesson from Manchester. Clinical Oncology (Royal College of Radiologists) 13:336–338

Munro A J, Sebag-Montefiore D 1992 Opportunity cost – a neglected aspect of cancer treatment. British Journal of Cancer 65:309–310

O'Rourke N, Edwards R 2000 Lung cancer treatment waiting times and tumour growth. Clinical Oncology (Royal College of Radiologists) 12:141–144

Palda V, Llewellyn-Thomas H A, MacKenzie R G et al 1997 Breast cancer patients' attitudes about rationing postlumpectomy radiation therapy: applicability of trade-off methods to policy-making. Journal of Clinical Oncology 15:3192–3200

Priestman T J, Bullimore J A, Godden T P et al 1989 The Royal College of Radiologists' fractionation survey. Clinical Oncology (Royal College of Radiologists) 1:39–46

Sackett D L 2000 The sins of expertness and a proposal for redemption. British Medical Journal 320:1283

Sackett D L, Rosenberg W M C, Muir Gray J A et al 1996 Evidence based medicine: what it is and what it isn't. British Medical Journal 312:71–72

Schrijvers C T, Mackenbach J P, Lutz J M et al 1995 Deprivation and survival from breast cancer. British Journal of Cancer 72:738–743

Scottish Executive 2001a Cancer in Scotland: action for change. Available: www.show.scot.nhs.uk 2 Aug 2001

Scottish Executive 2001b Cancer scenarios: an aid to planning cancer services in Scotland in the next decade. Available: www.show.scot.nhs.uk 2 Aug 2001

Scottish Intercollegiate Guidelines Network 1997 Colorectal cancer: a national clinical guideline recommended for use in Scotland vol.16 Scottish Intercollegiate Guidelines Network, Edinburgh

3

The treatment trajectory

Mary Wells

INTRODUCTION

For most people, the concept of radiation is a difficult one to understand. Images of the effects of Hiroshima and Chernobyl inevitably link exposure to radiation with an invisible and mysterious sense of danger. Signs and symbols used to warn people of the hazards of ionising radiation can also invoke fear and apprehension. Many patients hold fundamental misconceptions about radiation despite the knowledge that radiotherapy treatment is given in a controlled environment, by experienced and specialist healthcare professionals, specifically to cure or control disease and symptoms. As Rotman et al (1977) pointed out (p. 744), 'Few therapeutic modalities in medicine induce more misunderstanding, fear and anxiety than the use of radiation in cancer treatment'. Unfortunately, many healthcare professionals also misunderstand the therapeutic use of radiotherapy, and this is not helped by the fact that radiotherapy departments are usually some distance from the main body of the hospital, and are thus viewed as separate entities.

The majority of patients receiving radiotherapy attend as outpatients, and the increasing centralisation of services has resulted in many patients travelling long distances for treatment. Those who require inpatient care may be admitted to a dedicated radiotherapy ward, but many hospitals do not have enough designated oncology beds and are forced to mix patients undergoing radiotherapy treatment with surgical patients. Care tends to be, of necessity, concentrated on the acute surgical patients rather than the 'walking wounded' radiotherapy patients. Even in specialist oncology units, the focus of care is frequently on patients undergoing chemotherapy, whose nursing needs may appear to be more obvious or more immediate. The shortage of therapy radiographers and specialist nurses in radiotherapy departments inevitably means that the emphasis of patient care is often on the technical aspects of treatment (Wells 1998a). Inadequate numbers of clinical

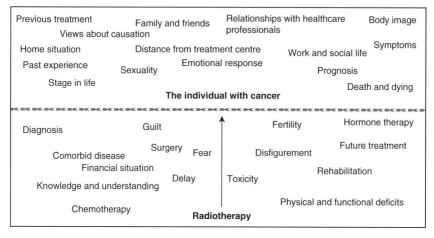

Figure 3.1   The context of the radiotherapy experience.

oncologists in the UK result in a need for many patients to be followed up in surgical clinics, where the experience and consequences of radiotherapy cannot be fully
understood. These factors all contribute to the tendency for radiotherapy services,
to focus on the episode of treatment itself, rather than to incorporate an holistic
approach to the care of patients with cancer who are undergoing radiotherapy as
part of their treatment trajectory.

Although the primary purpose of attendance or admission to a radiotherapy
department is for a course of radiotherapy treatment, there is a need to recognise
that individuals may already be facing a complex range of physical and emotional
challenges as a result of their cancer diagnosis. Radiotherapy takes place in a
context; it is not an isolated event, and its impact must be understood within the
overall experience of cancer, or the treatment trajectory (Fig. 3.1).

THE NEEDS OF PATIENTS AT COMMENCEMENT OF RADIOTHERAPY

When patients are referred to a radiation oncologist, they could be at any stage
of the cancer trajectory. Some individuals may not even have had a diagnosis of
cancer confirmed at this point, others may have already had surgery and/or
chemotherapy and require adjuvant radiotherapy, and a number may be returning
for palliative treatment.

Although it is obvious to those working in radiotherapy departments that individuals in each of these groups will require different doses and different fractionation schedules, non-specialist staff and patients do not always appreciate that
effective radiotherapy can be given as a single treatment, or as a course of treatment lasting up to 6 weeks. It can be particularly confusing for patients to understand that an equivalent dose can be given in a number of different ways for the
same disease. Some patients assume that 'more is better', and perceive that a long

course of treatment is likely to be more effective, but others interpret the need for weeks of treatment as meaning that their cancer is more serious than someone who is only having a short course of treatment. Of course, neither is strictly true, but patients themselves make assumptions about the meaning of treatment which are not only incorrect, but may cause them unnecessary worry. It is vital that healthcare professionals working in radiotherapy departments take care to assess individual assumptions and beliefs about treatment so that patients can fully understand the specific nature of their own radiotherapy.

The process of initial referral to commencement of treatment incorporates a number of stages, as seen in Figure 3.2. All of these stages may be subject to separate delays, making the overall time from initial symptoms, screening or referral potentially lengthy.

For a proportion of patients, for instance, those with early laryngeal cancers, radiotherapy may be the primary and sole treatment. For these individuals, the treatment episode is relatively short and clearly defined, although delays in diagnosis may have already prolonged the experience. Others, however, may have undergone neoadjuvant chemotherapy, surgery or primary chemotherapy and, for them, radiotherapy can be the final insult. The side effects of other treatments may continue to be troublesome; the patient is still adjusting to a life-changing diagnosis and is often weary of hospitals and treatment. The impact of starting a radical course of radiotherapy on top of the effects of chemotherapy or surgery can be huge, and it is important that the entirety of that experience is recognised. However, the language used by healthcare professionals can sometimes underemphasise the significance of what the patient is going through. For example, Costain Schou & Hewison (1999) found that patients having adjuvant therapy were commonly told that their 4–5-week radiotherapy was 'just a precaution'. As they point out, this message may offer reassurance to some extent, but could also

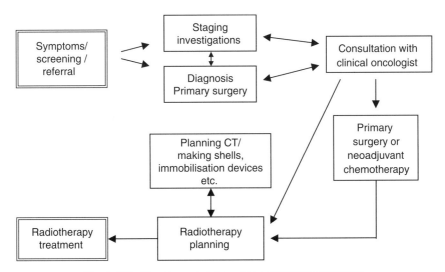

Figure 3.2   The stages leading up to radiotherapy treatment.
CT, computed tomography.

make it more difficult for patients to legitimise their anxieties and problems during treatment.

THE SIGNIFICANCE OF TIME

Recent government targets have encouraged earlier referral to cancer specialists, but may have inadvertently ensured that when patients are diagnosed with cancer, they may wait longer for treatment to start. Many patients find it extremely worrying to know they have a cancer growing inside them, for which treatment cannot be given for several weeks. Administrative delays or poor communication from the radiotherapy department can exacerbate this situation.

Cancer treatment can also profoundly interfere with the way in which people use their time. Frankenberg (1993) describes the 'waiting culture' of medicine, where patients lose control of their own time as it becomes governed by imposed appointments and delays. More specifically, Thorne (1986) describes the results of a survey conducted within a radiotherapy department, illustrating the loss of control, frustration and anxiety that waiting for treatment appointments produced. Patients in this survey highlighted the importance of staff acknowledging their presence, of their need to be kept informed, and of the potential for the environment to make a difference to the waiting experience. These findings were echoed by the Clinical Oncology Patients' Liaison Group (1999), which emphasised that some patients prefer not to be seated immediately next to other sick patients, and that the facilities provided in waiting areas can reduce the stress of waiting.

The scheduling of treatment can also be a source of stress. It may be assumed that patients who have their own transport are able to attend for treatment at any time of day. In reality, however, many patients have to collect children from school, maintain specific work schedules or rely on friends and relatives who can only provide transport at certain times of the day. The centralisation of services may also increase the practical, psychosocial and physical burden for those patients who have to travel long distances for their treatment (Payne et al 2000). It is difficult for radiotherapy departments to be totally flexible about treatment times, but there is a need for consideration of patients' circumstances so that, as far as possible, treatment can be arranged to fit in with personal commitments, and the pressures imposed by travelling to and from the treatment centre are minimised.

TREATMENT PLANNING

Before starting radiotherapy, all patients must have their treatment planned or simulated. However, the complex process of planning can be difficult for patients and non-specialist staff to appreciate. One common source of misunderstanding is the length of time required to complete the planning process, including the fact that there is usually a delay before treatment can start. Although this may be due to the availability of treatment slots, a period of several days is often required so that treatment calculations can be made, detailed treatment plans be drawn up and films checked.

Many plans can be produced from X-rays taken in the simulator itself, but for complex plans, CT scans may be necessary. Nicolaou (1999) provides a succinct overview of the technical aspects of this process. The planning process usually takes between 15 min and an hour, and can be an uncomfortable and lengthy experience if the patient is in any pain, or has to adopt an unusual position. This is usually the first time that patients have experienced the sensation of lying under a treatment machine, and some are alarmed by the size of the machine and the highly technical nature of the experience. As Sporkin (1992) comments (p. 36), 'during simulation, patients will be exposed to a series of new and unfamiliar procedures'. The focus of the planning session has to be on technical accuracy, but unfortunately this can result in a somewhat dehumanising experience for the patient. One patient with breast cancer and partial deafness recently described how traumatic she had found the planning process for radiotherapy, as she had to lie still with her head turned to the side of her good ear, so that she could hear nothing that was said. She was aware of the machine rotating, her arm and head being moved and of X-rays being taken, as well as people 'darting in and out of a darkened room', but she did not feel able to participate in the experience in any way. She explained that she did not understand what was going on, and felt she had no control over the situation.

Prior to the simulation session, some patients will require specific preparation such as catheter insertion (to ensure an empty bladder for pelvic radiotherapy), or the making of an immobilisation shell (for brain tumour and head and neck cancer patients). The experience of having a beam directional shell (BDS) made can be distressing, particularly for patients who are claustrophobic or who have breathing difficulties. Although mould room technicians are usually skilled in the preparation and education of patients for this procedure, there are aspects of the experience that can still be an unpleasant surprise for patients. During the making of the shell, the patient's face and neck are partially covered in plaster of Paris, which feels warm, flexible and wet on contact with the skin, but hardens as it dries. There are usually two stages to this process, to enable the back and front of the head to be cast separately. Impressions of the plaster cast are used to create a perspex shell, which is moulded perfectly to that individual's head. At simulation, the finished clear plastic shell is placed over the patient's face, and this may involve securing a press-stud mechanism at each side. Although patients are often prepared for the sensation of their face being covered, the noise of the press-studs being secured for the first time can be an unpleasant surprise. A number of patients have described feeling as if they being nailed into a coffin, bolted down or strapped in. As John Diamond pointed out, 'Had you told me that I would spend 15 minutes a day thus constrained I'd have told you about my small claustrophobia problem and tried not to vomit in your lap at the thought. But even claustrophobia becomes routine' (Diamond 1998, p. 106).

During simulation, the treatment area is defined using skin marks or tattoos, and for some patients this is an undignified experience which makes them feel 'branded' or marked. One breast cancer patient explained what she had done at the end of her treatment:

Washed all the marks off my chest – took a bit of time but I'm happy they're not there any more.

Interestingly, there is no published research exploring the experience of radiotherapy planning for the patient.

INFORMATION NEEDS PRIOR TO TREATMENT

In the last 25 years, there has been increasing recognition of the many myths and misconceptions held by patients about radiotherapy, as well as the level of anxiety engendered by this treatment. Studies have shown that patients are often ill-prepared for radiotherapy, express unmet needs for information and do not expect the severity or duration of side effects (Eardley 1985, 1986). A seminal study carried out in the 1970s interviewed 50 patients twice during radiotherapy, and found that more than 60% were experiencing mild or moderate anxiety or depression prior to starting radiotherapy treatment (Peck & Boland 1977). Most believed that they would not have needed radiotherapy if their surgery had been successful, and many had either received no information or had been given incorrect and negative information from friends and family. When asked what worried them most about treatment, the majority expressed concern about the machines, the radioactivity, having to take their clothes off, being exposed for any length of time and being burnt or scarred. When interviewed after the end of treatment, many expressed a sense of alarm about aspects of the environment such as the size of the machines, the thickness of the walls, the sounds during treatment, and the experience of lying 'under' the machine.

Although this study was conducted in the 1970s, it is still relevant today. Some patients are still frightened about the safety of machines, and fearful of the perceived dangers of the radiation. Misinformed healthcare professionals can also reinforce fears about radioactivity: they may not understand how external beam radiotherapy works, and what happens to patients receiving it. Terms commonly used in the past, such as 'radiation burns' and 'radium treatment', conjure up images of damage or hurt being inflicted, and these images are hard to dispel. Recent studies confirm that patients continue to be worried about radiation safety, damage to the body and side effects of treatment. Adverse media publicity only serves to fuel such concerns (Hammick et al 1998).

Because the radiation itself cannot be seen or felt, the provision of sensory information about the environment in which radiotherapy takes place is essential. Patients need to know what they will hear, see, feel, taste and smell. Although there are usually no specific tastes or smells associated with treatment, patients who are required to bite on a mouthpiece to immobilise the jaw may taste or smell the solution used to sterilise the mouthpiece. Patients should be prepared for the fact that the treatment table is hard and narrow, that the gantry will rotate around them and the bed may be moved up and down. They need to know that there may be a buzzing or ticking sound from the machine during treatment, and that they will be alone in a dimmed room, although watched through closed circuit television or a window and intercom system. If it is not explained, some patients may be alarmed by the fact that their treatment is given from many different angles. One intelligent young woman undergoing radiotherapy to the breast and axilla had assumed that the doctors had decided to treat her back as well, as she had not appreciated that her treatment had been planned using a five-field technique, which included a posterior field. Anxiety in radiotherapy patients can be high, and a lack of information about what to expect during radiotherapy can add to psychological distress (Frith 1991).

Factors such as gender and age can influence the degree to which the emotional and information needs of patients with cancer are met. McNamara (1999) used a postal questionnaire to elicit the information needs of patients a week before their radiotherapy planning appointment: 199 out of 297 patients responded (67%). More than 80% of patients had been given information about their treatment, but there were discrepancies in the degree of information and support received by different groups. Nearly a third of all patients indicated that they would have liked more support at home before starting radiotherapy. Patients with breast cancer were more likely to have been given information on their radiotherapy treatment, were more likely to have been seen by a nurse and were less likely to want further information than those with lung cancer, of whom 51% desired more information. Other studies have confirmed that patients with breast cancer are more likely to be provided with information than other groups (Jones et al 1999).

In McNamara's (1999) study, younger patients were also more likely to have received information about treatment, and young female patients were more likely to have seen a nurse. It could be that patients who are younger and/or female tend to seek support more than older and/or male patients do (Hammick et al 1998). Carlisle (1999) suggests that men may experience higher levels of stress than women, and proposes that healthcare professionals should be trained to recognise signs of stress so that early interventions are possible.

It can be assumed that patients' needs for information and emotional support prior to radiotherapy are centred around the treatment itself, but many patients will arrive in the radiotherapy department with fundamental misconceptions or lack of knowledge about their diagnosis or prognosis. The degree of uncertainty and hope experienced by patients during radiotherapy may influence the degree to which patients adjust after completion of treatment (Christman 1990). A recent study by Koller et al (2000) illustrates the problem of misconception in relation to expectations of treatment. Fifty-five inpatients with a variety of diagnoses were asked to complete a set of questionnaires before and after the end of their course of radiotherapy. Thirty-six of these patients were undergoing palliative treatment, and the remainder were receving adjuvant or primary curative radiotherapy. Their quality of life was measured using the European Organisation for Research and Treatment Quality-of-life Questionnaire (EORTC-QLQ C30) (Aaronson et al 1993), and expectations were assessed using a checklist relating to expectations of healing, reduction in tumour size or growth, prevention of relapse or metastases, pain and symptom relief and psychological improvement. All patients receiving palliative radiotherapy had been told that treatment would not cure them, but would help to 'lessen the burden of their illness'. Despite this, more than half these patients appeared to have expectations that treatment would cure them, and nearly two-thirds expected their treatment to alleviate pain or emotional distress. Post-treatment questionnaires demonstrated that expectations were not always met. At the end of treatment, patients' perceptions of the success of treatment were significantly less positive; only 26% still expressed the expectation that healing would occur ($P < 0.001$). Overall, there were no significant differences between pre- and post-treatment quality of life, although side effects known to be related to radiotherapy were more pronounced after treatment, e.g. nausea and vomiting, loss of appetite, diarrhoea. However, those patients who did not have their expectations of healing fulfilled, demonstrated a considerable drop in global quality of life. The authors acknowledge that having an optimistic attitude may be an important coping strategy, but they also highlight the need to foster realistic expectations through consistent and open communication during the treatment process.

THE EXPERIENCE OF TREATMENT

Following a lengthy planning appointment, many patients are surprised at how quickly their radiotherapy treatment is given, and how little they actually *feel* during treatment. Patients are usually told that they will not feel anything at the time of treatment, but some describe a warm, tingly sensation immediately after radiotherapy, and studies have shown that certain symptoms such as fatigue are experienced to a greater extent soon after each treatment (Smets et al 1998). Again, there are no studies which specifically look at what it actually *feels* like to have radiotherapy treatment.

Although the experience of radiotherapy is recognised as being stressful, research studies have generated differing results about patterns of anxiety and stress. Munro & Potter's study (1996) of 110 on-treatment patients found that anxiety, worry and depression were more common at the beginning of radiotherapy, and that by the end of treatment, physical symptoms were more prominent. A small interview study (Carlisle 1999) found no differences in anxiety ratings before and at completion of radiotherapy, but found that perceived stress had decreased significantly by the end of treatment. Eakes et al (1996), however, found that most of the 50 patients in their study experienced either the same or an increased level of emotional difficulty by the end of treatment. They concluded that the experience of radiotherapy was itself a source of emotional distress. Given the complexity of the treatment context, it is likely that a wide spectrum of anxieties and stresses can affect patients, and that individuals experience a range of emotional responses and crises at different times (Lamszus & Verres 1995).

As Frank (1991) states, cancer 'leaves no aspect of life untouched'. Figure 3.1 illustrates the many aspects of having cancer which can influence the experience of radiotherapy. During treatment, needs also change over time. It is clear tha the planning and initial treatment phase is a time of considerable uncertainty and anxiety, and it is at this stage that most radiotherapy departments concentrate their efforts so as to provide specific opportunities for giving information and support. As treatment progresses, patients continue to have regular contact with staff, but the way in which services are organised may not always provide adequate opportunity to explore the real impact of radiotherapy for the individual.

One difficulty is that many patients are reluctant to ask for help, and may underemphasise symptoms, not wanting to take up professionals' 'valuable' time. An early study by Mitchell & Glicksman (1977) interviewed 50 patients undergoing radiotherapy and found that none of them would discuss emotional problems with the radiographers, whose main role they perceived as operating the machine. A more recent study of patients with head and neck cancer after completion of radiotherapy illustrated that the treatment environment does not always empower patients to reveal their concerns (Wells 1996). One explained:

> *When you go in for your radiotherapy, they always ask, how do you feel, but that's the standard how do you feel, and they are getting the machine ready anyway...*

It is clear that perceptions of staff as busy or preoccupied with the task in hand can prevent patients from asking for help when they need it.

Equally, patients may make light of physical and emotional problems as they do not feel they are important enough, or they do not want to complain. One patient revealed,

> *The people you get having radiotherapy would all be people who are trying to make the best of the situation ... you want to be positive ... you want to feel fine so you play down how you really feel ... anyway, everybody knows that when you have radiotherapy you don't feel well*

(Wells 1995).

A combination of the high-tech environment, pressures of staff time and tendency for patients to 'play down' their problems may all contribute to a situation in which a friendly, but somewhat superficial, relationship develops. John Diamond (1998) illustrates this well (p. 105): 'At 4.10 a [radiographer] would call my name and I'd stroll into a barn-sized room with its irradiating machine in the middle of it. One of the three [radiographers] would offer a cheery 'How are you then?' and I'd say 'Well, since you ask, I've got cancer' and it is a tribute to their saintliness that even those [radiographers] who'd heard this tired gag six or seven times never smacked me in my irradiated teeth'.

Wells' study exposed a number of other factors that appeared to affect the degree to which patients admitted how they really felt. Several interviews demonstrated that patients had difficulty legitimising treatment-related symptoms, as they perceived these as minor compared with the 'big thing' (i.e. the cancer), which was being treated. They also seemed to feel that if something was really a problem, someone else would have noticed it and done something about it. Accounts of the treatment experience revealed that symptoms tended to creep up in an insidious way and that this made it harder to articulate specific needs. As one man said,

> *It happens so gradually that it sort of infiltrates slowly and you don't realise how ill you are feeling ... you don't realise it's waiting for you to say ...*

(Wells 1995).

Another common phenomenon is that patients rationalise that others are worse off than they are. Most of those who undergo radical radiotherapy encounter a range of other patients having treatment at the same time, and many exchange stories during their daily contacts. For some, this can be a very positive source of support, and the tendency to make comparisons with others can be a helpful coping strategy, as it emphasises their own health or strength. Others, however, find it traumatic to be exposed to fellow patients who are sick or who have had radiotherapy before, as it overtly demonstrates the potential for treatment to fail. The perception that these patients are worse off can also discourage patients from expressing the difficulties they are experiencing, as they feel they should not waste professionals' time when others' needs are greater (Wells 1998a).

This problem can be magnified once treatment is over. As Bury (1991) pointed out, patients at this stage may fear that their 'share of attention is used up', believing that others who are still having treatment are more deserving of attention. This was illustrated by a woman with breast cancer who, 1 month after her radiotherapy finished, said

> *... the girls said just ring, but you can't because you're dragging them away from people who need them more than you, you've had your treatment.*

Although patients can experience considerable fatigue, unexpected emotional difficulties and the loss of a 'safety net' during this time, (Graydon 1994, Walker et al 1996, Ward et al 1992) the needs of patients after treatment is complete are relatively unexplored. Chapter 4 further addresses this important issue.

The need to understand the entirety of the cancer experience and the treatment trajectory as a whole is emphasised by Hinds & Moyer's (1997) study of support during radiotherapy. They interviewed 12 patients and five family caregivers to ascertain their support needs during treatment. Findings illustrated the impact of radiotherapy on all aspects of life, and confirmed that patients are not merely concerned with treatment procedures and side effects. Patients and carers identified five main aspects of the radiotherapy experience through which they needed support (Table. 3.1).

Hinds & Moyer point out that there is a discrepancy between what patients and healthcare professionals perceive as supportive. They found that patients identified family and friends as their main sources of support. Supportive behaviours fell into three main areas: being there, giving help and giving information and advice. Support appeared to be less connected with meeting a specific need, and more to do with the *way* in which it was provided. Although patients accepted brusque and unhelpful attitudes from staff as unsurprising, without specifically identifying these as unsupportive, they did, however, notice and appreciate nurses who made a special effort and were 'ungrudging' in their actions.

Table 3.1 Support needs identified by patients and carers during radiotherapy (Hinds & Moyer 1997)

Need for support	Examples
Making the decision to undergo cancer treatment so soon after a diagnosis	Whether to have treatment at all, and if so, where and when
Undergoing the first treatment	Being treated away from home in unfamiliar surroundings, not knowing what to expect, lacking information, feeling vulnerable, being worried about the machines
Managing the indignities and experience of radiotherapy	Lying in awkward treatment positions, feeling exposed, missing meals because of treatment times, coping with the pain and discomfort of side effects
Coping with the inconvenience of treatment	Travelling to and from the treatment centre, arranging and waiting for transport, delays, equipment breakdown, being away from home, not being able to look after the house and garden
Dealing with longer-term considerations	Coming to terms with a potentially terminal illness, coping with changing emotions and perceptions of the situation

Patients' comments demonstrated that they needed different types of support at different times during treatment, and that support from healthcare professionals was most likely to be valued when it occurred within the context of a relationship. As the authors point out, the provision of support within such a relationship affirms feelings of worth, helps to maintain identity and ensures that the person is treated as a person rather than as a recipient of treatment. They also emphasise the need for staff to protect patients from the inadequacies of the treatment system by ensuring that practical difficulties are minimised, such as disruption to meal times, daily routines and responsibilities.

IMPROVING THE EXPERIENCE OF TREATMENT FOR THE INDIVIDUAL

If we are to improve the experience of patients undergoing radiotherapy treatment, we must ensure that care is based on the specific needs of individuals, and not on general assumptions about what patients need and want. Issues such as assessment, involvement in decision-making, information provision and development of 'patient-friendly' services are fundamental to this approach. A comprehensive and holistic assessment should take into account what patients know already, what they still want to know, how they are affected by pre-existing symptoms, emotional concerns, family and work problems and what concerns they have about the specific risks attached to their treatment. The use of a needs assessment tool or quality-of-life instrument may provide a basis for individualised assessment, and a number of authors have tested this approach. Maher et al (1996) used the EORTC QLQ C30 and the Hospital Anxiety and Depression (HAD) questionnaire to assess physical and emotional symptoms in 269 patients attending for radiotherapy treatment (72% of all patients in a 2-month period). They found that the scores of 40% people indicated abnormal levels of anxiety and depression. Higher levels of emotional distress appeared to correlate with higher symptom scores and lower functional scores. Some patients improved by 1 month after completion of radiotherapy, but others did not, indicating that new cases of anxiety and depression can occur after treatment is over.

Dennison & Shute (2000) take a more pragmatic approach to needs assessment, using a simple checklist distributed by outpatient clinic receptionists to elicit whether patients had concerns or worries about their illness, treatment, symptoms, finances, support, relationships, self-image and other aspects. Completed checklists were reviewed by the outpatient nurses prior to consultation with the doctor, so that appropriate assessment, support and referral to specialists could be instigated. The checklist also assisted the doctors in quickly identifying issues of concern for patients, and was well evaluated by patients, who found that it improved communication and relationships with staff, giving greater potential for involvement.

Involvement in decision-making

There is a trend towards increased involvement in decision-making about treatment, but there are still many unanswered questions about the degree to which informed decisions can truly be made by patients, based on the information they receive from healthcare professionals in radiotherapy departments. As a recent *Effective Health Care Bulletin* points out, 'Patients cannot express informed preferences about their care, choose to be involved in shared decision-making, or indeed choose not to participate, unless they are given sufficient and appropriate information' (NHS Centre for Reviews and Dissemination 2000, p. 3).

Radiotherapy incidents such as the overtreatment of patients in Exeter (Exeter Health Authority 1988) and the investigation into brachial plexus injury following complaints by the Radiation Action Group Exposure (RAGE) (Bates & Evans 1995) have raised public anxiety about radiotherapy, and increased professionals' concern about litigation. The RAGE movement in particular has forced staff to reconsider the accuracy of information given to patients about side effects. This is problematic, as there may be a difference between the attitudes of patients and oncologists in terms of the perceived significance of acute and late toxicity. A survey by Turner et al (1996) found that the majority of long-term survivors of Hodgkin's disease rated short-term side effects at least as important as or more important than late effects with respect to influencing choice of treatment. Patients may be more concerned about how they are going to feel immediately after treatment, whereas oncologists are more concerned about late effects. Some staff appear to believe that telling patients about potential side effects makes it more likely that they will experience them, and there is sometimes a fine line between full disclosure of information about treatment and discouraging the patient entirely from pursuing a course of advisable treatment.

It is increasingly common, but not standard practice, to ask patients to give written consent to treatment. The issue of eliciting written consent prior to radiotherapy is a complex one. It would be considered totally unethical not to request patient consent for surgery or clinical trial participation, yet many radiotherapy departments do not routinely ask for written consent. One ethical view is that taking part in research and having treatment are essentially different, in that the basic premise underlying conventional treatment is the intention to benefit the individual, and that such benefit is assumed to outweigh any disadvantage by both patient and doctor (Gillon 1989). The difference between consenting to surgery as opposed to radiotherapy is perhaps less clear. A recent report from the Royal College of Radiologists (1999), however, recommends that all patients should give written consent prior to treatment with radiotherapy or cytotoxic or biological response-modifying anticancer drug treatment. The report specifies that such consent must be obtained by a suitably qualified doctor who understands the risks of the proposed treatment, following discussion of all common side effects and any potentially serious effects (unless these are exceedingly rare). The complexity of this issue is discussed further in Chapters 2 and 14.

Information provision

The basis of informed consent is the provision of adequate information which in itself appears to offer a number of benefits to the patient. In the 1980s and early 1990s, several US studies reported the positive effects of information on self-care behaviours, side effects and anxiety (Dodd 1987, Hagopian 1991, Johnson et al 1988,

Weintraub & Hagopian 1990). Although studies assessing the effect of information on self-care and side effects do not adequately address the impact on the *whole* person undergoing treatment, they do demonstrate the potential for staff to improve aspects of well-being through the provision of individualised information and education.

Despite evidence to demonstrate that information is beneficial to patients, some healthcare professionals still take the view that patients do not desire honest and accurate information about their cancer or its treatment. Written patient information materials also tend to give an overoptimistic view, emphasising benefits and glossing over risks and side effects (Coulter et al 1999). A survey of 2331 outpatients across the UK found, however, that 87% of people preferred to be given as much information as possible about their illness, whether it was good or bad (Jenkins et al 2001).

Porock's work (1995) suggests that preparatory education, which combines both sensory and procedural information, is an important component of support, and that its provision can reduce anxiety during treatment. Weintraub & Hagopian (1990) found that patients allocated to receive specific nursing support and information during radiotherapy experienced less anxiety throughout, although their symptom profiles were more severe towards the end of treatment. Although the sample size was small, the study suggests that nurses may be able to reduce the emotional burden of treatment for patients, *despite* worsening side effects. The reporting of more severe side effects in the nursing group could indicate that information and support from nurses has no impact on reducing symptoms, or alternatively may suggest that nursing support raises awareness of symptoms and encourages patients to be honest about how they feel. Further research is required into the impact of information, using broader outcome measures such as psychological well-being, quality of life, functional status or patient satisfaction.

Verbal and written information

A number of studies have looked at the type of information patients prefer, and the most suitable mode of delivery of that information. Johnson (1996) has written widely on the information needs of patients undergoing radiotherapy. Her work is based on a model of self-regulation theory, which proposes that patients cope with stressful experiences through regulation of two different coping mechanisms: emotional and functional responses. She believes that the way in which the individual understands the stressful experience affects the regulation of this dynamic coping process. In other words, those who prefer to use concrete objective information to help predict and understand a stressful experience (i.e. the functional responders) will value interventions that strengthen their ability to cope in this way. Those who respond emotionally (i.e. the emotional responders) will be more likely to seek emotional comfort in order to reduce their vulnerability and help them cope. Once emotionally comfortable, the functional aspects of coping can then be addressed.

This model may help practitioners to consider the ways in which patients respond to their illness and its treatment, so that information and support can be tailored to their needs. Individuals require different levels of information at different times in their treatment trajectory, and it is vital that their preferences and requirements are elicited at an early stage so that appropriate information can be provided in a timely fashion.

Most studies of information preferences have, however, looked at the acceptability of different types of information from the point of view of a general sample of patients, rather than by attempting to tailor information to the coping styles of individuals. Fieler et al (1996) investigated the information preferences of 134 patients who had completed radiotherapy for cure or local control of cancers of the head and neck, lung, breast or prostate. Patients were asked to prioritise four different types of information, giving their first and second choices. The largest proportion (42%) chose concrete objective information about the possible side effects of treatment, when to expect them and how long they would last. This type of information was also the most common second choice (32%), although 29% opted for wanting to know how to deal with side effects. One-third of patients preferred to know how radiotherapy kills cancer, but few prioritised information on physical tests and examinations. Patients' reasons for their preferences centred on mental preparation, relief of anxiety and increased understanding.

Hinds et al (1995) found that patients commencing radiotherapy treatment tended to prefer verbal information backed up by written material and that they were most likely to identify the doctor as their main source of information. Preferences for information were similar at the end of treatment, although a greater proportion of patients mentioned written information at this time. Porock (1995) illustrates that patients prefer to be given information without having to ask questions, and Hammick et al (1998) reinforces the finding that patients are more positive about information received from individuals (particularly doctors) rather than through written leaflets.

It is interesting that, although patients do identify nurses and radiographers as sources of information and support, they seem to be more likely to emphasise the doctor's role in the provision of information and emotional support. A large survey by Slevin et al (1996) found that the three most important sources of emotional support were registrars (73%), family (73%) and consultants (63%), with other healthcare professionals lagging behind. These findings do reinforce the value patients place on information and contact with their doctor, but also suggest that nurses and other professionals may not be adequately addressing patients needs, or that their role is not clear to most patients. It is vital that nurses and radiographers are able to articulate their contribution to patient care so that it can be evaluated more effectively in future studies.

Although good practice dictates that up-to-date written information should be available and that it should be accompanied by verbal explanation, this is not always easy to achieve. Edwards & Campbell (1998) highlight the difficulties involved in producing high-quality written information leaflets. There are also dilemmas about *where* these leaflets should be available to patients. Some radiotherapy staff feel uncomfortable about patients accessing leaflets in non-specialist areas, where general staff are unlikely to have the knowledge to answer questions or allay fears. However, as Eardley (1988) identified, many patients express a desire for information about radiotherapy to be available in other areas so that they have some idea of what to expect before they get to the department. There is huge potential for developing stronger links with general practice surgeries, district and practice nurses, staff in cancer units and general wards, so that consistent information can be provided in a timely fashion and specialist advice sought where necessary. Managed clinical networks may assist the development of such links at a strategic level, but it is vital that communication channels are also strengthened on a day-to-day basis. Equally, it is important that patients' views and experiences are used to develop meaningful information resources (Coulter et al 1999). Christman et al (2001) describe how the study of patients' symptoms during pelvic radiotherapy is an essential component of the development of relevant preparatory information for this patient group. Local audits, focus groups, published research papers and reports from associations such as the National Cancer Alliance (1996) can provide crucial insights into the experience of patients, which can then be incorporated into the information provided by the radiotherapy centre.

Audiovisual information

The limitations of the written word have encouraged many researchers and practitioners to explore alternative methods of providing information for patients, mainly using videos and tapes. Hagopian (1996) randomised 75 patients receiving radiotherapy to two groups: the first received standard information, the second also received an informational audiotape. Patients completed a knowledge test and side effects profile. Hagopian found that those who listened to the audiotape were more knowledgeable about radiotherapy and side effects, and used more self-care measures.

Two recent studies have evaluated the effectiveness of videotaped information about radiotherapy (Harrison et al 2001, Thomas et al 2000). Both studies randomised more than 200 patients to receive either written information alone or a video as well the standard written information. Both used the HAD scale (Zigmond & Snaith 1983) to assess effectiveness, supplemented by an additional questionnaire assessing satisfaction (Thomas et al 2000) or 'worry about radiotherapy' (Harrison et al 2001). The first study found that patients in the video group were substantially more satisfied with the information they had received than those in the non-video group. Their anxiety and depression scores had also significantly improved by the time they were 3 weeks into treatment, whereas the anxiety scores of the non-video group had not improved and the depression scores were significantly higher (Thomas et al 2000). The second study (Harrison et al 2001) assessed patients more frequently: at recruitment, start of treatment, completion of treatment and 6 weeks later. Although general anxiety had decreased in both groups by the last day of treatment, there were no significant differences between the groups. However, when anxiety levels were measured 6 weeks after radiotherapy, those of the 'written information only' group had increased to pre-treatment levels whereas those of the videotape group had continued to fall. The authors suggest that videotaped images of longer-term survivors of cancer may provide reassurance for patients who have recently completed therapy.

The development of computerised information and education for patients is also being explored. Numerous sources of information are now available on the internet, and there are some excellent sites (for example, those listed at the end of this chapter) from which patients and healthcare professionals can access high-quality information about cancer and radiotherapy. Internet support groups are also becoming more popular. Some internet sources are, however, of dubious quality and the sheer amount and range of information available can overload and confuse certain individuals. Jones et al (1999) point out that finding information on the internet can be difficult and that more thought is needed about its role as a primary information source for patients. As Klemm & Nolan (1998) comment, the use of the internet for the education and support of patients also raises a number of ethical and legal issues, concerned with confidentiality, consent and copyright.

The use of touch-screen computerised information packages in clinical departments offers huge potential for patients to be better informed and educated about their treatment. Although some patients do not have the computer skills, simple step-by-step programs could enable them to access individualised information about their treatment at their own speed. Jones et al (1999) demonstrate the potential for computer programs to enable patients to access a combination of personal and general medical information. They compared a personalised computerised information system, linked to a summary of the patient's medical records, with a general computer system or set of written information booklets. A total of 525 patients undergoing radiotherapy were randomised into the study and outcomes were measured at the start of treatment, 3 weeks into treatment and 3 months later. The cost analysis indicated that the introduction of an electronic patient record would make the personalised information system no more expensive to run than a general system. Patients who were given access to personal information were more likely to score highly on patient satisfaction. Those who received written booklets only were more likely to feel overwhelmed by the information given and those who received general information only were significantly more likely to be anxious 3 months after treatment finished.

Other studies have also found that the provision of general information can be disadvantageous. Dunn et al (1993) provided general information tapes to patients and found that they were likely to inhibit recall of specific consultations. The importance of personalising information does appear to be important to patients who want to be treated as individuals. Jones et al (1999) found that 80% of patients preferred a 10-min consultation with a specialist nurse or radiographer to computer or booklet information. These studies demonstrate the need to provide adequate opportunity for one-to-one dialogue throughout the treatment trajectory as well as to facilitate the involvement of patients in discussions about their care.

PROVIDING PATIENT-FRIENDLY SERVICES

The lay members of the Clinical Oncology Patients' Liaison Group (1999) have recently produced recommendations for making services more patient-friendly, illustrating the need to consider the patient's perspective more carefully in the planning and delivery of care. These recommendations contain many helpful practical suggestions for improving the experience of patients attending the department (Box 3.1).

The messages in this booklet are remarkably simple, but the fact that a lay group of people who had experienced radiotherapy felt a need to write it illustrates that services are not always patient-friendly. It is vital that we elicit the views of local 'users' of treatment through greater involvement in decision-making, audit and research so that we can provide truly responsive services.

Box 3.1 Recommendations from the Clinical Oncology Patients' Liaison Group (1999) for making your radiotherapy service more patient-friendly

- Improving the reception area and welcome procedure to ensure that first impressions are positive and do not alienate patients
- Facilitating pre-treatment visits to the department, providing information about side effects and radiotherapy personnel and ensuring that staff in cancer units have the knowledge and skills to provide adequate information for patients
- Recognition of the practical difficulties faced by some patients in order to travel to and from the department at a specific time of day
- Information and explanation about delays in treatment and waiting times for treatment
- Improvements to waiting areas to reduce exposure to 'public gaze' and provide better facilities for those waiting
- Provision of verbal, written and audiovisual information on the experience of treatment, procedures involved and staff in the department, in languages appropriate to the patient population
- Cooperation and communication within the multidisciplinary team to ensure that information and advice are consistent, and all relevant staff are informed about the treatment plan
- Ensuring privacy and dignity are maintained during radiotherapy and that adequate time and space are given to patients who need to undress
- Reducing unnecessary numbers of staff in a room at any one time
- Providing clear information about the need for skin markings and avoiding the use of the word 'tattoo', which is misleading and alarming
- Attending to patients' needs at the end of treatment when the sudden cessation of radiotherapy can induce feelings of loneliness and uncertainty, in addition to physical distress
- Actively seeking and considering patients' views in the provision of care

---

CONCLUSION

Radiotherapy is physically and emotionally demanding, and the invisible and high-tech nature of the treatment may cause particular anxiety for patients. Although the treatment itself can induce specific concerns, it forms only part of the overall experience of having cancer, and it is vital that professional carers attempt to understand the entirety of this experience. Patients are referred for radiotherapy with a wide variety of previous experiences, fears, concerns and physical problems, and their individual needs for emotional, practical and physical support must be assessed at an early stage. Radiotherapy treatment has the potential to cause disruption in all areas of life, and care provision must be directed towards minimising this disruption and alleviating treatment-induced problems within the context of the whole cancer experience.

Outpatient nurses, specialist nurses and radiographers play a key role in the initial assessment of patients and their continued input throughout treatment is crucial, given that the majority of patients attend on a daily basis for their radiotherapy. Particular emphasis should be placed on liaison and communication between outpatient staff, radiographers, doctors, ward nurses and community staff so that transitions between different areas of the healthcare system are managed smoothly.

Each stage of treatment may bring with it particular demands, and staff must anticipate and respond quickly to these demands so that patients' needs are met promptly, before further problems occur. Needs change throughout treatment, and adequate opportunity must be provided for individuals to voice their concerns in a confidential and supportive atmosphere. There is a need for the environment of care in radiotherapy departments to be reorganised so as to promote the development of therapeutic relationships with individual patients, and to ensure the provision of a patient-friendly service. This then establishes the basis for supportive care to be provided throughout the episode of radiotherapy and beyond.

AREAS FOR FURTHER RESEARCH AND DEVELOPMENT

- Multidisciplinary team working in radiotherapy departments
- Clarification and evaluation of roles of healthcare professionals in radiotherapy departments
- The experience of treatment planning and the delivery of treatment itself
- The evaluation of patients' experiences of the environment of care in which radiotherapy treatment is given
- Impact of centralisation on patients' experiences of treatment services
- Innovative methods of information and education and the evaluation of such methods
- The experience of completing and recovering from radiotherapy treatment
- Development and evaluation of alternative models of support for patients and relatives during treatment
- Development and evaluation of communication pathways between cancer centres, cancer units and primary care staff
- Involvement of patients in decision-making and the development of information resources.

FURTHER INFORMATION

---

1. CHIQ – The Centre for Health Information Quality website with link to Macmillan Directory, listing numerous patient information resources about aspects of radiotherapy http://www.hfht.org/chiq

2. National Cancer Institute – US website with many patient information and healthcare professional resources on all aspects of cancer http://cancernet.nci.nih.gov

3. Radiotherapy – US website with information about guidelines, organisational issues, links to journals and abstracts http://www.radiotherapy.com

4. Royal College of Radiologists – RCR publications on all aspects of standards in radiotherapy departments http://www.rcr.ac.uk

5. UK government cancer sites – links to NHS cancer plan, nursing and radiotherapy reports http://www.doh.gov.uk/cancer www.show.scot.nhs.uk/sehd/cancerinscotland/

6. Database of Individual Patient Experiences http://www.dipex.org/

REFERENCES

Aaronson H K, Ahmedzai S, Bergman B et al 1993 The European Organization for Research and Treatment of Cancer QLQ-C30: a quality of life instrument for use in international clinical trials in oncology. Journal of the National Cancer Institute 85:365–376

Bates T, Evans R 1995 Brachial plexus neuropathy following radiotherapy for breast carcinoma. Independent review. Royal College of Radiologists, London

Bury M 1991 The sociology of chronic illness: a review of research and prospects. Sociology of Health and Illness 13(4):451–468

Carlisle J 1999 An evaluation of perceived stress in radiation therapy patients. Radiation Therapist 8(2):119–129

Christman N 1990 Uncertainty and adjustment during radiotherapy. Nursing Research 39(1):17–47

Christman N, Oakley M G, Cronin S N 2001 Developing and using preparatory information for women undergoing radiation therapy for cervical or uterine cancer. Oncology Nursing Forum 28(1):93–98

Clinical Oncology Patients' Liaison Group 1999 Making your radiotherapy service more patient-friendly. Board of the Faculty of Clinical Oncology, Royal College of Radiologists, London

Costain Schou K, Hewison J 1999 Experiencing cancer. Open University Press, Buckingham

Coulter A, Entwistle V, Gilbert D 1999 Sharing decisions with patients: is the information good enough? British Medical Journal 318:318–322

Dennison S, Shute T 2000 Identifying patient concerns: improving the quality of patient visits to the oncology out-patient department – a pilot audit. European Journal of Oncology Nursing 4(2):91–98

Diamond J 1998 Because cowards get cancer too. Vermillion, London

Dodd M 1987 Efficacy of proactive information on self-care in radiation therapy patients. Heart and Lung 16:538–544

Dunn S M, Butow P N, Tattersall M H N et al 1993 General information tapes inhibit recall of the cancer consultation. Journal of Clinical Oncology 11:2279–2285

Eakes G, Rafkal S M, Keel E et al 1996 The cancer experience: responses of patients receiving outpatient radiotherapy. Journal of Psychosocial Oncology 14(3):19–30

Eardley A 1985 Patients and radiotherapy. 1. Expectations of treatment. 2. Patients' experiences of treatment. Radiography 51:324–326

Eardley A 1986 Patients and radiotherapy. 3. Patients' experiences after discharge. 4. How patients can be helped. Radiography 52(601):17–22

Eardley A 1988 Patients' views. Clear views. Health Service Journal 108(5608):30–31

Edwards S, Campbell J 1998 An information strategy for radiotherapy patients. Professional Nurse 13(7):456–458

Exeter Health Authority 1988 The report of the committee of inquiry into the incident in the radiotherapy department. Exeter Health Authority, Exeter

Fieler V K, Wlasowicz G.S, Mitchell M L et al 1996 Information preferences of patients undergoing radiation therapy. Oncology Nursing Forum 23(10):1603–1608

Frank A 1991 At the will of the body. Reflections on illness. Houghton Mifflin, Boston

Frankenberg R 1993 Time, health and illness. Sage, London

Frith B 1991 Giving information to radiotherapy patients. Nursing Standard 5(34):33–35

Gillon R 1989 Medical treatment, medical research and informed consent. Journal of Medical Ethics 15:3–5, 11

Graydon J 1994 Women with breast cancer: their quality of life following a course of radiation therapy. Journal of Advanced Nursing 19:617–622

Hagopian G 1991 The effects of a weekly radiation therapy newsletter on patients. Oncology Nursing Forum 18:1199–1203

Hagopian G 1996 The effects of informational audiotapes on knowledge and self-care behaviors of patients undergoing radiation therapy. Oncology Nursing Forum 23(4):697–700

Hammick M, Tutt A, Tait D et al 1998 Knowledge and perception regarding radiotherapy and radiation in patients receiving radiotherapy: a qualitative study. European Journal of Cancer Care 7(2):103–112

Harrison R, Dey P, Slevin N J et al 2001 Randomized controlled trial to assess the effectiveness of a videotape about radiotherapy. British Journal of Cancer 84(1):8–10

Hinds C, Moyer A 1997 Support as experienced by patients with cancer during radiotherapy treatments. Journal of Advanced Nursing 26:371–379

Hinds C, Streater A, Mood D 1995 Functions and preferred methods of receiving information related to radiotherapy. Cancer Nursing 15(5):374–384

Jenkins V, Fallowfield L, Saul J 2001 Information needs of patients with cancer: results from a large study in UK cancer centres. British Journal of Cancer 84(1):48–51

Johnson J E 1996 Coping with radiation therapy: optimism and the effect of preparatory information. Research in Nursing and Health 19(1): 3–12

Johnson J, Nil N M, Lauver D et al 1988 Reducing the negative impact of radiation therapy on functional status. Cancer 61: 46–51

Jones R, Pearson J, McGregor S et al 1999 Randomised trial of personalised computer based information for cancer patients. British Medical Journal 319:1241–1247

Klemm P, Nolan M 1998 Internet cancer support groups: legal and ethical issues for nurse researchers. Oncology Nursing Forum 25(4):673–676

Koller M, Lorenz W, Wagner K et al 2000 Expectations and quality of life of cancer patients undergoing radiotherapy. Journal of the Royal Society of Medicine 93:621–628

Lamszus K, Verres R 1995 Social support of radiotherapy patients in emotional stress and crisis situations. Strahlentherapie und Onkologie 171(7):408–414

Maher E J, Mackenzie C, Young T et al 1996 The use of the Hospital Anxiety and Depression Scale (HADS) and the EORTC QLQ-C30 questionnaires to screen for treatable unmet needs in patients attending routinely for radiotherapy. Cancer Treatment Reviews 22(suppl. A):123–129

McNamara S 1999 Information and support: a descriptive study of the needs of patients with cancer before their first experience of radiotherapy. European Journal of Oncology Nursing 3(1):31–37

Mitchell G, Glicksman A 1977 Cancer patients: knowledge and attitudes. Cancer 40(1):61–66

Munro A, Potter S 1996 A quantitative approach to the distress caused by symptoms in patients treated with radical radiotherapy. British Journal of Cancer 74:640–647

National Cancer Alliance 1996 Patient-centred cancer services? What patients say. National Cancer Alliance, Oxford

NHS Centre for Reviews and Dissemination 2000 Effective health care bulletin, vol. 6. Informing, communicating and sharing decisions with people who have cancer. NHS Centre for Reviews and Dissemination, York

Nicolaou N 1999 Radiation therapy treatment planning and delivery. Seminars in Oncology Nursing 15(4):260–269

Payne S, Jarrett N, Jeffs D et al 2000 The impact of travel on cancer patients' experiences of treatment: a literature review. European Journal of Cancer Care 9:197–203

Peck A, Boland J 1977 Emotional reactions to radiation treatment. Cancer 40:180–184

Porock D 1995.The effect of preparatory patient education on the anxiety and satisfaction of cancer patients receiving radiotherapy. Cancer Nursing 18(3):206–214

Rotman M, Rogow L, Delean G et al 1977 Supportive therapy in radiation oncology. Cancer 39:744–750

Royal College of Radiologists 1999 Good practice for clinical oncologists. Royal College of Radiologists, London

Slevin M, Nichols S E, Downer S M et al 1996 Emotional support for cancer patients: what do patients really want? British Journal of Cancer 74(8):1275–1279

Smets E M, Visser M R, Willems-Groot A F et al 1998 Fatigue and radiotherapy: (A) experience in patients undergoing treatment. British Journal of Cancer 78(7):899–906

Sporkin E 1992 Patient and family education. Nursing care. In: Dow K, Hilderley L, (eds) Radiation oncology. W B Saunders, Philadelphia, p 33–44

Thomas R, Daly M, Perryman B et al 2000 Forewarned is forearmed – benefits of preparatory information on video cassette for patients receiving chemotherapy or radiotherapy – a randomised controlled trial. European Journal of Cancer 36:1536–1543

Thorne S 1986 Waiting, the 'patient' experience. Canadian Journal of Radiography, Radiotherapy, Nuclear Medicine 17(1):44–46

Turner S, Maher E J, Young T et al 1996 What are the information priorities for cancer patients involved in treatment decisions? An experienced surrogate study in Hodgkin's disease. British Journal of Cancer 73(2):222–227

Walker B L, Nail L M, Larsen L et al 1996 Concerns, affect and cognitive disruption following completion of radiation treatment for localised breast or prostate cancer. Oncology Nursing Forum 23(8):1181–1187

Ward S E, Viergutz G, Tormey D et al 1992 Patients' reactions to completion of adjuvant breast cancer therapy. Nursing Research 41(6):362–366

Weintraub F, Hagopian G A 1990 The effect of nursing consultation on anxiety, side effects, and self-care of patients receiving radiation therapy. Oncology Nursing Forum 17(3):31–38

Wells M 1995 The impact of radiotherapy to the head and neck: a qualitative study of patients after completion of treatment. Centre for Cancer and Palliative Care Studies, Institute of Cancer Research, London

Wells M 1998a The hidden experience of radiotherapy to the head and neck: a qualitative study of patients after completion of treatment. Journal of Advanced Nursing 28(4):840–848

Wells M 1998b What's so special about radiotherapy nursing? European Journal of Oncology Nursing 2(3):162–168

Zigmond A, Snaith R 1983 The Hospital Anxiety and Depression Scale. Acta Psychiatrica Scandinavica 67:361–370

4

After treatment is over

Caroline Nicholson   Mary Wells

INTRODUCTION

As discussed in previous chapters, the supportive care of patients undergoing radiotherapy must consider the context in which treatment takes place. This not only requires recognition of events and experiences *before* treatment, but also acknowledges the needs of patients at the *end* of treatment, when reactions are at their peak, and day-to-day links with the hospital are severed (Wells 1998a). Despite advances in both the practice and research of radiotherapy as a treatment modality, the needs and experiences of patients posttreatment remain largely neglected by researchers and practitioners. In part, this may be explained by the general lack of emphasis on supportive care in the radiotherapy literature (Faithfull 2001). Additionally, it is fair to say that in most areas of health service delivery and enquiry, issues of community care have, historically, been dominated by those of the acute sector. However, it is also the ambiguity of the patient's status after completion of radiotherapy treatment that influences both the provision of care and the perception of patients' needs during this vulnerable time. Patients are neither acutely sick nor are they well: neither healthy nor cured. They may well be suffering side effects of treatment, but without requiring hospitalisation or a full package of care at home. They are not fully discharged from hospital, nor are they likely to be in frequent contact with hospital services. Often, they are not known to community services or aware of what these services can provide.

Since the implementation of the Calman–Hine report (Department of Health 1995) increasing emphasis is being placed on the primary sector to be the focus of care for all patients with cancer. Although the completion of acute treatment such as radiotherapy appears to be the obvious time for care to be transferred to community staff, this is not a process that occurs smoothly. Difficulties and delays in communication between hospital and community staff and a lack of understanding of roles inevitably result in poor discharge planning at the end of treatment (Eardley 1990). The number of patients undergoing radiotherapy who are seen by individual general practitioners and district nurses may be quite small, thus it is difficult for community staff to maintain up-to-date knowledge and expertise in this area. As a result, patients are often left to fend for themselves during a time of considerable uncertainty and persisting symptoms.

This chapter explores some of the conceptual and practical challenges associated with the postradiotherapy period as well as the planning and provision of care after treatment is complete. It begins by exploring the concept of transition, in order to shed light on the ambiguous nature of this period in the patient's treatment trajectory, as referred to earlier (Ch. 3).

THE TRANSITION FROM RADIOTHERAPY TO HOME

Transition is defined as 'the passage or movement from one state to the other' (Schumacher & Meleis 1994, p. 119). Indicators of a healthy transition include a subjective sense of well-being and quality of life, achievement in and comfort with a change in role, and a sense of well-being in relationships. These relationships can be conceptualised through family adaptation and integration with broader social networks and community (Schumacher & Meleis 1994). The transition(s) from radiotherapy patient to person on follow-up is accompanied by an enormous and varied number of challenges. Despite the positive aspects of finishing treatment, this transition can be associated with physical, psychological, social and spiritual difficulties, which are rarely acknowledged in the care that we provide. Although it must be recognised that every individual experiences these differently, their dimensions can be conceptualised in terms of these four areas, as seen in Figure 4.1.

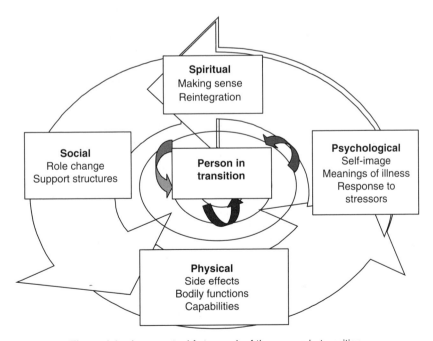

Figure 4.1   A conceptual framework of the person in transition.

Physical transitions

It is well known that the physical effects of radiotherapy tend to reach their peak as treatment ceases, and may not resolve for several weeksor even months afterwards. Walker et al's work (1996) highlighted persistent problems with fatigue, pain and trouble sleeping during the post-treatment period. Other studies have illustrated the distress associated with new or worsening side effects after treatment is over (Eardley 1986a, Faithfull 1995, Wells 1998a). Although acute side effects often decrease over the subsequent 3 months, this is not always the case. Symptoms such as fatigue can last for many months and others, such as radiation enteritis, can cause chronic difficulties, profoundly affecting quality of life (Faithfull 2001). As Chapter 10 illustrates, the effects of radiotherapy to the head and neck may result in permanent changes to salivary function, and late effects may appear months to years after treatment is given. It is clear that the side effects of radiotherapy present an ongoing challenge for patients post-treatment, yet many are unprepared for the nature and duration of symptoms experienced (Eardley 1986b). A number of reasons may explain why this is the case, including:

- Inadequate assessment and information prior to, during and after treatment
- An inability to receive information at the time due to a focus on the immediate task of managing the treatment
- Incongruence between a person's expectations of completing treatment and the reality of the recovery and rehabilitation process.

Wells (1998a) suggests that these problems are exacerbated by a tendency for patients to normalise their situation. In her study some patients felt that any side effects were minimal compared to the larger issue of the cancer and that this made them unlikely to seek help in managing symptoms. Another explanation for this tendency may be the cultural imperative to move quickly out of the sick role and remain positive and independent in the light of a cancer diagnosis (Sontag 1989, Stacey 1997).

Wells' study (1998a) highlighted the unpredictability of symptoms after completion of treatment, and found that patients needed the confidence that symptoms were improving to encourage them to resume normal activities. However, the side effects of treatment may result in bodily changes or functional capabilities which require specific rehabilitative care. Such changes may include local swelling and lymphoedema, difficulties in eating, drinking or speech due to dry mouth, sexual problems as a result of pelvic radiotherapy or bladder or bowel dysfunction resulting in pain and urgency on micturition or defecation. Although the acute severity of symptoms has often subsided by the time patients attend their first follow-up appointment, the functional problems left behind may still be causing patients considerable difficulty. Yet the follow-up appointment rarely provides the opportunity to address such rehabilitation needs. As one patient's story illustrates, even concerns framed as 'little' are not easily acknowledged in this setting:

When I went to see Mr H [surgeon], oh I can't remember how long ago it was, I'd just been out of hospital [the centre, following implanted wire treatment] maybe a couple of weeks. But you see he just seemed very busy and tired, and kept putting his hand on the doorknob and I kept asking another question! And then he'd turn round and answer me but, I felt as if I didn't have, enough time, to talk about little things, which probably were not important, but I came out feeling quite angry with him ... just how long would it take for my, breast to seem ... it still seems swollen, how long would it take that to disappear. Swimming, things like swimming you know, things you can use on your skin, diet, you know you should have, still continue with more of a high-protein diet, to boost your blood cells or, you know, little things

(Costain Schou & Hewison 1999).

The Clinical Oncology Patients' Liaison Group (1999) have emphasised the importance of providing information for patients on skin care, diet and exercise at the end of treatment, as well as contact details for healthcare professionals who will be able to answer questions. Without such guidance, it is not uncommon for patients to appear in the follow-up clinic 4–6 weeks after treatment, asking if it is safe to resume routine activities such as using deodorant, shaving or eating a normal diet.

Psychological transitions

Despite the severity and impact of physical symptoms after treatment is over, many patients do not access specialist advice or care from the treatment centre, and few are referred to community services, usually because of the perception that they are 'walking wounded' rather than acutely unwell (Wells 1998b). If physical problems after radiotherapy are underestimated, then the emotional distress and potential threat to a person's sense of self are often hidden to an even greater extent. Studies have shown that emotional problems, including anxiety and depression, are not uncommon at this time (Eardley 1986a, Ward et al 1992, Wells 1998a). Although this may seem counterintuitive, the perceived relief of treatment ending may be replaced by fear of the future, worry over possible relapse and the overwhelming challenge of incorporating a cancer diagnosis and its treatment into the rest of life. The transition from cancer patient to cancer survivor is a precarious one and, arguably, may never be complete. Persistent or new side effects may trigger thoughts of cancer or precipitate negative emotional responses (Hinds & Moyer 1997, Walker et al 1996). Ambivalence about the discontinuation of treatment and the withdrawal of intensified support can also hamper this process (Christman 1990).

Ward et al's (1992) research into patients' responses to completion of radiotherapy found that patients' perception of their illness is an important indicator of whether they become depressed following treatment. This perception was of much greater significance than the objectively defined stage of disease progression in determining the person's affective response. Such findings challenge us to elicit and work with the meanings patients place on their illness (Popay & Williams 1994). This process must be initiated at an early stage, so that a therapeutic relationship can be built up during the treatment process, and patients become confident enough to express their feelings in a supportive environment. To this end, the following questions may guide the assessment of meaning and perceptions of treatment with a patient who is undergoing radiotherapy.

- What does this treatment mean to you?
- What are your feelings about the treatment?

- What has already changed?
- What do you think might change as a result of having the treatment?
- What do you want of me?

Patients can sometimes be surprised by the fact that they feel emotionally vulnerable after treatment finishes. A combination of psychological and practical support may be most appropriate. As the Clinical Oncology Patients' Liaison Group (1999) points out (p. 20):

Treatment represents a major commitment on the part of patients. After a period of such intense activity and support, patients often become distressed, uncertain and lonely. Although one phase of the treatment comes to an end, it remains very much an unfinished episode for the patient. Reassurance is very important, but some practical advice can also be helpful.

Social transition

The transition from a patient 'on-treatment' to a patient who is recovering at home is a profound social as well as personal process. The change of focus from treatment, disease and the cancer clinic to the attempted resumption of normal activities can lead to a sense of loss and bewilderment. Additionally, the sense of isolation after being separated from the secure environment of the hospital may be felt acutely.

> And after the radiotherapy is finished, you shouldn't need to have any more contact but you do. I felt that everything had been taken away. Although coming back here had been a tiring routine I felt safe, I knew I could ask … What you need is a gradual weaning away from your dependency. I can't be isolated in feeling like this … a gradual weaning off and I wouldn't have felt so bereft
>
> (Wells 1994, cited in Faithfull 2001).

Izod (1996) described how hard it was to complete treatment for his testicular cancer, saying:

> For the previous 6 months, cancer, the treatment, and particularly the staff at the hospital had been the dominant factor in my life. And then all of a sudden nothing. I had been sucked in by the system as an ill person, treated by it and now it was spitting me out as a healthy person, but I was left with a very big hole.

These quotes illustrate the way in which the treatment centre can become a person's community in its broadest sense. Orr (1992) suggests that the traditional definition of community as the location in which the patient lives is unhelpful, and that a person's community is a much more complex and fluid entity. Orr's re-examination of the concept incorporates the activities, resources and demographic structure of a population as well as the feelings, sense of solidarity and belonging that a community engenders. The intensity of shared experiences in clinic may lead people to feel more at home in the hospital than in their own family or locality. Costain Schou & Hewison (1999, p. 38) also explore this phenomenon, describing the social world of the clinic in which many of the social barriers common in a general social context no longer apply. Their interviews with patients attending for cancer treatment illustrate the security and familiarity provided by the treatment centre, and explain why the completion of treatment may not be easy.

The sudden cessation of the daily routine of travelling to and from the radiotherapy department can also be a difficult adjustment to make. Despite the inconvenience, days are punctuated by a specific event, and the loss of such purpose can leave patients with time on their hands to consider how much life has changed. As one patient remarked: 'It was the first time I really had the time to think about it' (Wells 1998a). The sense of being unsafe and isolated once at home can be further heightened by changes in social role. An increased dependence on others to carry out simple social tasks such as shopping can lead to a change in family roles and structure. Sometimes complete role reversal can take place, resulting in a loss of self-esteem and self-worth for the individual who used to be responsible for such tasks.

Further social transitions may also be necessary. Eardley's (1986b) study revealed a number of hidden costs of radiotherapy treatment, including loss of earnings and increased expenditure on food and heating. Adjustments to lifestyle may be essential for a patient recovering from cancer, but the financial implications of such change are often unrealistic for someone who is not earning or faces an uncertain employment future. Information regarding financial support and referral to a social worker may ease this burden for some patients. It is important that this issue is raised sensitively during treatment, as many patients will not perceive their financial problems to be of concern or relevance to healthcare professionals, preventing them from asking for help or advice. Although this could be due to a desire for privacy, it may also be because it does not occur to patients that help or advice is available for such problems. It is therefore imperative that we, as healthcare professionals, initiate this dialogue.

The ability to regain the sense of self that can be lost as a result of cancer treatment (Wells 1998a) depends to an extent on patients' ability to master new roles and integrate into their present community (Schumacher & Meleis 1994). Health professionals may be instrumental in working with patients and families to identify and validate patients' coping strategies, rebuild confidence and explore ways in which they can readapt to their social world outside the hospital.

Identifying local resources to create an alternative to the safe community of the clinic may aid this transition. These may include opportunities for sharing experiences of treatment, such as support groups, or building up a different set of shared experiences, for instance with the family, local organisations or interest groups. For some patients, the provision of information may take away feelings of powerlessness. Information resources to prepare patients for what to expect during and after treatment can take many forms, as described in Chapter 3. Individuals may favour different kinds of information, and their preferences must be established early on, so that the appropriate and specific resources are available to them once they have completed treatment. Some patients may need considerable support to adjust to the fact that their expectations of recovery are incongruous with reality. The assessment of individual expectations, goals and priorities at an early stage is fundamental to successful rehabilitation after treatment is over. Members of the multidisciplinary team, such as the occupational therapist, physiotherapist and dietician, can greatly contribute to this process.

Spirituality/finding meaning

To a large extent the work of finding meaning is inherent in all the transitions discussed so far. However, the importance of the need to make sense of the experience cannot be overemphasised. It may be that such work can only begin following treatment, as patients negotiate how the illness sits in relation to the rest of their life (Radley 1993, Williams 1984). The need for patients to evaluate and be heard is vital if reintegration is to take place. Healthcare professionals may be called upon to listen to the same story numerous times in order for it to make sense for the patient. For this reason, referral to appropriate community staff for ongoing support may be fundamental to the process of reintegration. Other strategies that may support this process include keeping diaries to elicit patients' experiences (Wells 1998a), telephone follow-up systems, drop-in clinics and raising the awareness of patients, family and professionals to the importance of this work.

FACTORS INFLUENCING HEALTHY TRANSITION

If the aim of the health professional is to assist in a healthy and smooth transition, consideration of the factors that influence the quality of the transition experience is vital. These include:

- Meanings: what meaning does the patient/family give to the disease, treatment and potential factors arising from it?
- Expectations: what does the person/family expect to happen? How do they expect professionals to behave and, conversely, how do we as professionals expect the patient to behave?
- Level of planning: how prepared is the person/family/community for the transition? What resources are available?
- Level of knowledge and skill: what skills, knowledge or practical intervention may help in this process?
- Emotional and physical well-being: what physical and emotional problems does the patient have as a result of treatment, and what support, coping strategies and resources does the patient and family have or need in order to alleviate these? What needs for rehabilitation does the patient have, and how might the multidisciplinary team address these?

Such considerations are a huge challenge to all involved in the care of radiotherapy patients. Clearly such a process should begin at diagnosis and accompany patients along their journey. Indeed, it is questionable that such work can be effective if left until the person has completed treatment.

In order to ensure that patients have sufficient support once treatment is over, nurses and therapy radiographers need to be aware of the local services available. Questions to consider include:

- Who is the general practitioner and where is she/he based? Some thought should be given as to how it is best to communicate and at what time of day – some services break in the afternoon as they provide an evening surgery.

- Does the district nursing service need to be involved? If so, what support and care can be provided? Are nurses available at night and how is it best to communicate with them? If services are not set up prior to discharge, does the patient know how to make contact, and what services are available should the need arise at home? Can patients refer themselves or what are the procedures for referral? If the service is already involved, how are district nurses kept informed while the patient is on treatment? Some patients may carry their own case notes, which can greatly assist with communication and continuity of care.
- How will links between the hospital, general practitioner (GP) and patient be maintained once treatment is over? It is vital that communication is maintained both ways: hospital staff also rely on GPs and district nurses to inform them of any important changes or issues facing the patient at home.
- What other services are available to patients and carers in their area? Information about support groups and other voluntary services are found in Cancerlink's (1999) Directory of Self-help and Support or should be available from social work departments, Macmillan nurses or hospital palliative care teams.

When planning a patient's ongoing community care following discharge from radiotherapy, healthcare professionals must consider the wider definitions of community discussed earlier. How will links with the community be maintained, who needs to be involved and what information and resources do patients require to assist them in their recovery? Patients may well maintain contact with fellow patients once treatment is over but, as previously mentioned, they are often reluctant to 'bother' hospital staff, whose time they believe should be reserved for those who are still having treatment (Wells 1998a). The timing of follow-up appointments may not coincide with patients' symptoms or concerns, and the environment in clinic may not be conducive to providing the level of support required. The assumed benefits of traditional follow-up (detection of recurrence, improved quality of life and survival) are, in any case, increasingly being questioned (Brada 1995) and it is now recognised that alternative methods of post-treatment follow-up or support may be more effective. In the radiotherapy setting, telephone clinics, helplines or drop-in clinics staffed by nurses or radiographers may ensure that patients' needs are identified and that they themselves can access professional support and advice once they are at home. A number of different telephone services have been described in the literature (Booker et al 2001, Collins 2001, Rose et al 1996), all of which provide the opportunity for symptoms to be identified, further care to be initiated and communication with the patient and community to be maintained. Booker et al (2001) found that 96% patients were satisfied with this type of service, many commenting that the telephone clinic was less stressful and more convenient than attending an outpatient clinic.

Regular assessment of patients' needs and optimum management of radiotherapy-related problems *throughout* treatment can ensure that patients are prepared for the post-treatment period and do not experience the 'loss of a safety net', as described by Ward et al (1992). Information and advice about how to manage post-treatment symptoms must be reiterated during and at the end of treatment, and adequate prescriptions given so that appropriate medications are available when and if the patient needs them. It may be that new or stronger medications are prescribed towards the end of treatment, and it is vital that the GP is made aware of such changes so that he or she can titrate doses according to the patient's symptoms once treatment is over. Some patients may require practical support to aid activities of daily living, or to help with skin care, mouth care or incontinence problems, for example. Others may benefit from the loan of equipment, for instance a nebuliser to alleviate a dry nose, mouth and throat, or a liquidiser to ease eating after radiotherapy to the head and neck. District nurses may be an invaluable source of support, advice and help with all these problems. However, they can only provide such support if adequately informed about patients' needs. When Wengstrom & Haggmark (1998) asked radiotherapy nurses to identify and rank nursing problems experienced in caring for this group of patients, the most frequently mentioned problem was poor follow-up postdischarge, including insufficient time to talk to the primary healthcare team about concerns over a patient.

Part of the problem is that hospital and community staff often lack awareness of each other's roles and contributions. Given the fact that recent changes in government policy place primary care services at the centre of cancer care provision, we must find ways of improving understanding and collaboration between staff in primary and secondary care settings. Specialist nurses and therapy radiographers have a responsibility to educate and liaise with staff in cancer units and primary care so as to facilitate and enhance their contribution to post-radiotherapy care. Strategies could include establishing specific links with community liaison nurses or Macmillan nurses, providing opportunities for rotation between primary and secondary care, or promoting educational initiatives for staff working in both settings.

Communication with the GP must be initiated at an early stage, so that any post-treatment problems can be resolved promptly, and are not left until the patient's follow-up appointment (Eardley 1990). Given that GPs cannot be expected to maintain up-to-date knowledge of all cancer treatments and how they affect patients, it is the responsibility of staff within the cancer centre to keep them informed and educated about patient care. In a pilot study of on-treatment review for a group of patients with head and neck cancer, GPs frequently reported, several weeks after the end of treatment, that they had not been informed that their patient had even *commenced* radiotherapy (Wells personal communication). Although investment in secretarial resources might well resolve such issues, it is vital that we consider other ways of addressing communication problems. Where protocols for the management of radiotherapy-induced symptoms or information leaflets for patients are available, these should be shared with relevant community staff. Electronic communication systems and shared-care records may provide a way forward, but where these are not in place, hospital staff must ensure that they liaise with community personnel *before* patients are discharged.

CONCLUSION

The framework of transitional theory has been used to conceptualise patients' needs for care and support after radiotherapy treatment is over. This is often a challenging period in the lives of people with cancer, not just because of the effects of treatment, but also because the process of returning to normal is extremely complex. Successful transition depends on adequate preparation of patients for what lies ahead, as well as attention to specific rehabilitative needs. Additionally, timely and appropriate communication between the radiotherapy centre and the community is essential. It is vital that we recognise that the completion of treatment represents an uncertain new beginning for many patients, and that this is reflected in the physical, psychological, social and spiritual care that we provide.

FURTHER INFORMATION

Cancerlink
http://www.cancerlink.org

CHIQ – The Centre for Health Information Quality website with link to Macmillan directory listing documents containing information about support groups and cancer information
http://www.hfht.org/chiq

Macmillan Cancer Relief
http://www.macmillan.org.uk

REFERENCES

Booker J, Cowan R A, Logue J P et al 2001 Evaluation of a nurse-led telephone clinic in the follow-up of patients with prostate cancer. Clinical Oncology (Royal College of Radiologists) 12(4):273

Brada M 1995 Is there a need to follow up cancer patients? European Journal of Cancer Part A General Topics 31(5):655–657

Cancerlink 1999 Directory of self-help and support 1999. Cancerlink, London

Christman N 1990 Uncertainty and adjustment during radiotherapy. Nursing Research 39(1):17–20

Clinical Oncology Patients' Liaison Group 1999 Making your radiotherapy service more patient-friendly. Board of the Faculty of Clinical Oncology, Royal College of Radiologists, London

Collins D 2001 Telephone follow-up clinics. Macmillan Voice 17:11–12

Costain Schou K, Hewison J 1999 Experiencing cancer. Open University Press, Buckingham

Department of Health 1995 A policy framework for commissioning cancer services: a report by the expert advisory group on cancer to the chief medical officers of England and Wales. (The Calman–Hine report). Department of Health, London

Eardley A 1986a Expectations of recovery. Nursing Times 82(17):53–54

Eardley A 1986b After the treatment's over. Nursing Times 82(18):40–41

Eardley A 1990 Patient's needs after radiotherapy. The role of the general practitioner. Family Practice 7(1):39–42

Faithfull S 1995 'Just grin and bear it and hope that it will go away': coping with urinary symptoms from pelvic radiotherapy. European Journal of Cancer Care 4(4):158–165

Faithfull S 2001 Radiotherapy. In: Corner J, Bailey C (eds) Cancer nursing: care in context. Blackwell Science, Oxford, p 222–261

Hinds C, Moyer A 1997 Support as experienced by patients with cancer during radiotherapy treatments. Journal of Advanced Nursing 26:371–379

Izod D 1996 The patient's perspective. Plenary paper given at the 9th International Conference on Cancer Nursing, 12–18 August, 1996, Brighton, UK

Orr J 1992 The community dimension. In: Luker K, Orr J (eds) Health visiting towards community health nursing. Blackwell Scientific, Oxford, p 43–72

Popay J, Williams G 1994 Lay knowledge and the privilege of experience. In: Gabe J, Kellaher D, Williams G (eds) Challenging medicine. Routledge, London, p 118–139

Radley A (ed.) 1993 Worlds of illness: biographical and cultural perspectives on health and disease. Routledge, London

Rose M A, Shrader-Bogen C L, Korlath G et al 1996 Identifying patient symptoms after radiotherapy using a nurse-managed telephone interview. Oncology Nursing Forum 23(1):99–102

Schumacher K, Meleis A 1994 Transitions: a central concept in nursing. Image Journal of Nursing Scholarship 26(2):119–127

Sontag S 1989 Illness as metaphor. Aids and its metaphors Penguin, Harmondsworth, Middlesex

Stacey J 1997 Teratologies: a cultural study of cancer. Routledge, London

Walker B, Nail L, Larsen L et al 1996 Concerns, affect and cognitive disruption following completion of radiation treatment for localised breast or prostate cancer. Oncology Nursing Forum 23(8):1181–1187

Ward S, Viergutz G, Douglas T et al 1992 Patients' reactions to completion of adjuvant breast cancer therapy. Nursing Research 41(6):362–366

Wells M 1998a The hidden experience of radiotherapy to the head and neck: a qualitative study of patients after completion of treatment. Journal of Advanced Nursing 28(4):840–848

Wells M 1998b 'What's so special about radiotherapy nursing?' European Journal of Oncology Nursing 2(3):162–168

Wengstrom Y, Haggmark C 1998 Assessing the problems of importance for the development of nursing care in a radiation therapy department. Cancer Nursing 21(1):50–56

Williams G 1984 The genesis of chronic illness: narrative reconstruction. Sociology of Health and Illness 6:175–200

5

The radiobiological basis of radiation side effects

Douglas Adamson

INTRODUCTION

Radiation therapy for patients has been used for just over 100 years, being introduced soon after the discovery of X-rays by Roentgen in 1895, of radioactivity by Becquerel in 1896, and the isolation of radium by Curie in 1898. These scientists noticed early in their work that radiation was capable of inducing biological side effects which could be severe and permanently damaging. In the last 100 years, a new science – radiobiology – has emerged, combining the disciplines of physics, biology and mathematics to explain how radiotherapy works. Understanding this subject provides a basis for answering questions such as 'Why does my treatment take so long?' and 'Why can't I miss a few days of treatment?' as well as explaining why different doses and schedules of radiotherapy are used, and why it is sometimes combined with other treatments such as chemotherapy.

In recent years, the study of molecular biology has increased understanding of how cells function and proliferate and why cancer cells arise. Using the information from resources such as the sequence of the entire human genome will allow the development of drugs that affect specific growth pathways in cells – a very different mode of action to the treatments employed in the twentieth century. While these new compounds are unlikely to cure cancer when used alone, they may reduce the number of side effects and dramatically alter the way current treatments work. Exciting possibilities include targeting treatment at the tumour by exploiting biological differences between cancer cells and normal cells, or modulating the cell pathways of normal cells to reduce radiotherapy side effects. Knowledge of radiobiology underpins an understanding of the rationale for new strategies, research trends and novel treatments. Perhaps most importantly, such knowledge is essential to helping patients understand the treatment that is being offered and the side effects it causes. This chapter is an introduction to – not a comprehensive review of – radiobiology, but there are many textbooks (see Further Information) that cover topics not explained here, such as linear energy transfer (LET), relative biological effectiveness (RBE), neutron therapy and radiation protection, to name but a few. However, the topics in this chapter will provide a flavour of why this subject is important to being able to help patients understand their treatment.

THE SCOPE OF RADIOBIOLOGY

Radiobiology is the study of how radiation affects the function of cells, both normal and malignant. Radiobiologists attempt to explain the observed effects of radiation treatment and guide new treatment strategies for the future. Equations can be used to describe numerically what is seen experimentally (for instance, the number of cells surviving a given dose of radiation). Such mathematical models are commonly used in radiobiology to predict what will happen if the treatment is given in different ways, although no model will give accurate predictions for every situation. Mathematical modelling is therefore very useful in radiobiology, although it cannot safely replace clinical investigation when a new radiotherapy treatment is proposed. In the future, it may be possible for radiotherapy treatment to be tailored for each individual by examining tumour or normal tissue in the laboratory by means of *predictive assays* and using a model to estimate the dose required to destroy the tumour or the dose that will be tolerated by the normal tissues in the treatment field. The radiobiologist is also interested in discovering what determines tumour response to radiation. Some factors that have been found to be important are the amount of oxygen available to the tumour, the ability of tumours to grow faster (repopulate) during cytotoxic treatment and mechanisms of repair of radiation-induced damage in both normal cells and in tumours. All these are discussed later in this chapter. Before considering how ionising radiation works in the treatment of cancer and how it causes side effects, it is important to understand something about the cells on which it has its effect and think about the nature of ionising radiation itself.

Cell growth

To understand how cells are affected by radiation, we must first remind ourselves how cells control growth and metabolism. Cells vary greatly in shape, size and function to allow them to perform their role. With a few exceptions, all have a central dense structure called the nucleus that contains the chromosomes, composed primarily of deoxyribonucleic acid (DNA), containing the genetic blueprint of the organism. Surrounding the nucleus is the cytoplasm where all the cellular processes necessary for life take place. The cell is bounded by a plasma membrane, the integrity of which is crucial for the cell to function normally. The genetic code contained in the DNA provides each cell with the information it needs to stay alive, divide to form new cells, increase its size and perform its function. This information is *transcribed* into ribonucleic acid (RNA), which leaves the nucleus as messenger RNA before being *translated* into proteins by organelles in the cytoplasm, called ribosomes. Some of these proteins form the structural elements of the cell or facilitate movement, but others allow the cell to communicate with its neighbours, sense its environment, respond to toxic insults (including radiation) and maintain normal cellular functions.

A cancer cell has damage to its DNA that prevents normal function, although many characteristics of the normal cell from which it arose may be retained. It is this similarity to normal cells that makes it difficult to find cytotoxic treatments that kill tumour cells without damaging normal ones too. There are many genes that produce proteins to monitor the DNA for damage and repair any they find. If the damage cannot be repaired, the cell may self-destruct through the process of apoptosis, a programmed cell death that causes the cell to break up in an ordered way (Tamm et al 2001). However, if the damage to the DNA genetic code is repaired incorrectly, the cell may survive but function abnormally. It may lose the function of genes that normally cause the cell to stop dividing (tumour-suppressor genes), sustain damage to genes such as growth factors that subsequently drive cells to keep dividing indefinitely (activated oncogenes) or may produce abnormal proteins that allow excessive cell motility and therefore promote metastasis. Cancer cells are therefore damaged cells that have lost their normal control mechanisms. However, because they retain most of the features of normal cells, the immune system cannot easily detect and destroy them.

Radiation and the cell cycle

The way cells grow may be described by the concept of the cell cycle (Fig. 5.1). Those that are resting and not dividing may be thought of as having left the active cell cycle – a phase defined by the term G_0. Those cells that are dividing

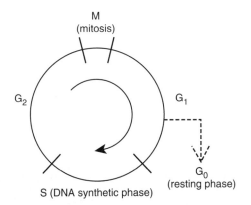

Figure 5.1 The phases of the cell cycle. The intervals of apparent inactivity are labelled G_1 and G_2. (Reproduced with permission from Hall 2000.)

must double their DNA content in order to create two new cells (DNA synthesis phase or S-phase) before dividing by mitosis (M-phase). Both these phases are preceded by gaps (G_1 before S-phase and G_2 before M-phase) during which time the cell is preparing for division and may have time to repair any areas of damage in its DNA. Cells may leave the cell cycle and enter G_0, or may leave the resting G_0 phase and enter the cell cycle to increase cell numbers.

The cell cycle is important because cells have varying sensitivity to radiation-induced damage depending on what stage of the cycle they are at. Cells can be irradiated experimentally at different stages of the cell cycle and a graph plotted of how well they survive as the dose is increased. Those cells in mitosis are much more sensitive to radiation than those at the end of S-phase. Therefore the more cells of a tissue or tumour that are in M-phase, the more damage would be expected for a given dose of radiation (Fig. 5.2).

Atomic structure and different types of radiation

The chemical elements that make up the cells of the body are composed of atoms. An atom has a *nucleus*, composed of particles called protons and neutrons, and has

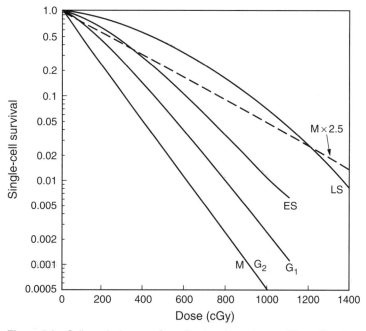

Figure 5.2 Cell survival curves for cells at various stages of the cell cycle. The survival curve for cells in mitosis is steep and has no shoulder. The curve for cells late in S-phase is shallower and has a large initial shoulder. G_1 and early S-phases are intermediate in sensitivity. The broken line is a calculated curve expected to apply to mitotic cells under hypoxia. ES, early S-phase; M, mitosis; LS, late S-phase. (Reproduced with permission from Sinclair 1968.)

a positive electrical charge. Orbiting the nucleus are *electrons*, which are small negatively charged particles balancing the positive charge of the nucleus and making the atom overall electrically neutral. Atoms can combine with each other to form *molecules*. For example, two atoms of hydrogen combine with one of oxygen to form a water molecule (H_2O). An *ion* is an atom that is not electrically balanced (neutral) because the number of negatively charged electrons in its orbit does not equal the number of positively charged protons in the nucleus (neutrons carry no charge). Loss of electrons creates an ion with a positive electrical charge; gain of electrons creates an ion with a negative charge. *Ionisation* can occur if enough energy is supplied to an electron to allow it to escape from orbit around the nucleus, and this process is important in radiation treatment (hence the term *ionising radiation*).

Ionising radiation may take several forms. It may consist of particles (bits of atoms, such as electrons, protons or neutrons) or may be *electromagnetic radiation*, such as X-rays and gamma-rays (γ-rays). Both these two forms of radiation are used for therapy. Perhaps the commonest form of radiotherapy is that of X-ray photon therapy. X-rays have properties shared by radio waves, visible light and microwaves, and all form part of the electromagnetic spectrum (Fig. 5.3).

The radiation used for treatment has a very short wavelength and a high frequency, and is similar to the type of radiation used to obtain X-ray films, but is much more penetrating. It is usually produced by linear accelerators, which bombard metal targets with a stream of electrons to produce X-rays, but it is also emitted from the nuclei of radioactive elements such as cobalt-60, when it is then termed gamma-radiation.

Reactive subatomic particles can be used to produce the same beneficial effects (and side effects) seen with electromagnetic radiation such as X-rays and γ-rays. There are sometimes advantages to using particulate radiation over X-rays, as different forms of radiotherapy deliver energy to tissues in distinct ways. Superficial tumours can be treated by electrons, which do not have the same penetrating power as photons and may spare normal tissues beneath the tumour. Another example would be the intravenous injection of the radioactive liquid strontium-89, which is taken up by bone metastases and delivers a dose of radiotherapy discretely to each metastatic tumour deposit, causing less severe side effects than wide-field, external beam radiotherapy. Other subatomic particles may be used for specialised forms of treatment and, although there are differences in how well they penetrate tissues, the principal mechanisms of therapeutic effect are the same.

Radiation dose

Different units can be used depending what aspect of radiation is being measured. *Absorbed dose* is one encountered commonly in relation to clinical treatment. This is measured in the SI unit of the gray (Gy), although the older unit, the rad (100 rad = 1 Gy) is still occasionally seen. The Gy is a measure of how much energy has been deposited in a given volume of tissue (or other material) and is equal to joules per kilogram. When radiotherapy regimens are described, the dose per fraction will be given in Gy (although cGy are also popular, as they are equal to the older rad).

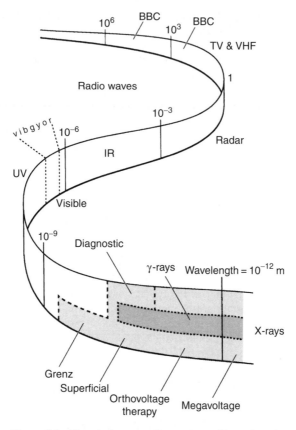

Figure 5.3 The electromagnetic spectrum. (Reproduced with permission from Bomford & Kunkler 2002.)

HOW DOES RADIATION WORK?

One of the most important targets of ionising radiation is the DNA, the material that contains the genetic information necessary for all aspects of survival and function of the cell. Radiation also causes damage to other molecules in the cell, such as the fats in membranes and proteins, but damage to the genetic material in the nucleus is thought to be of particular significance.

When X-rays are absorbed in tissue, the energy they carry is transferred to electrons that are then able to escape from their usual orbits and cause chemical reactions within the cell (Fig. 5.4). These energetic electrons are called *recoil electrons* and are responsible for the damage produced by X- and γ-rays. Ionising radiation produces damage in two distinct ways – by *direct* or *indirect* action on important chemical structures within the cell. The radiation may deliver energy *directly* to the atoms making up the DNA, changing its chemical structure and

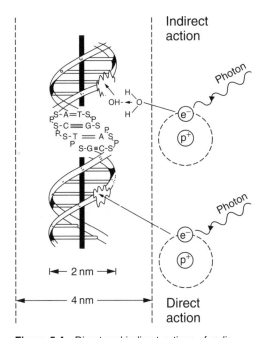

Figure 5.4 Direct and indirect actions of radiation. The structure of DNA is shown schematically. In direct action a secondary electron resulting from absorption of an X-ray photon interacts with the DNA to produce an effect. In indirect action the secondary electron interacts with, for example, a water molecule to produce a hydroxyl radical (OH·), which in turn produces the damage to the DNA. The DNA helix has a diameter of about 20 Å (2 nm). It is estimated that free radicals produced in a cylinder with a diameter double that of the DNA helix can affect the DNA. Indirect action is dominant for sparsely ionising radiation, such as X-rays. S, sugar; P, phosphorus; A, adenine; T, thymine; G, guanine; C, cytosine. (Reproduced with permission from Hall 2000.)

leading to abnormal function. As has been discussed, DNA controls all cellular functions and any damage to it may lead to either cell malfunction or cell death. The structure of DNA is that of a double helix formed by two strands of DNA linked by the molecules called bases. It is the four different bases that specify the genetic code and they are supported by a backbone of sugar and phosphate molecules. The four bases are particularly sensitive targets for radiation. On the other hand, indirect action of ionising radiation does not initially damage DNA and other critical structures. Instead it acts elsewhere in the cell, particularly on water molecules in the presence of oxygen, to create pairs of ions that are unstable – called *free radical ions*. These free radical ions can in turn produce very reactive atoms lacking an electron but which are electrically neutral, termed *free radicals*. The *radiolysis* of water (breaking down of water by radiation) produces such a cascade of free radical ions and free radicals. The reactive nature of these unusual species drives them to combine quickly (in about one-thousandth of a second or less) with other atoms, causing chemical change and damage. During the radiolysis of water, free aqueous electrons and hydrogen radicals may combine with oxygen to form more stable radicals that can prove very damaging to biological structures. Therefore, the presence of oxygen enhances the damaging effect of certain types of radiation, which have a significant effect through indirect damage (the oxygen effect).

DNA damage by radiation

Ionising radiation may cause either single or double strand breaks in the DNA, by the direct and indirect actions discussed above. Single strand breaks are often rectified by the cell's damage-sensing and repair mechanisms, which have evolved over millions of years to respond to environmental insults. Double strand breaks (damage to both strands of the DNA helix at the same level or clusters of damage within the proximity of a few bases) are much more difficult to repair and usually cause the cell to die (Fig. 5.5).

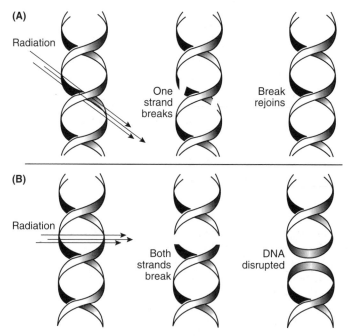

Figure 5.5 Damage to DNA may be (A) temporary and reparable or (B) it may be irreparable and have serious long-lasting effects. (Reproduced with permission from Wootton 1993.)

Cell death

Surprisingly, only a few cells (such as lymphocytes and germ cells of the reproductive system) die immediately after radiation damage and before they are able to complete a cell division. Such *interphase* death is unusual. Most cells effectively treated by radiation continue to divide a few times before succumbing during cell division. Such *mitotic death* is the commonest way for radiotherapy to sterilise tumours. The only tumour cells that may cause a recurrence of cancer following radiotherapy are those with clonogenic potential (a clone is a group of cells all formed from a single parent cell). In experimental work, a clonogenic cell is arbitrarily defined as one capable of forming colonies of 50 or more cells following radiation treatment. When considering the outcome of radiotherapy, we therefore have to review our usual definition of cell death. Tumour cells which are unable to produce significant progeny following treatment may be thought of as dead, even though they continue to show signs of metabolism or even cell division. This mode of death explains why the rate of tumour shrinkage will depend on how often the cells divide, as most cells die during the mitosis phase. A slow-growing tumour may take many months to shrink following radiotherapy. If assessment is performed too soon following radiotherapy, it may be thought that the treatment has been ineffective when there is still significant shrinkage of the tumour to occur. This explains why patients may still be aware of a lump after the end of treatment. In appropriate cases, patients will need reassurance that the radiotherapy 'continues to work' after the course is finished and that the tumour may continue to shrink for many weeks following the treatment. Some normal cells do, however, die within a very short time of receiving a dose of radiation. Lymphocytes are extremely sensitive to radiation and die during the interphase stage. It is common to see a rapid fall in the lymphocyte count in the peripheral blood of patients undergoing radiotherapy (Fig. 5.6). The sensitivity of the germ cells of the gonads means that side effects such as infertility or sterility occur at very low doses of radiation compared with the doses needed to destroy the hormone-producing cells of the same organ.

The normal tissue surrounding the tumour relies on stem cells within it to replace the cells that are constantly being lost. Stem cells may be thought of as specialised cells, the role of which is simply to create more cells that can then go on to perform other functions. Gradual stem cell loss coupled with other changes caused by radiation treatment will become apparent as some of these cells succumb to a mitotic death. The delay in destruction of cells of normal tissue, unavoidably irradiated with the tumour, means that the side effects of radiotherapy may occur days, weeks or many months after the radiation dose is given. The timing of side effects is partly dependent on the rate at which the cell population that has been irradiated normally divides. For example, radiation to the gut, an organ with a high proliferation rate, produces side effects within hours, while damage to the central nervous system may take months or years to become apparent. One paradoxical effect of radiotherapy is that it may damage a normal cell enough to disrupt its function but not enough to kill it. This is the basis of radiation-induced malignancies following treatment, which, although rare, does mean that caution has to be used when considering radiotherapy for benign disease.

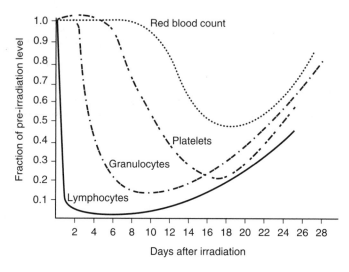

Figure 5.6 The pattern of depletion and recovery of the principal circulating elements of the blood following an intermediate dose of total-body radiation. The curves are purely illustrative. The time at which the nadir occurs is a combination of the radiosensitivity of the stem cells and the lifetime of the mature functional cells. (Reproduced with permission from Hall 2000.)

Fractionation

Patients can sometimes find it difficult to understand why an overall course of radiotherapy treatment can take so long, and why it is divided into so many apparently short daily treatments. Fractionated radiotherapy refers to radiotherapy treatment given in many small, equal doses rather than all in one go. It has the advantage of allowing higher total doses to be given safely and enables preferential destruction of tumour cells by capitalising on the small differences between tumour cell and normal tissue responses to radiation.

The factors that modify the response of both malignant and normal tissues to fractionated radiotherapy may be remembered as the four Rs of radiobiology:

1. Repair of radiation-induced damage within cells
2. Repopulation of the irradiated area by surviving cells
3. Redistribution of cells within the cell cycle
4. Reoxygenation of the tumour (Withers 1975).

Repair and repopulation are factors that tend to overcome the effect of radiation and are present in tumours as well as normal tissue. Tumours may exhibit an accelerated repopulation response to radiotherapy, that is, they start to proliferate *faster* in response to the initial cell loss caused by the treatment. Redistribution and reoxygenation are factors that increase the cytotoxic effect of radiation and occur in normal, as well as malignant, tissue.

Damage repair

Sublethal damage

Sublethal damage repair is a concept used to explain the finding that less cell killing occurs when a given dose of radiation is delivered in two or more fractions given with a time gap than when the same dose is given in one go. Not all cells have the same capacity to repair damage, and it is obviously to the patient's advantage if the normal tissue is better than the tumour at recovering from the treatment. The rate of repair for a given tissue has a significant bearing on how it responds to radiation and what side effects are seen.

It has been estimated that half the DNA damage that is *sublethal* will be repaired after 30–90 min in most tissues. This type of repair is important for late-responding tissues (see below) and it is therefore critical to leave sufficient time between fractions to allow for such repair. In practice, if more than one fraction is being given daily, the fractions should be 6 h apart if potentially catastrophic late side effects are to be avoided. Clinically, researchers have tried very short treatment intervals, such as 2 h, combined with multiple fractions per day. However, as the mathematical theory would predict, the morbidity owing to the late effects is high (Nguyen et al 1985).

Potentially lethal damage

Potentially lethal damage is a term used to explain the laboratory finding that cells that are not dividing appear to survive a given dose of radiotherapy better than those that are actively proliferating. This effect can be seen by irradiating cells in vitro and then allowing them to continue to grow at 37°C or cooling them to 20°C to arrest their growth. A larger fraction of the cells cooled after irradiation survive, suggesting that the pause in proliferation allows the damage to be repaired more effectively than when the cells continue to divide.

Repopulation

When tissue or tumour is damaged by radiation, cells that are not dividing, i.e. those in G_0, enter the cell cycle to replace the cells destroyed by treatment. Tumours that show accelerated repopulation will not be cured if the destruction of malignant cells does not keep pace with the increasing rate of their production. It has been realised for many years that repopulation is important in determining the outcome of radiotherapy (Withers et al 1988), particularly for tumours such as those of the head and neck (Overgaard et al 1988). These tumours often grow faster after radiotherapy starts, as the repopulation process takes hold. Treatment delay may therefore have disastrous consequences if repopulation has been stimulated but subsequent treatment delivery is insufficient to keep up with the new mode of growth of the tumour. It has been estimated that extending a planned course of treatment by 1 week may decrease the cure rate by 13% (Dische 1995a). This explains why it is crucially important that patients do not take time off during radiotherapy and why twice-daily treatments are sometimes given to compensate for gaps due to public holidays or machine breakdowns. Until recently, radiotherapy was given at most once every working day, 5 days a week. Increasing awareness that certain tumours repopulate faster than others has led to the development of accelerated radiotherapy regimens, in which the total dose of radio therapy is delivered in a shorter period of time than previously, often combined with hyperfractionation (giving several fractions in a day), which allows a higher total dose to be given without causing severe late effects. These techniques are explained in more detail in the section on Fractionation schedules, below.

Reoxygenation

It was recognised in the mid twentieth century that the effectiveness of radiotherapy is dependent on how much oxygen is available to the tissue being irradiated (Gray et al 1953). The amount of oxygen available depends on factors such as blood supply to the tissue concerned and whether the patient is anaemic. Interestingly, there does seem to be an association between anaemia and poor response to radiotherapy, even when factors such as stage of disease are taken into account (Dische 1995b). There is some controversy over whether correcting anaemia through blood transfusion prior to treatment improves response. Studies are under way evaluating the potential for erythropoietin to enhance the oxygen-carrying capacity of the blood and therefore improve the outcome of radiotherapy, but results are not yet available (Lutterbach & Guttenberger 2000).

Normal tissues have a delicate network of capillaries that supply oxygen to all areas. Tumours, because of their abnormal growth characteristics, quickly outgrow their blood supply and have large areas that are hypoxic. In addition, new and abnormal blood vessels are induced in tumours by the process of angiogenesis, and the combination of antiangiogenic treatments with radiotherapy may improve treatment results in the future (Siemann et al 2000). Tumours may therefore be chronically hypoxic, but can also suffer from intermittent bouts of acute hypoxia when the blood vessels supplying them close down temporarily (Brown & Giaccia 1998). Areas of the tumour that are hypoxic are less responsive to radiotherapy, because less of the damaging reactive oxygen species can be formed in areas where the oxygen tension is low. Such hypoxic cells interfere with the efficacy of chemotherapy (Denny 2000), as well as radiotherapy (Fig. 5.2). Fractionation allows time for the tumour to regress and become more responsive to treatment, as areas that were previously hypoxic gradually become oxygenated as they move closer to the blood vessels (Fig. 5.7).

Redistribution of cells in the cell cycle

As cell loss occurs in the treated area, cells that were previously quiescent (in G_0 phase) start to divide and will therefore move into phases of the cell cycle in which they are more sensitive to radiation-induced killing. Cells are most resistant to ionising radiation in S-phase and maximally responsive in M and late G_2. Prolonged fractionation means that cells have a greater chance of being in a sensitive phase of the cell cycle at some point during treatment than if all the radiation is given in a single dose.

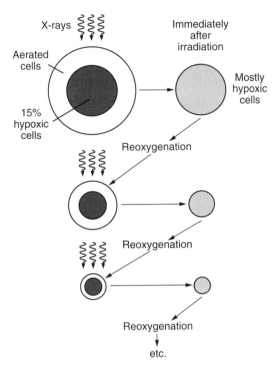

X-rays

Aerated cells

15% hypoxic cells

Immediately after irradiation

Mostly hypoxic cells

Reoxygenation

Reoxygenation

Reoxygenation

etc.

Figure 5.7 The process of reoxygenation. Tumours contain a mixture of aerated and hypoxic cells. A dose of X-rays kills a greater proportion of aerated than hypoxic cells, because they are more radiosensitive. Immediately after irradiation, most cells in the tumour are hypoxic. But the preirradiation pattern tends to return because of reoxygenation. If the radiation is given in a series of fractions separated in time sufficiently for reoxygenation to occur, the presence of hypoxic cells does not greatly influence the response of the tumour. (Reproduced with permission from Hall 2000.)

ACUTE AND LATE RADIATION SIDE EFFECTS

The typical side effects of radiotherapy can be subdivided into early and late depending when they appear in relation to treatment, although it is important to realise that both early and late reactions can occur in the same tissue. Some tissues, such as skin, mucosa and bone marrow, can react very rapidly to radiation treatment and will show signs of toxicity (erythema, ulceration and peripheral blood changes) during the course of radiation. Stem cells within the tissue are responsible for producing new cells that can then differentiate to perform specific functions, and the production of such daughter cells can be increased when required. If radiotherapy involving the skin destroys more epidermal cells than can be produced by the stem cells, then the deficit can be partly made up by migration of healthy cells into the damaged area. Once the rate of cell death exceeds these compensatory mechanisms, the skin will start to break down, causing moist desquamation. Such side effects, although unpleasant, are rarely life-threatening but can be severe enough to cause interruption of the course of radiotherapy. They usually resolve completely within days or weeks of stopping treatment.

Late-responding tissues, such as the spinal cord and kidney, have capacity for extensive repair (see above), but only if the radiotherapy is given in small enough doses with large enough gaps between each fraction. These tissues show no immediate effect of the radiation therapy. However, damage still occurs during treatment and becomes manifest in the following months and years. Such radiation-induced side effects can be devastating and much of the radiotherapy-planning process is aimed at reducing the risk of late complications (in addition to ensuring adequate dose to the tumour). Late radiation effects on the kidney produce declining function leading to severe renal impairment and the risk of hypertension; on the brachial plexus result in debilitating arm pain associated with loss of function (see Ch. 14); and on bone result in osteoradionecrosis, which may be difficult to distinguish from metastatic disease in later years (see Ch. 18). This late damage, unlike acute damage, is never fully repaired. Late damage may be related to damage to the connective tissue of the organ, causing abnormalities such as fibrosis. Another important site of late damage may be to the vascular supply of the tissue, and telangectasia (abnormal visible capillaries in the skin) are a late effect of skin treatment, developing months or years after radiotherapy. The seriousness of late side effects of radiation therapy is also dictated by how the tissue functions, particularly if one part of an organ is dependent on another. For example, if the chain of communicating nerve fibres in the spinal cord is badly damaged at one level by radiation, even if the area involved is quite small, then this will result in paraplegia. Conversely, the kidney comprises many identical functional units, and a large proportion of kidney tissue can be destroyed before the effect on renal function becomes obvious, as the undamaged areas are not dependent on the damaged ones and can still fulfil their physiological role. More detailed information on late effects can be found in Chapters 14, 18 and 19.

Analogy of tissue repair

To summarise some of the radiobiological concepts explored in this chapter, a useful analogy to the clinical problem of allowing enough time for repair of normal tissues during radiotherapy would be that of workmen (the cells) carrying rocks (the radiation) to a place of work. Although the loads (the dose per fraction) would tire the workers, they would recover between each trip and be able to continue with their work unless the weight of the load was increased to a certain threshold. The critical threshold would vary between each worker, but once it was reached they would sustain injuries that would interfere with their ability to do the job. Certain workers (the cells of late-responding tissues) may be more susceptible to heavy loads and be prone to getting injuries so severe that they produce permanent disability (late effects). Similar injuries might occur when a normally manageable load is carried back and forth too frequently, without sufficient rest periods (fractions given too close together). The likelihood of permanent injury would therefore be dependent on both the total load (total dose) and the load per trip (dose per fraction), and how susceptible the worker was to this type of injury (which tissue is being treated). However, the amount of general tiredness experienced (acute effects) would depend mainly on the size of the job or the total load (total dose).

Sometimes irradiated tissue may look normal until a second insult reveals its lack of capacity to respond to further damage, owing to late covert damage. An example of this would be unusually severe pancytopenia (reduction in all the cellular elements of the blood) after chemotherapy in a patient who has previously had large areas of bone marrow irradiated. Surgery to irradiated tissue may result in a much higher rate of complications, not only because of impaired healing properties but also because of the permanent fibrotic changes making the surgery more difficult. Another factor thought to be important in producing these side effects is the damage to blood vessels caused by radiation which in turn compromises the supply of nutrients and oxygen to the affected tissues.

RADIOSENSITIVITY AND CELL SURVIVAL CURVES

When cells are examined under laboratory conditions, measurements can be made to determine the proportion of cells of a particular type that survive different doses of ionising radiation. The results of such experiments can then be plotted semilogarithmically (i.e. the dose against the log of the surviving fraction). The proportion of cells surviving decreases as the dose increases and, if the points of the plot are joined with a smooth line, a curve is produced.

Several different equations have been used to describe the results obtained experimentally. Although none is completely faithful to what is seen, the *linear quadratic model* (Fig. 5.8) is perhaps one of the most useful, as it gives a close approximation to the killing effect of the smaller doses of radiation that are typically used in radiotherapy. This model relies on the concept that cell death may result either from a single lethal event (the linear component) or from the addition of two independent sublethal events (the quadratic component). The linear component is described by a factor alpha (α) and the quadratic by beta (β). If these two values are determined experimentally and the ratio obtained, a mathematical description can be made of how a given tissue will respond to treatment:

$$S = e^{\alpha D - \beta D^2}$$

where S is the fraction of cells that survive a dose D, and e is the base of natural logarithms. The α/β ratio for a particular tissue is the dose at which the linear (α) and the quadratic (β) components of cell killing are equal. Tissues that display early reactions to radiation, such as gut or skin and tumours, tend to have a high α/β ratio (e.g. 10 Gy), whereas tissues that show little initial damage, but show radiation-induced late effects months or years later, tend to have a low α/β ratio (e.g. 2 Gy).

Mention has been made of cellular repair mechanisms, such as the proteins that scout over the DNA looking for damage and which stop the cell from proceeding through the cell cycle while repair mechanisms are activated. The degree to which

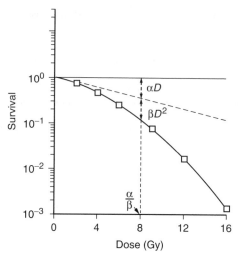

Figure 5.8 Shape of survival curve for mammalian cells exposed to X-rays. The fraction of cells surviving is plotted on a logarithmic scale against dose on a linear scale. The experimental data are fitted to a linear quadratic function. There are two components of cell killing: one is proportional to dose (αD), the other is proportional to the square of the dose (βD^2). The dose at which the linear and quadratic components are equal is the ratio α/β. The linear quadratic curve bends continuously but is a good fit to experimental data for the first few decades of survival. (Reproduced with permission from Hall 2000.)

a cell can repair itself depends on the dose of radiation given, and how long it is before another dose (fraction) of radiotherapy is given. Of importance is that both tumour cells and normal tissues undergo repair following radiation therapy. The success of treatment depends in part on whether the normal tissues can repair themselves faster and more fully than the tumour cells before a further dose of radiation is given. Cell killing by radiation is logarithmic and not linear. This means that a given *proportion* rather than a given number of cells are killed with each fraction of radiation administered. For example, if a radiation fraction kills 50% of the cells treated, then the same dose will destroy 1000 cells in a tumour composed of 2000 cells, but only 10 cells in a tumour composed of 20 cells. This effect is amplified by fractionated therapy. If 65% of the cells of a late-responding tissue survive every fraction of radiotherapy compared with 55% of the tumour cells, then the relative survival of normal compared to tumour cells over a course of treatment of 30 fractions is $(65/55)^{30} = 150$ times greater.

In summary, the way the radiotherapy is delivered is important in determining the risk of developing side effects. Acute effects tend to be related to the total dose of radiotherapy and the length of time over which the treatment is delivered.

The late effects are also dependent on total dose, but are very dependent on the dose per fraction. Small doses per fraction allow a much greater total dose to be delivered to a late-responding tissue than when the same total dose is given with larger doses per fraction (i.e. with fewer treatments). Palliative radiotherapy (designed to relieve symptoms but not to cure the tumour) may therefore be given quickly in a few fractions, minimising the distress and inconvenience to the patient. However, the maximum total dose that can be given safely is less when the treatment is given over many weeks and the scope for retreating an area such as the spinal cord (e.g. when spinal metastases occur in a previously treated site) is severely limited. Conversely, if a large dose is needed to cure a tumour, it must be given in many small fractions in order to avoid late effects. The realisation of the importance of such tissue responses has stimulated research into new fractionation regimens such as accelerated and hyperfractionated radiotherapy.

FRACTIONATION AND ADJUVANT TREATMENTS USED WITH RADIOTHERAPY REGIMENS

CHART and other non-standard radiotherapy regimens

Accelerated radiotherapy refers to giving conventional fraction sizes and total dose, but treating more often, e.g. sometimes twice a day, so that the treatment is completed in a shorter time than usual. It is designed to overcome accelerated repopulation of tumours. Hyperfractionation describes the reduction in dose per fraction in an attempt to reduce late side effects as has been mentioned above. Continuous hyperfractionated accelerated radiotherapy (CHART) is the combination of both these techniques in the one treatment and was pioneered at Mount Vernon Hospital, UK, in collaboration with the Gray laboratory (Saunders et al 1997). A radical treatment was delivered in only 12 days, by giving three fractions a day, with a 6-h interval between each fraction. The accelerated treatment produced much more severe acute effects but did not seem to increase late effects (although there was initial concern about unexpected toxicity to the spinal cord). There is little doubt that it has a significantly better tumour control rate, although implementing CHART would cause considerable working practice changes for most departments.

Fractionation schedules and biologically effective dose

Why am I getting different treatment from other people with the same disease?

Patients will speak to others and obtain information from the internet about different treatments for the same disease. This may lead them to believe that they are getting more or less treatment than someone else being treated in their own or another centre. Radiotherapy schedules for the treatment of the same tumour at the same stage may, at first sight, appear to vary quite considerably. Regimens for the treatment of a bone metastasis include 10 Gy single fraction, 20 Gy in five fractions over one week and 30 Gy in 10 fractions over 2 weeks. It might appear that the shortest regimen delivers only one-third of the treatment of the longest one.

However, it must be remembered that the effect of radiotherapy is dependent not just on the total dose, but also on the time over which that dose is given. Each of the three regimens above gives a similar treatment effect – indeed, the effect is so similar that many centres have adopted shorter palliative regimens in order to deliver treatment more efficiently and reduce the time the patient has to be in hospital. In addition to having a similar treatment effect, each one of the above fractionation schedules delivers a high dose per fraction and this means that the tolerance dose is reached rapidly and the scope for further treatment to the same area is limited, despite the fact that a relatively small total dose has been given.

Radical (curative) regimens also differ. Some centres, notably the Christie Hospital in Manchester, UK, use relatively short courses (e.g. 3 weeks) giving a lower total dose with a higher dose per fraction. Centres in the south of England and in the USA use longer schedules (6 weeks) aiming for a high total dose and a dose per fraction of around 2 Gy. Other centres opt for the middle route with typical treatments lasting 4 weeks. These different regimens were devised in the first half of the twentieth century and were designed to dovetail with the resources available in a given area and the numbers of patients who required treatment. Which regimen is the best? The reply to this question depends mainly on where the person answering learnt about radiotherapy! One difficulty in answering this question is that there have been few randomised trials directly comparing each of these regimens with the other, making it difficult to compare treatment outcomes of each regimen.

One useful concept that has been developed since the 1980s is that of biologically effective dose (BED), reviewed in Jones et al (2001). This again uses mathematical modelling to give an estimate of the change in dose per fraction needed when, for example, changing from a 30-fraction treatment to a 20-fraction treatment. The BED is calculated using the linear quadratic equation and estimates how the treatment delivery must change in order to deliver the same tumour kill. The calculation can be made more complex by allowing for tumour repopulation and other factors. One of the pitfalls of this method is that it is not always clear what some of the values for the modelling equation should be. For instance, it is well known that although tumour/ratios are said to be high, that is, in the same range as those seen for early-responding tissues, their true range does in fact vary quite considerably (Jones & Dale 1999). The important message to remember is that it is *how* the radiotherapy is delivered, not just what total dose is given, that determines the tumour response and side effects. In addition, seemingly different treatment regimens may have a similar biological effect.

Tolerance dose and therapeutic index

What are the risks of serious side effects from my radiotherapy treatment?

Tolerance is a concept that is useful when deciding what dose of radiation may be delivered to certain organs or areas of the body. A tolerance dose may be thought of as one that will result in some side effects, but also an acceptable number of cures. This concept explains why radiotherapy is not without risk and helps patients understand why side effects are unavoidable with current treatment regimens. Tolerance of a particular organ cannot be predicted accurately in an individual, because radiation damage is a random process and the factors such as degree of oxygenation of the tissue or ability of the tissue to undergo repair vary *between* individuals and even within the *same* individual at different times. The idea of tolerance dose is therefore a statistical one. A dose can be determined that will produce significant side effects in a given proportion of patients, although it will be impossible to predict which individual will get these complications. Attempts have been made to develop laboratory tests to predict which patients are most at risk. Some researchers have used in vitro laboratory tests, such as studying growing fibroblasts from biopsies of patients' skin, to estimate the risk of late toxicity. Although not all investigators have found this particular test to be useful (Peacock et al 2000), other in vitro methods have been investigated (Brock & Tucker 2000). Barber et al (2000) found (in contrast to some previous work) that chromosome abnormalities induced in patient blood samples could be used to predict acute, but not late, radiotherapy reactions. The degree of risk for any complication needs to be balanced against the risk of similar damage if the tumour is not controlled, and the morbidity of the expected side effect. For example, more risk of radiation myelopathy with subsequent paraplegia would be taken for a tumour which threatens the viability of the spinal cord than would be the case for the dose of radiotherapy given to the spinal cord incidentally when treating a lung cancer. The potential seriousness of any given side effect is often taken into account when a tolerance dose is being considered. Generally, a 5% risk of myelopathy and paraplegia would be unacceptable, but a 5% risk of permanent skin changes might be considered acceptable. One of the difficulties about treating critical areas such as the spinal cord with radiation is that it is not established with certainty what a 'safe' dose is (Fowler et al 2000, Macbeth 2000).

The therapeutic index is the difference in the amount of damage the radiation causes to the tumour compared with the normal tissues for any given dose. As can be seen from Figure 5.9A, as the dose increases, the likelihood of cure increases, but so does the normal tissue damage. Low doses cause virtually no severe side effects but produce few cures; high doses cure many tumours but lead to an unacceptable rate of serious side effects. The radiosensitivity of the tumour determines how many complications arise from treatment for a given number of cures (Fig. 5.9B). For most treatments, Goldilocks doses (not too hot; not too cold) have been arrived at by experience over many decades to allow the highest cure rate without too many unacceptable late side effects.

Given the wide variation in how different people respond to radiation, it is likely that a universally safe dose would be so low as to cure no one. Careful treatment planning and delivery limit the volume of tissue irradiated, reducing severe side effects and permanent damage to the patient. However, the anatomy and physiology of the organ are also important determinants of how much radiation can be delivered safely, and must be considered along with radiobiology and treatment volume if side effects are to be avoided (Hopewell & Trott 2000).

Chemotherapy

Patients with certain tumours may receive combination chemoradiotherapy or adjuvant chemotherapy, the timing of which can be particularly important. Cytotoxic chemotherapy is complementary to radiation in that it treats the whole body (apart from certain sites, such as the brain, which are partly protected from drug penetration), whereas radiotherapy is generally a localised treatment.

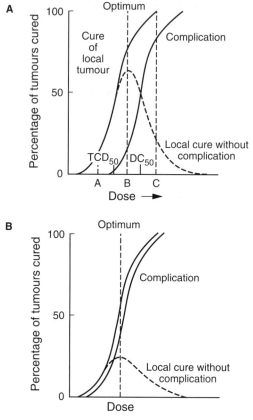

Figure 5.9 Theoretical dose–effect relationships for the percentage of local control of one particular type of tumour and the appearance of complications in the irradiated normal tissues. (A) Tumour of average radiosensitivity; (B) to a more radioresistant tumour than (A), cure without complication is possible only for a small proportion of tumours. At A, cure without complication; B, the optimal dose; C, cure of all the tumours but with a high proportion of complications. TCD$_{50}$, dose to cure 50% of the tumours. DC$_{50}$, dose resulting in a complication in 50% of the patients. (Reproduced with permission from Tubiana et al 1990.)

Chemotherapy can be used to treat micrometastatic disease while the primary tumour is treated with radiation. A strength of employing both treatments is that many drugs work well in parts of the cell cycle in which radiation is less effective, such as S-phase. Cytotoxic chemotherapy is mainly used as an adjuvant treatment. It rarely produces cure when used without surgery and radiotherapy, with the exception of the treatment of certain tumours arising from the gonads and haemopoietic system, when it is extremely effective.

Combining chemotherapy and radiotherapy to try to harness the benefits of both is an attractive concept. However, it must be remembered that the patient will have to suffer the toxicities of both treatments. The challenge therefore is not just to add chemotherapy to an established radiotherapy regimen and accept increased side effects for a marginal improvement in outcome. The same improvement in outcome might be achievable by simply giving a larger dose of radiotherapy. The challenge is to use both treatments synergistically. Some of the questions that should be asked before combining these two modalities are:

- Can the addition of chemotherapy improve the outcome of treatment compared with radiotherapy alone, without causing unacceptable side effects?
- Can the addition of chemotherapy allow a lower dose of radiation to be used, without compromising outcome, while reducing the level of unacceptable side effects?
- Can chemotherapy enhance the effect of radiotherapy either by sensitising tumour cells to the radiation or by killing cells that are resistant as a result of the stage of the cell cycle they are in or because they are hypoxic?
- Can chemotherapy improve the outcome of treatment by killing cells outwith the radiation field?

There are pitfalls to combining these two treatments. Drugs that are specifically toxic to the organ being irradiated (e.g. bleomycin and the lung) and drugs that may sensitise normal tissue to radiation (e.g. Adriamycin) should be used with great care when combined with radiotherapy. It is clear from experimental work that very different side effects may be obtained from combining chemotherapy and radiotherapy, depending on whether the drug is given before, after or during radiation. Often the greatest side effects are seen when radiation is given very close to chemotherapy, either before or after, or when radiation is given during administration of the drug (chemoradiotherapy). Although the idea of using sophisticated schedules of chemotherapy and radiation simultaneously in an attempt to produce a synergistic effect is attractive, much of the improvement seen is probably owing to a simple additive effect of the two treatments. There is ample evidence that chemotherapy combined with radiotherapy in the treatment of non-small cell lung cancer alters the course of the disease, but the magnitude of improvement is similar to that seen when CHART is used instead of conventional radiotherapy (Jassem 2001). However, there is evidence that the addition of chemotherapy to radiotherapy and surgery in diseases such as head and neck cancer may save the patient from extensive surgery, such as laryngectomy, and that chemoradiotherapy does have the potential to improve survival rates significantly when compared to radiotherapy alone (Lamont & Vokes 2001).

Brachytherapy and continuous, low-dose-rate radiotherapy

Brachytherapy is the use of radioactive sources (radioisotopes) to deliver radiotherapy to a specific area in close proximity to the treatment source. This method is used in intracavitary treatments to treat gynaecological malignancies and in interstitial therapy, when the radioactive material is implanted directly into the tumour, either permanently or temporarily. The dose rates (i.e. the number of cGy delivered per min) in both these therapies may vary but, if the radiation is delivered slowly enough, then this therapy may be thought of as an extreme form of hyperfractionation, killing cells by directly lethal events but allowing maximal repair of sublethal damage, thereby sparing late-responding tissues. Brachytherapy may therefore be useful in situations where previous radiotherapy has been given and there is concern about the effect on late-responding tissues, or where a large total dose needs to be delivered to improve the prospect of tumour control. Although, in general, lowering the dose rate means that a higher total dose must be used to produce the same effect on the tumour, a paradoxical effect may occur in certain dose ranges whereby lowering the dose rate allows tumour cells to proceed to a radiosensitive part of the cell cycle, increasing the number destroyed by the treatment.

Radiosensitisers and hypoxic cytotoxins

Certain drugs augment the effect of radiotherapy and such compounds are known as radiosensitisers. Despite the apparent attractiveness of using these drugs to increase the likelihood of cure, it must be remembered that the effectiveness of radiotherapy exploits the differences between the susceptibility of the tumour and of the dose-limiting normal structures nearby to survive the damage the treatment produces. A radiosensitiser that increases the susceptibility of both tumour and normal tissue equally may not produce any therapeutic gain. Radiosensitisers act by becoming incorporated into the DNA (e.g. iododeoxyuridine) and making it susceptible to radiation attack, or by mimicking the effect of oxygen (e.g. drugs related to the antibiotic metronidazole).

A slightly different therapeutic approach is to use compounds, termed bioreductive drugs, which have a greater cytotoxic effect in cells that are hypoxic. This has the advantage of selectively attacking tumour cells that are relatively radiation-resistant. Mitomycin C is one such bioreductive drug, although the increased cytotoxic effect it produces in hypoxic cells is not particularly large. Radiosensitisers have been used experimentally for many years in an attempt to improve treatment outcome, although they have not been successful enough to enter routine clinical use. Radiosensitisation is not the preserve of chemotherapy agents, as other drugs used commonly in cancer treatment, such as the antiemetic metoclopramide, have also been shown to be radiosensitisers.

Radioprotectors

Any compounds that scavenge free radicals (such as glutathione or thiol-containing amino acids) are capable of ameliorating the adverse side effects of radiotherapy. Obviously, the effect of a radioprotector must be greater in normal tissue compared with a tumour for it to be of any therapeutic benefit. Amifostine is a drug that shows promise in sparing tissues such as salivary glands from radiation damage. However, it is unclear at present just how useful drugs like this will be clinically (Lindegaard & Grau 2000).

CONCLUSION: THE FUTURE

There has been a massive increase in the amount of knowledge in the past decade about how cell function is controlled at the molecular level. The opportunities for novel treatments are tantalising, but have so far not come of age. Standard therapy has improved, but there have not been the paradigm shifts that were predicted from the results of initial laboratory science. Interestingly, when significant clinical advances (such as CHART) are made, they are not rapidly adopted for a variety of political, economic and other reasons. Gene therapy raises the possibility of sensitising cancer cells to radiation by restoring the expression of damaged genes or inserting genes that produce cytotoxic products when activated by radiation. Powerful techniques such as gene assay technology, which can examine the change in expression of huge numbers of genes from one sample, mean that the number of genes known to play a role in the response to radiation will increase (Hanna et al 2001), perhaps allowing predictions to be made about how a tumour will respond to treatment. This raises perhaps the most interesting question for the next decade: can we predict how an individual with cancer will respond to treatment and tailor the treatment accordingly? At present, there are major obstacles to be overcome. The first is that predictive assays have not proven to be as useful clinically as had been hoped, although certain laboratories have had extremely encouraging results (West et al 1991). These techniques are often invasive, fickle and time-consuming. However, it may become possible to improve treatment significantly in the future by individualising it, if suitable methods are found. This might allow the dose of radiation to be increased if we can predict that a patient's tissues are resistant to late side effects or screen for patients who are unusually sensitive to radiation treatment, reducing the suffering and side effects that some currently experience as a result of radiotherapy.

FURTHER INFORMATION

Withers H R 1992 Biological basis of radiation therapy for cancer. Lancet 339:156–159
A lucid, concise summary of the key ideas in radiobiology.

Hall E 2000 Radiobiology for the radiologist, 5th edn. Lippincott Williams & Wilkins, Philadelphia
A comprehensive, single-author book with flowing style. Many other general radiobiology textbooks are excellent, among them:

Steel G G (ed.) 1993 Basic clinical radiobiology. Edward Arnold, London

Tubiana M, Dutreix J, Wambersie A (eds) 1990 Introduction to radiobiology. Taylor & Francis, London

Sumner D, Wheldon T, Watson W 1991 Radiation risks. Tarragon Press, Glasgow
A simple introduction into the basic physics and biology of radiation damage.

Price P, Sikora K 1995 Treatment of cancer. Chapman & Hall, London, chs 1–7
A more comprehensive introduction to the principles underlying cancer therapy, including radiobiology.

Darnell J, Lodish H, Baltimore D 1995 Molecular cell biology, 3rd edn. Scientific American Books, New York
Extensive information on all aspects of cell biology.

REFERENCES

Barber J B P, Burrill W, Spreadborough A R et al 2000 Relationship between in vitro chromosomal radiosensitivity of peripheral blood lymphocytes and the expression of normal tissue damage following radiotherapy for breast cancer. Radiotherapy and Oncology 55(2):179–186

Bomford C K, Kunkler I H (eds) 2002 Walter and Miller's textbook of radiotherapy, radiation physics, therapy and oncology, 6th edn. Churchill Livingstone, Edinburgh, p 16

Brock W A, Tucker S L 2000 In vitro radiosensitivity and normal tissue damage. Radiotherapy and Oncology 55(2):93–94

Brown J M, Giaccia A J 1998 The unique physiology of solid tumors: opportunities (and problems) for cancer therapy. Cancer Research 58(7):1408–1416

Denny W A 2000 The role of hypoxia-activated prodrugs in cancer therapy. Lancet Oncology 1(1):25–29

Dische S 1995a Clinical radiobiology. In: Price P, Sikora K (eds) Treatment of cancer, 3rd edn. Chapman & Hall Medical, London, ch 5, p 63

Dische S 1995b Clinical radiobiology. In: Price P, Sikora K (eds) Treatment of cancer, 3rd edn. Chapman & Hall Medical, London, ch 5, p 67

Fowler J F, Bentzen S M, Bond S J et al 2000 Clinical radiation doses for spinal cord: the 1988 international questionnaire. Radiotherapy and Oncology 55(3):295–300

Gray L H, Conger A D, Ebert M et al 1953 The concentration of oxygen dissolved in tissues at the time of irradiation as a factor in radiotherapy. British Journal of Radiology 26:638–648

Hall E 2000 Radiobiology for the radiologist, 5th edn. Lippincott/Williams & Wilkins, Philadelphia

Hanna E, Shrieve D C, Ratanatharathorn V et al 2001 A novel alternative approach for prediction of radiation response of squamous cell carcinoma of head and neck. Cancer Research 61(6):2376–2380

Hopewell J W, Trott K-R 2000 Volume effects in radiobiology as applied to radiotherapy. Radiotherapy and Oncology 56(3):283–288

Jassem J 2001 Combined chemotherapy and radiation in locally advanced non-small-cell lung cancer. Lancet Oncology 2(6): 335–342

Jones B, Dale R G 1999 Mathematical models of tumour and normal tissue response. Acta Oncologica 38(7):883–893

Jones B, Dale R G, Deehan C et al 2001 The role of biologically effective dose (BED) in clinical oncology. Clinical Oncology (Royal College of Radiologists) 13(2):71–81

Lamont E B, Vokes E E 2001 Chemotherapy in the management of squamous-cell carcinoma of the head and neck. Lancet Oncology 2(5):261–269

Lindegaard J C, Grau C 2000 Has the outlook improved for amifostine as a clinical radioprotector? Radiotherapy and Oncology 57(2):113–118

Lutterbach J, Guttenberger R 2000 Anemia is associated with decreased local control of surgically treated squamous cell carcinomas of the glottic larynx. International Journal of Radiation Oncology, Biology, Physics 48(5):1345–1350

Macbeth F 2000 Radiation myelitis and thoracic radiotherapy: evidence and anecdote. Clinical Oncology (Royal College of Radiologists) 12(5):333–334

Nguyen T D, Demange L, Froissart D et al 1985 Rapid hyperfractionated radiotherapy. Clinical results in 178 advanced squamous cell carcinomas of the head and neck. Cancer 56(1):16–19

Overgaard J, Hjelm-Hansen M, Vendelbo Johansen L et al 1988 Comparison of conventional and split-course radiotherapy as primary treatment in carcinoma of the larynx. Acta Oncologica 27:147–152

Peacock J, Ashton A, Bliss J et al 2000 Cellular radiosensitivity and complication risk after curative radiotherapy. Radiotherapy and Oncology 55(2):173–178

Saunders M, Dische S, Barrett A et al 1997 Continuous hyperfractionated accelerated radiotherapy (CHART) versus conventional radiotherapy in non-small cell lung cancer: a randomised multicentre trial. Lancet 350:161–165

Siemann D W, Warrington K H, Horsman M R 2000 Targeting tumor blood vessels: an adjuvant strategy for radiation therapy. Radiotherapy and Oncology 57(1):5–12

Sinclair W K 1968 Cyclic X-ray responses in mammalian cells in vitro. Radiation Research 33:632–643

Tamm I, Schriever F, Dörken B 2001 Apoptosis: implications of basic research for clinical oncology. Lancet Oncology 2(1):33–42

Tubiana M, Dutreix J, Wambersie A (eds) 1990 Introduction to radiobiology. Taylor & Francis, London

West C M L, Davidson S E, Hendry J et al 1991 Prediction of cervical carcinoma response to radiotherapy. Lancet 338:818

Withers H R 1975 The four R's of radiotherapy. Advances in Radiation Biology 5:241–271

Withers H R, Taylor J M G, Maciejewski B 1988 The hazard of accelerated tumour clonogen repopulation during radiotherapy. Acta Oncologica 27(2):131–146

Wootton R 1993 Radiation protection of patients. Cambridge University Press, Cambridge

6

Assessing the impact of radiotherapy

Sara Faithfull

INTRODUCTION

The earlier chapters in this book describe how cancer therapy affects not only the cancer cells but also the normal tissues of the person receiving treatment. This unintentional damage to normal tissues is often termed toxicity. Assessment of toxicity is made for several reasons: firstly to estimate the biological effect of treatment on tissues, and secondly to set therapeutic limits for cancer treatment. Until recently, interest in radiation toxicity has focused on tolerance to treatment and specific late side effects in relation to potential dose-limiting complications.

The need to make decisions about the effectiveness of cancer treatment by weighing up the pros and cons of different treatment modalities is one of the principal reasons for assessment. This requires a broad holistic approach. In addition to exploring observed toxicity, assessment should incorporate patients' own perception of their illness, its emotional consequences and the daily inconveniences of coping with treatment. These outcomes need to be measured against the different radiotherapy treatment techniques in use (Bentzen 1998). A vast array of assessment tools and quality-of-life indicators exists for those working in oncology today. Despite the variety of measurement tools available, however, there is little consistency in outcome assessment between radiotherapy centres or even between clinical oncologists within a centre. Outcomes of treatment have traditionally been evaluated in terms of mortality, pathophysiological processes, radiological, clinical and laboratory assessments, but these indicators only provide rough guides of treatment effectiveness. A broader and more detailed assessment of treatment impact has been a growing area of concern. Inadequate assessment and poor documentation have so far presented a major problem for those trying to evaluate the effectiveness and impact of radiation therapy. This chapter presents a broad view of the assessment of side effects of radiotherapy not only from the more traditional stance of observed toxicity, but also from the patient's perspective of the impact of treatment.

ASSESSING EARLY AND LATE TOXICITY

The biological effects of therapeutic radiation on normal tissues have, since the earliest days of radiotherapy, posed many problems for clinicians. Over the past 100 years we have learned:

- That acute effects must be differentiated from late effects
- That in contemporary radiotherapy it is usually late effects, rather than acute effects, which are dose-limiting
- That clinical and scoring systems imperfectly reflect the extent of any underlying biological damage
- That tolerance is a poorly defined concept, with problems of subjectivity and reproducibility
- That the functional structure of a tissue is important in determining the incidence and severity of late effects
- That the factors involved in determining normal tissue damage and their relationship with radiation-induced symptoms are more complex and intricate than originally imagined
- That non-healing acute reactions may become permanent and are called consequential late effects.

Toxicity data are currently collected by a variety of means, but the principal criteria of radiation-induced toxicity are based on signs, physiological indicators or observations of a patient's clinical problems. In 1979 the World Health Organization introduced its advice for reporting the results of cancer treatment, which included the toxicity criteria related to side effects, although these were more specifically aimed at chemotherapy. The National Cancer Institute also developed the common toxicity criteria (CTC) (Trotti et al 2000), which were designed to allow a better comparison of side effects between different cancer therapies and across clinical trials (Dische et al 1989, Dische 1999, Seegenschmiedt 1998). Although useful, these broad categories do not distinguish clearly between the site-specific effects of radiotherapy treatment. In radiotherapy, there has always been a distinction between acute and late toxicity and this is reflected in specific assessment criteria. The late morbidity scoring criteria were developed in the late 1970s by one of several committees of the Radiation Therapy Oncology Group (RTOG), in response to the need to improve the consistency of toxicity scoring. Investigators from the European Organisation for Research and Treatment of Cancer (EORTC) also wanted to monitor variations in effects on normal tissues and their criteria were combined with those of the RTOG to form today's assessment criteria (see Appendix 6.1). Scores range from 0 (the absence of radiation effects) to 5, which indicates that toxicity has led to the patient's death (Cox et al 1995). The RTOG/EORTC criteria have become a standard method for presenting toxicity data. The acute radiation toxicity scoring criteria were developed in 1985 as a complement to the late effects scoring criteria. More detailed observer criteria, incorporating signs, investigations, treatment and results, have since been developed (Table 6.1). Despite the advantages of scoring systems that generate a greater

Table 6.1 Toxicity assessment criteria tools

Assessment strategy	Critique
WHO CTC version 2 (Trotti et al 2000)	Version 2 of the WHO scale includes items specifically for the recording of acute side effects from radiotherapy. Although originally designed for chemotherapy, it has been adapted for wider treatment toxicity; however, it does not incorporate the wide range of radiation reactions
RTOG/EORTC classification of radiation morbidity (Cox et al 1995)	These criteria have been used extensively in clinical studies over the past 30 years in the classification of radiation morbidity. The scales cover all areas of the body and deal separately with acute and late reactions
Franco-Italian glossary (Chassagne et al 1993)	This scoring system has been developed over 15 years for reporting both acute and late complications for the treatment of gynaecological cancer. Acute and late symptoms are included together and the scoring system has a detailed clinical and subjective assessment of symptoms
LENTSOMA (Pavy et al 1995, Rubin 1995)	This scoring system was published in 1995. Scoring criteria are given for each body area. The system is highly detailed and there is a separation between signs, symptoms, treatment and investigations. The problem with these scoring criteria is that considerable judgement is required to allocate grades
Oncology Nursing Society: assessment of radiation effects (Bruner et al 1998)	This scoring system, published in 1994, is based on eight site-specific forms. Symptoms are scored according to severity. This is not widely used in the UK

WHO, World Health Organization; CTC, common toxicity criteria; RTOG, Radiation Therapy Oncology Group; EORTC, European Organization for Research and Treatment of Cancer; LENTSOMA, late effects normal tissues/subjective/objective/management/analytic

picture of toxicity, they have not been widely utilised in practice (Overgaard & Bartelink 1995).

The variety of assessment tools now available means that there is opportunity for clinical oncologists, therapy radiographers and nurses to improve the assessment of radiation toxicity. However, there are several problems with the use of existing assessment criteria in radiotherapy. Unless these are standardised and explicitly related to treatment techniques, duration and timing, they are relatively meaningless. In a review of radiotherapy studies published in 1985, Dische and colleagues (1989) found that only 6% of studies used standard systems for assessing radiotherapy toxicity. Out of 83 studies reviewed, 16 did not mention morbidity and 29 gave only anecdotal accounts. Out of the 38 studies that provided incidence figures, 65% gave no grading, 13% used a previously described grading system, whilst 21% used their own system. In a repeat of the exercise in 1997, Munro (1997) found that, out of 80 consecutive clinical studies of radiotherapy published, only 10% used standard systems of reporting toxicity, 26% of studies had no toxicity information and 22% had only narrative accounts. Out of the 41 studies that reported incidence of morbidity, 19 different systems for assessment were used. It appears that toxicity reporting remains poor, and that the basis for comparison between studies is weak. This becomes critical when trying to review research systematically and make judgements about the efficacy of interventions (Overgaard & Bentzen 1998). Bentzen (1998) goes further to suggest that radiotherapy outcome studies should be considered incomplete if toxicity is not included.

One of the problems with objective scoring systems is that there is considerable variation in how these criteria are applied. Physicians may interpret the extent of symptoms differently and thus the reliability of scores may be compromised (Dische 1999). The lack of sensitivity of such simplistic assessments means that only gross changes are reflected in toxicity scores. The more detailed scoring systems incorporate a range of both objective and subjective assessment, but scores must still be interpreted with care, as any variations may reflect differences in symptom management as well as true toxicity. This problem was illustrated in the continuous hyperfractionated accelerated radiotherapy (CHART) randomised trial where there was good correlation within each trial centre, between the severity of morbidity recorded on both arms of the study, but there was considerable variation in scores between one centre and another (Griffiths et al 1999). The sensitivity of these criteria assessments for detecting toxicity presents a problem when there is a low number of late complications. In this case, large numbers of patients are required to detect small differences between therapies. One of the difficulties is that some of the symptoms of late toxicity are closely associated with disease progression and therefore it is difficult to distinguish symptoms as a result of radiotherapy from those that were pre-existing or those that have developed with advancing disease. Also the latency period of such late effects means that a proportion of patients may have died prior to assessment. If toxicity incidence is based on a percentage of survivors only, it may reveal an unrealistically low incidence of actual side effects. It has been suggested, therefore, that late toxicities are reported as actuarial estimates (analysing morbidity patterns for the total population) to reflect this mortality (Pedersen et al 1993).

An additional problem is that any new system of recording toxicity means that recent records cannot be compared to previous records, resulting in a reluctance to use newer scoring criteria (Dische et al 1989). Another limitation is that observer-rated toxicity scores may underreport side effects. There is evidence in the literature that substantial differences exist in the reporting of symptoms between physician, patient, nurse and lay carers (Parliament et al 1985). All these difficulties compromise the validity of toxicity assessments in relation to radiotherapy treatment.

Little prospective evaluation of radiotherapy outcomes has meant that complication and survival rates have been based on data provided by individual centres or single trials, with reported late toxicities ranging from 5% to 20% (Tan et al 1997). The implications of poor toxicity assessment for clinical evaluation are highlighted in the recent national audit of treatment outcomes of women treated in the UK for gynaecological cancer (Denton et al 2000). The national audit team revealed many difficulties in retrospectively reviewing toxicity. Researchers found that 9% of survival data was not available and that complication status was not known for 6% of patients. Two of the cancer centres approached did not have data at all for patients treated during the audit year (1993). Data on surgical outcomes were even scarcer. The lack of information on symptoms, disease progression and toxicity scores meant that it was not possible to compare treatment outcomes. There appeared to be, however, a relatively low rate of occurrence of toxicity, highlighting that late side effects are fairly rare and usually not life threatening (Hunter 2000). The audit demonstrates how poorly toxicities are recorded, therefore illustrating the potential inaccuracy of relying on retrospective data review. It also presents a worrying picture of how little is known about the outcomes of gynaecological treatment. Considering that £200 million is spent in the UK on cervical screening alone and a substantial amount more on therapy, this lack of information on treatment outcomes reflects poorly on our healthcare system.

It is clear that there is no one right way to document observer-rated toxicity. Despite the flaws of many of the assessment systems, the provision of *any* toxicity data for clinical evaluation is better than none. It is particularly important that toxicity associated with new treatments is monitored carefully. However, it needs to be remembered that most scoring systems grossly simplify morbidity and are unable to reflect the personal experience of symptoms or illustrate the ways in which side effects impact on people differently. Radiotherapy assessments should, therefore, incorporate a subjective element.

SUBJECTIVE NATURE OF SYMPTOMS

The subjective nature of symptoms is clearly illustrated by the way in which the reporting of side effects differs between individuals. This is one of the problems with observer-rated toxicity assessment tools. In reality, symptoms are cues to be interpreted, signalling changes in our bodies that reflect disease (Helman 1996). Consequently they are very subjective and are based on cultural interpretation of the individual's perception of physical illness and its impact on functioning. How 'distressing' a symptom is depends on outward signs of illness, the experience of symptoms and beliefs about what they mean. The interrelatedness of these dimensions means that it is difficult to assess one without reflecting some of the other elements. For example, the distress caused by a certain symptom may reflect an individual's belief about what that symptom means and the degree of threat it may pose. In a study of men's experiences of pelvic radiotherapy, one man thought his symptoms of pain and reduction in urinary flow were due to his penis shrinking, and this belief contributed to his anxiety (Faithfull 2000). Individuals vary widely in how they understand their symptoms and this understanding is reflected in whether patients are distressed by their symptoms, how far self-care strategies are employed and whether help is sought (Kleinman 1980). Symptom distress therefore represents an intricate interaction of physical, social and emotional forces and not merely a level of symptom severity (Fig. 6.1).

People experience and interpret symptoms in culturally determined ways (Kagawa-Singer 1993). A number of sociological studies have identified the factors that influence their interpretation, and this is an interesting area for further reading (Bury 1991, Kleinman 1980, Radley 1994). This phenomenon may not just be related to individuals' country of origin, but can also be intertwined with their level of education, social status, age, gender and personal resources. These cultural

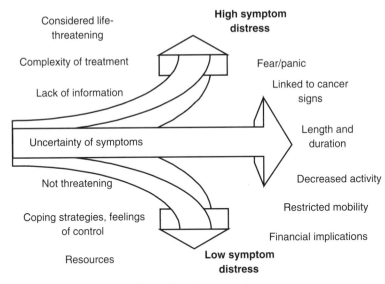

Figure 6.1   Symptom distress.

interpretations need to be considered when using symptom assessment tools such as questionnaires from differing countries. It is also important to consider how people from diverse backgrounds may respond to clinical assessments and questioning.

Recognising illness is a process that requires triggers, either through family or peer pressure, or as a response to disability. This recognition may not represent a logical decision-making process, evaluating what a symptom means to the individual, but is based more on the *context* of symptom occurrence (Radley 1994). Different symptoms will have different implications depending on how individuals see themselves (Verbrugge & Ascione 1987). Those suffering from a chronic illness often ignore their symptoms and delay seeking healthcare because they view symptoms as an inevitable consequence of disease or treatment (Giardino & Wolf 1993). Stigmatising or unsightly symptoms, particularly in head and neck or pelvic cancers, may be under-reported. The physical and emotional changes experienced as a result of radiotherapy often occur in clusters and can be very unpredictable. Wells (1995) found that this made it difficult for people to judge the seriousness of symptoms and be able to assess when to seek help.

The attribution of symptoms has been well explored in relation to delay in the diagnosis of cancer (Andersen & Cacioppo 1995), but not in relation to treatment effects. An acute symptom such as bleeding is frightening, and often considered a bad sign, therefore help is sought quickly. Less obvious symptoms may remain hidden. Individuals may report what they feel the doctor wants to hear, because they do not want to appear to complain or make a fuss. They may also doubt their own appraisal of symptoms and seek confirmation from health carers (Mishel 1981). For example, patients may believe that complaining of treatment-related symptoms distracts the doctor from taking care of the cancer (Ward et al 1993).

Health professionals may reinforce this tendency by making light of symptoms, saying that they have seen worse or that it is an accepted effect of therapy (Waxler 1980). Identifying patients' feelings about what is considered normal is therefore complicated by the above factors. This requires a shift in assessment focus to include meanings and beliefs, and a broader appreciation of what a symptom is and how it is defined. Self-assessment represents a way in which this can be accomplished.

SELF-ASSESSMENT OF SYMPTOMS

The assessment of symptoms is complicated by the fact that different people call symptoms different things. For example, fatigue is often termed anything from exhaustion to tiredness. However, there are three basic commonalities, an understanding of which promotes good symptom assessment. Firstly, all symptoms represent a common core of distressing events that happen to people, and we can use the same or similar methods for measuring different symptoms. For example, from our own personal experience we know when we have a cold and how we feel about it, as well as being able to make judgements about how severe it is and whether or not the symptoms are interfering with our lives. Patients with cancer use the same process. By accessing their own judgements and perceptions, we can effectively use self-assessment to understand their symptoms. Secondly, we should focus on what patients tell us. Recognising and legitimising symptoms is an important first step to being able to understand the implications of the illness experience. Thirdly, we need to plan and use systems in the clinical environment if we are to assess symptoms effectively. During a clinic visit, it may be left up to patients to mention if they have a particular symptom, but they may not have a way of describing the changes they are experiencing as a result of treatment, or may feel they are insignificant and as such unimportant. If there is no structure to the assessment or clinical history, there is more chance that personality, language and communication style will inhibit the recognition of symptoms. Standardising some of the questions and using tools for assessment can dramatically reduce variations in assessment technique. As a recent study by Fellowes and colleagues (2001) illustrated, patients need to be asked about specific symptoms, as they themselves may not be clear as to what counts as a side effect which requires mentioning.

Despite symptoms being multidimensional experiences, they can be evaluated in terms of specific characteristics (Fig. 6.2). The impact of symptoms may be described in terms of the frequency, severity and distress associated with the symptom experience. Although surveys have often assessed symptoms in terms of prevalence (occurrence and severity), more detailed descriptors such as distress reflect how bothersome the symptom is to that individual. This is more relevant in the clinical setting where often the distress of a symptom may be more difficult to manage than its severity. Research has identified the variability of these symptom characteristics in influencing distress (Tishelman et al 2000). Portenoy and colleagues (1994a), in a study of 215 cancer patients, found that variations in symptom severity and frequency of 32 symptoms assessed were not correlated with corresponding distress levels. They concluded that the mere report of a symptom

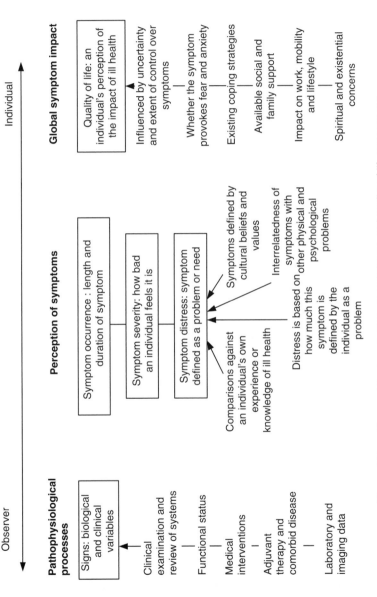

Figure 6.2 Measurable aspects of signs, symptoms and quality-of-life assessment.

does not necessarily indicate the level of suffering experienced. The impact of symptoms can also be exacerbated by many other phenomena. The presence of symptom clusters, defined as three or more symptoms (Dodd et al 2001), such as that experienced with radiotherapy, can also provide a 'cocktail' effect that can make such morbidity worse. Given et al (2001) found that the occurrence of three or more symptoms correlated with the extent of distress. The relationship between these factors is often non-linear. This is illustrated in the assessment of pain where increases in severity were not associated with an equal impact on function (Serlin et al 1995).

Distress implies physical or mental strain imposed by worries or other stresses, as well as a notion of suffering. Confusion arises as to whether distress most closely reflects psychological morbidity, such as anxiety or depression, or whether it is a way of expressing how difficult or troublesome a symptom may be. There have been attempts to characterise this suffering from cancer treatment by using global scores. Assessments such as quality-of-life tools (McClement et al 1997) incorporate symptoms as a major descriptor.

QUALITY OF LIFE AND ITS RELATIONSHIP WITH SYMPTOMS

Quality of life is usually described in terms of four dimensions: physical, psychological, social/role functioning and symptoms (King et al 1997). It is a complex concept covering many areas (Van Dam 1986), and capturing its essence is difficult, as its value and perception often vary from person to person. Quality-of-life assessment incorporates not only the functional and physical aspects of illness but also individuals' perceptions of well-being and a basic level of satisfaction with their condition (Bowling 1997). In other words, it is a global representation of an individual's health. Most investigators of quality of life distinguish between health-related quality of life (HRQOL) and subjective health, referring to patients' own perceived quality of life. These two assessment strategies for quality of life focus on different aspects. HRQOL, while also patient-based, looks at external forces that might change quality of life, such as the occurrence of symptoms and their perceived impact on health and functional states. Instruments used to study HRQOL generally examine a variety of domains which are believed to influence quality of life, as well as global perceptions of function and well-being (MacDonald 2000). Several cancer-specific HRQOL measures have been developed, such as the EORTC and Functional Assessment of Cancer Therapy (FACT) tools, and these are explored in Table 6.2. One criticism of these HRQOL tools is that decisions regarding which symptoms are more important or cause more distress are weighted in the scoring of the questionnaires, therefore patients' own perceptions of what is difficult or bothersome may not be represented (Schou & Hewison 1999). Patient perceived quality-of-life tools such as Schedule for the Evaluation of Individual Quality of Life (SEIQoL) and patient-generated index of quality of life (PGI) (Table 6.2) come from a different theoretical stance in that these assessment techniques ask patients to identify aspects *they* feel are important for their quality of life.

The multidimensional construct of quality of life is useful in assessing both the positive and negative influences of cancer and its treatment on perceived

Table 6.2 Quality-of-life instruments

Instrument	Critique
EORTC QLQ C30 plus additional site-specific cancers such as lung, gynaecological, prostate, head and neck and breast cancer (Aaronson et al 1993)	Self-completion questionnaire with questions organised around areas of functioning such as cognitive, emotional, social and role functioning. Likert-based scoring system. Higher scores represent better functioning. Incorporates specific questions for symptoms where higher symptom scores represent increased symptom severity. Includes a global quality-of-life question. The problem with this tool is that it requires scoring and is therefore not easily utilised or interpreted in clinical practice
SEIQoL (Macduff 2000, Waldron et al 1999)	This tool is based on a semistructured interview format and may be completed by both patients and general populations. It is completed in three stages: first, listing five areas of life judged to be most important in assessing quality of life; second, rating current status on a visual analogue scale as a continuum, from as good as could be or as bad, and then third, rating overall quality of life. This quality-of-life assessment is sensitive and responsive to change as it identifies the relative importance for individual specific concerns. The disadvantages are that it is time-consuming to complete in a clinical setting and the weighting and analysis of subsequent quality-of-life scores can be complex
PGI (Ruta et al 1994, Tully & Cantrill 2000)	This instrument is similar to the one above but has been developed for clinical practice, although it has not been validated in a general population. Although conceptually quite similar, the PGI has been found to be more reliable than SEIQoL. The major advantage of PGI is that this instrument can be used in postal surveys for research; however, this still remains a time-consuming assessment to administer and is still being developed further for clinical practice

EORTC, European Organisation for Research and Treatment; QLQ, quality-of-life question-naire; SEIQoL, schedule for the evaluation of quality of life; PGI, patient-generated index of quality of life.

well-being. Physical symptoms obviously contribute much to quality of life but these are merely components that increase or decrease distress. Cultural beliefs, meaning of illness and aspects of emotional and social well-being are key to influencing patients' perceptions of quality of life and these are much harder to assess. The multidimensional measurement of symptoms may provide the most information about the interactions between symptoms and quality of life. A study (Portenoy et al 1994a) of patients with cancer found that information relating to the impact of symptoms on quality of life was maximised by concurrent measurement of symptom distress.

SYMPTOM MEASUREMENT IN CLINICAL RESEARCH

In the past, symptom assessment has mainly focused on observer-rated toxicity; however, more recent recommendations for clinical trials suggest that researchers should also document side-effect duration. A growing number of studies are using concurrent multidimensional measures recording a broad spectrum of symptoms such as pain, fatigue and nausea. Exploring physical and psychological symptoms common to people with cancer can be achieved by several means, either through using simple checklists for the occurrence of symptoms, such as the Hospital Anxiety and Depression (HAD) scale or by using multidimensional symptom measures. Symptom checklists can be useful in that they provide a basis for recording whether problems are present or not. Osoba (1993) developed symptom checklists for use in patients with metastatic cancer of the head and neck and for patients with lung cancer. These site-specific questionnaires ask about the experience of symptoms during the past 2 days. Their aim was to assess patients prior to their clinic visit, thus forming a structured assessment, which would improve documentation and research. However, the four-point scales used are not very sensitive to change and have not been tested against other instruments for validity or reliability. Munro et al (1994) employed a useful system of cards to assess distress in radiotherapy patients; later this was transferred on to computerised self-assessment (Munro & Potter 1996). Patients identified which symptoms and concerns were most problematic and prioritised them. This system individualises patient assessment in a way that can also be quantified for clinical research purposes. The problem with most checklists is that they may identify whether symptoms are present but are unable to determine their frequency, severity and distress. Newer, well-validated multidimensional measures have superseded these methods, particularly in the assessment of multiple symptoms (Table 6.3).

One of the problems with these instruments is that they are only sensitive to the site-specific effects of radiotherapy if applied correctly. An example of how such validated instruments can miss important symptom effects is shown in the CHART study, which aimed to compare the effect of different fractionation regimes used for head and neck cancer on patients' physical and psychosocial symptoms. These two regimes were compared in 615 individuals at 10 time points during the course of treatment, using the Rotterdam symptom checklist and HAD scale. The conclusion was that those who received CHART had significantly worse acute side effects; those in the conventional treatment arm had a longer duration of symptoms, which were considered to offset these acute effects. However, the full range of site-specific side effects experienced by patients, such as sore mouth and skin problems, was not assessable using these tools. Although the study provided a wealth of subjective data, the lack of site-specific information may have influenced the results of the study and hence the conclusions. Careful consideration in clinical research does need to be given to the ability of an instrument to assess the dimensions and impact of symptoms in the specific population.

Alternatively, a more tailored approach can be employed in which a general screening instrument is supplemented by a specific assessment that captures information relevant to site-specific requirements. An example of such an approach is that of the EORTC quality-of-life core assessment used with a disease-specific module added (Aaronson et al 1988). The selection of measurement tools for

Table 6.3   Instruments for the self-assessment of symptoms

Instrument	Critique
Memorial symptom assessment scale (Portenoy et al 1994b)	Self-completion questionnaire that looks back over experiences of the past week. This instrument characterises 32 physical and psychological symptoms in terms of intensity, frequency and distress. The major groups identified in factor analysis are psychological issues classified as those of worrying, feeling sad and feeling nervous. The major physical areas are lack of energy, pain and feeling drowsy. The difficulty with this assessment is that the multiple ratings required for each symptom can make it less helpful as a clinical assessment
Rotterdam symptom checklist (deHaes et al 1990)	This 31-item scale asks patients to rate the extent to which a particular symptom bothered them during the past 3 days or past week. Possible answers include not at all, a little, quite a bit and very much. Symptoms on the checklist are lack of appetite, irritability, tiredness, depressed mood and nausea. This scale was designed to measure symptoms of cancer patients who participate in clinical research. An advantage of this scale is that it can be adapted for use with various patient groups by adding or deleting items. The major disadvantage is its length and its use of a rating scale based on verbal descriptors. Also the measure fails to evaluate some common symptoms that occur across cancer populations
Symptom distress scale (Holmes 1988, McCorkle & Young 1978)	The scale asks patients to rate the severity of the following 10 symptoms: nausea, mood, appetite, insomnia, pain, mobility, fatigue, bowel pattern, concentration and appearance. A total symptom distress score can be obtained by adding the scores for all 10 symptoms. The scale has been modified for patients with lung cancer. This scale is short enough for sick patients to complete but it may not capture adequately the intensity of symptom distress. It may also miss important site-specific effects

research must be guided by an understanding of the goals of the assessment and the practicality and acceptability of the instrument in that particular population. The burden and 'assessment fatigue' experienced by patients when they are required to complete multiple or complex questionnaires is increased when this is asked of them several times over treatment. This can lead to missing data and the subsequent inability to analyse certain time points. Measurement strategies that are brief and simple are the most effective, but these need to focus on anticipated patient problems, and must be balanced against the purpose of the assessment, the aims of the research and the timing of assessment when symptoms are likely to be at their worst.

ASSESSING SYMPTOMS IN THE CLINICAL AREA

Symptoms change over time, and this is especially relevant in radiotherapy practice. Symptom characteristics may change or distress levels may rise as more side effects occur or a patient's coping mechanisms alter. The factors already discussed influence such changes. This would suggest that longitudinal measurement of multiple symptom dimensions is essential in order to characterise accurately the long-term impact of symptoms. Symptom measurement is only one aspect of comprehensive assessment but the routine use of assessment tools for symptoms other than pain has not been systematically explored. This is unfortunate given the high levels of distress that fatigue or other symptoms can cause. Research in patients with breathlessness (Sarna 1998) has demonstrated that comprehensive symptom assessment can improve patient outcomes through careful ongoing monitoring and prompt intervention. The experience of pain assessment should be extrapolated to the measurement of other symptoms and Chapters 7–14 give suggestions for tools that might be appropriate. Problems of site-specific validity with checklists or multidimensional tools can be overcome when scales are complemented by sensitive communication during clinical examination. Table 6.4 highlights key areas for assessment when reviewing patients during radiotherapy and when they return for follow-up. Assessment checklists can help to focus staff's attention on symptom assessment (Dennison & Shute 2000). More detailed measures can also be used as a means of reviewing the quality of patient care or the barriers to symptom control.

CHALLENGES IN RADIOTHERAPY ASSESSMENT

There are significant attitudinal and practical challenges to bringing about comprehensive assessment of radiotherapy patients in the clinical setting. The large volume of patients undergoing radiotherapy at any one time makes routine assessment ambitious. The potential conflict between the demands of routine clinical practice and research necessitates the identification of core assessment criteria for the recording of patient outcomes and the evaluation of treatment. This is a multidisciplinary responsibility. The assessment of specific problems faced by those undergoing palliative and curative treatment requires skill and experience. There is a need to set up organisational structures that support systematic assessment by nurses, radiographers and doctors who are appropriately trained.

If we are to establish patient-centred care then the starting point must be thorough and comprehensive assessment. If a clinician is to ascertain a correct diagnosis, facilitate expression of the meaning and subjective nature of symptoms experienced and be able to plan effective interventions that meet an individual's specific needs, then thorough assessment is crucial. In order to carry out such assessment, theoretical knowledge is required: healthcare professionals need to understand radiotherapy side effects, treatment delivery and the physical and psychological impact of treatment. However, analytical and intuitive methods of thinking are also necessary. These are often described as 'perceptual awareness', where *knowing how* (theoretical knowledge) and *knowing that* (practical knowledge) work to complement each other (Benner & Wrubel 1989, Polyana 1962). Rather than thinking about symptoms in a one-dimensional way, such an approach

Table 6.4   Table of core values of radiotherapy on-treatment assessment

Core value	Related assessment
Emotional and physical assessment	Detailed assessment of current symptoms and factors that exacerbate or ameliorate them Explore whether symptoms existed prior to radiotherapy and, if so, have they worsened? Explore individuals' understanding of their cancer and subsequent radiotherapy treatment. This should include discussion of the meaning of symptoms and feelings about their health and future Which symptom or concern is causing most anxiety, concern or distress at the current time? Are symptoms connected in how they occur or in the distress experienced?
Informational assessment	Has information been provided on potential effects of treatment and how the patient can recognise symptoms when they occur and when to seek help? Ascertain if contact numbers and information on services available, both within the hospital and at home, have been provided Assess what the patient is finding most difficult about the radiotherapy treatment
Instrumental assessment	What medications is the individual taking and would these influence potential side effects? Assess knowledge of self-care strategies that help or improve patient's symptoms Physical examination if appropriate Does the patient require aids such as incontinence pads or nutritional supplements?
Family and social support	Available support from family and friends Impact of symptoms on work and social life Assess support from other areas such as the church, minister or self-help group

requires skills to draw together connections between physiological changes and the important contextual factors that influence symptom severity or distress.

There is some scepticism in medicine about the value and importance of patients' own perceptions of symptoms as valid outcome measures. The traditional preference for physiological outcomes allows easier measurement, but does not provide the breadth of assessment for holistic care. The adoption and implementation of subjective assessment tools has been held back by a lack of evaluation and lack of comparison with objective tools in terms of validity and reliability. Measuring outcomes in nursing research is problematic (Avis 1995, Bond & Thomas 1991); healthcare providers are often unfamiliar with the range of tools and assessment techniques available, and many view formal assessment as purely a research initiative. It is essential that we improve our familiarity with these tools and incorporate systematic assessment into our delivery of clinical care.

The implementation of systems which enable the routine screening of radiotherapy patients does have resource implications. Young & Maher (1992) provide insight into the dilemmas of screening patients for anxiety and depression routinely at the start of radiotherapy. They found that referrals to the radiographer counsellor increased dra-matically during the period in which assessments were being made. However, a recent study evaluating nurse-led care found that making a detailed assessment of male patients prior to radiotherapy for pelvic cancer actually reduced usage of health services. Outcomes were improved because symptoms could be addressed early. This had a beneficial impact on resources, with fewer inpatient admissions and outpatient appointments compared to those receiving conventional care (Faithfull et al 2001).

Assessment requires the setting of priorities, identifying those most in need of healthcare or support. Some patient populations are especially difficult to assess, particularly patients who are confused or who have language barriers or cognitive impairment. These types of problems may limit the patient's ability to participate in the assessment process, and may make subjective measurement tools inappropriate. Healthcare professionals working in radiotherapy need to consider the practicality and relevance of available assessment tools and instigate systems which are also flexible enough to accommodate the needs of the individual.

SUMMARY AND CONCLUSION

There are significant challenges to bringing systematic toxicity assessment to the radiotherapy clinic. The diverse nature of patients' problems arising from their treatment and illness necessitates broader assessment than existing tools allow. It is important, however, that assessments incorporate a site-specific focus, relevant to the treatment site. Despite existing challenges, there are substantial benefits to be gained from undertaking symptom assessment during routine clinic visits. Frank (1991) in his autobiographical account of experiencing cancer and critical illness reflects how important it is for health carers to understand the wider experience of symptoms and treatment. He says that:

> Those who provide treatment give patients cues as to the emotions that are appropriate to express. Because patients are dependent on medical staff, they tend to accept these cues ... continuing suffering threatens them, so they deny it exists. What they cannot treat, the patient is not allowed to experience. Physicians and nurses often forget that when treatment runs out, there can still be care. Simply recognising suffering for what it is, regardless of whether it can be treated, is care (p. 100).

Sensitive and informed assessment provides the basis for such care.

SUMMARY OF KEY CLINICAL POINTS

• Monitoring of radiotherapy side effects is important for the assessment of biological effects on an individual, to set therapeutic limits for cancer treatment and to identify areas of need for patients and families.
• Actuarial rates need to be reported instead of crude rates for late toxicity to give a more realistic risk of the potential for side-effect occurrence.
• Assessment provides the basis for treatment decisions. A checklist can help guide assessment and provide a focus for routine clinic visits.

- Systematic site-specific assessment during radiotherapy is essential.
- Objective scores and measurement scales are important; however, subjective data from the patient's perspective are also required.
- Quality-of-life measurement is a useful adjunct to routine assessment but needs to be used carefully in the clinical setting. Patient-focused quality-of-life instruments based on individual needs (such as PGI or SEIQoL) are being developed.
- No assessment tool is perfect for radiotherapy patients and more work is required in the evaluation of multidimensional symptom assessments in the radiotherapy setting.
- It is essential to recognise the complexity of side effects and how they change over time.

AREAS FOR FURTHER RESEARCH

- The development and evaluation of a radiotherapy-specific checklist that could aid clinicians in the outpatient setting towards rapid assessment of patients' needs
- Development and testing of valid and reliable measures of assessment for site-specific radiotherapy side effects that would be suitable for evaluating healthcare interventions
- Evaluation of the impact of comprehensive radiotherapy assessment on patient outcomes
- Studies to explore the interface between patients' subjective assessment of symptoms and existing objective measurements.

REFERENCES

Aaronson N, Bullinger M, Ahmedzai S 1988 A modular approach to quality of life assesment in cancer clinical trials. In: Scheurlen H, Kay R, Baum M (eds) Recent results in cancer research, vol. 111 Springer-Verlag, Berlin, p 231
Aaronson N, Ahmedzai B, Bergman M et al 1993 The European Organisation for Research and Treatment of Cancer QLQ-C30: a quality of life instrument for use in international clinical trials in oncology. Journal of the National Cancer Institute 85:365–376
Andersen B, Cacioppo J 1995 Delay in seeking a cancer diagnosis: delay stages and psychophysiological comparison processes. British Journal of Social Psychology 34:33–52
Avis M 1995 Valid arguments? A consideration of the concept of validity in establishing the credibility of research findings. Journal of Advanced Nursing 22:1203–1209
Benner P, Wrubel J 1989 The primacy of caring: stress and coping in health and illness. Addison-Wesley, California
Bentzen S 1998 Towards evidence based radiation oncology: improving the design, analysis, and reporting of clinical outcome studies in radiotherapy. Radiotherapy and Oncology 46:5–18
Bond S, Thomas L 1991 Issues in measuring outcomes of nursing. Journal of Advanced Nursing 16:1492–1502
Bowling A 1997 Measuring health: a review of quality of life measurement scales. Open University Press, Milton Keynes
Bruner D, Iwamoto R et al 1998 Manual for radiation oncology nursing practice and education. Oncology Nursing Press, Pittsburgh
Bury M 1991 The sociology of chronic illness: a review of research and prospects. Sociology of Health and Illness 13:451–468
Chassagne D, Sismondi P, Horiot J et al 1993 A glossary for reporting complications in gynaecological cancers. Radiotherapy and Oncology 26:195–202

Cox J, Stetz J, Pajak T 1995 Toxicity criteria of the Radiation Therapy Oncology Group (RTOG) and the European Organisation for Research and Treatment of Cancer (EORTC). International Journal of Radiation Oncology, Biology and Physics 31:1341–1346

deHaes J, van Knippenberg F, Neijit J 1990 Measuring psychological and physical distress in cancer patients: structure and application of the Rotterdam Symptom Checklist. British Journal of Cancer 7:6–9

Dennison S, Shute T 2000 Identifying patient concerns: improving the quality of patients' visits to the oncology out-patient department – a pilot audit. European Journal of Oncology Nursing 4:91–98

Denton A, Bond S, Mathews S et al 2000 National audit of the management and outcome of carcinoma of the cervix treated with radiotherapy in 1993. Clinical Oncology 12:347–353

Dische S 1999 Revealing morbidity. Radiotherapy and Oncology 53:173–175

Dische S, Warburton M, Jones D et al 1989 The recording of morbidity related to radiotherapy. Radiotherapy and Oncology 16:103–108

Dodd M, Miaskowski C, Paul S 2001 Symptom clusters and their effect on the functional status of patients with cancer. Oncology Nursing Forum 28:465–470

Faithfull S 2000 Supportive care in radiotherapy: evaluating the potential contribution of nursing. PhD thesis. London University, London

Faithfull S, Corner J, Myer L et al 2001 Evaluation of nurse-led care for men undergoing pelvic radiotherapy. British Journal of Cancer 18:1853–1864

Fellowes D, Fallowfield L, Saunders C et al 2001 Tolerability of hormone therapies for breast cancer: how informative are documented symptom profiles in medical notes for 'well tolerated' treatments? Breast Cancer Research Treatment 66:73–81

Frank A 1991 At the will of the body. Reflections on illness. Houghton Mifflin, Boston

Giardino E, Wolf Z 1993 Symptoms: evidence and experience. Holistic Nurse Practice 7:1–12

Given C, Given B, Azzouz F et al 2001 Predictors of pain and fatigue in the year following diagnosis among elderly cancer patients. Journal of Pain and Symptom Management 21(6):456–460

Griffiths G, Parmar M, Bailey A 1999 Physical and psychological symptoms of quality of life in the CHART randomized trial in head and neck cancer: short-term and long-term patient reported symptoms. British Journal of Cancer 81:1196–1205

Helman C 1996 Culture, health and illness. Butterworth-Heinemann, Oxford

Holmes S 1988 Use of a modified symptom distress scale in assessment of the cancer patient. International Journal of Nursing Studies 26:69–79

Hunter R 2000 Morbidity in radiotherapy practice. Clinical Oncology (Royal College of Radiologists)12:345–346

Kagawa-Singer M 1993 Redefining health: living with cancer. Social Science and Medicine 37:295–304

King C, Haberman M, Berry D et al (1997) Quality of life and the cancer experience: the state of the knowledge. Oncology Nursing Forum 24:27–41

Kleinman A 1980 Patients and healers in the context of culture. University of California Press, Berkeley

MacDonald B 2000 Quality of life in cancer care: patients' experiences and nurses' contribution. European Journal of Oncology Nursing 5:32–41

Macduff C 2000 Respondent generated quality of life measures: useful tools for nursing or more fool's gold? Journal of Advanced Nursing 32:375–382

McClement S, Woodgate R, Degner L 1997 Symptom distress in adult patients with cancer. Cancer Nursing 20:236–243

McCorkle R, Young K 1978 Development of a symptom distress scale. Cancer Nursing 1:373–378

Mishel M 1981 The measurement of uncertainty in illness. Nursing Research 30:258–263

Munro A 1997 Assessing radiotherapy toxicity. (Personal communication.)

Munro A, Potter S 1996 A quantitative approach to the distress caused by symptoms in patients treated with radical radiotherapy. British Journal of Cancer 74:640–647

Munro A, Biruls R, Griffin A et al 1994 Distress associated with radiotherapy for malignant disease: a quantitative analysis based on patients' perceptions. British Journal of Cancer 60:370–374

Osoba D 1993 Self-rating symptom checklists: a simple method for recording and evaluating symptom control in oncology. Cancer Treatment Reviews 19:43–51

Overgaard J, Bartelink H 1995 About tolerance and quality. An important notice to all radiation oncologists. Radiotherapy and Oncology 35:1–3

Overgaard J, Bentzen S 1998 Evidence based radiation oncology. Radiotherapy and Oncology 46:1–3

Parliament M, Danoux C, Clayton T 1985 Is cancer treatment accurately reported? International Journal of Radiation Oncology, Biology, Physics 11:603–608

Pavy J, Denekamp J, Letscher J 1995 Late effects toxicity scoring: the SOMA scale. Radiotherapy and Oncology 35:11–15

Pedersen D, Bentzen S, Overgaard J 1993 Reporting radiotherapeutic complications in patients with uterine cervical cancer. The importance of latency and classification system. Radiotherapy and Oncology 28:134–141

Polyana M 1962 Personal knowledge. Routledge and Kegan Paul, London

Portenoy R, Thaler H, Kornblith A et al 1994a Symptom prevalence, characteristics and distress in a cancer population. Quality of Life Research 3:183–189

Portenoy R, Thaler H, Kornblith A et al 1994b The memorial symptom assessment scale: an instrument for the evaluation of symptom prevalence, characteristics and distress. European Journal of Cancer 30A:1326–1336

Radley A 1994 Making sense of illness: the social psychology of health and disease. Sage, London

Rubin P 1995 Late effects of normal tissues (LENT) consensus conference. International Journal of Radiation Oncology, Biology, Physics 31:1035–1036

Ruta D A, Garratt A M, Leng M et al 1994 A new approach to the measurement of quality of life. The Patient Generated Index

Sarna L 1998 Effectiveness of structured nursing assessment of symptom distress in advanced lung cancer. Oncology Nursing Forum 25:1041–1048

Schou K, Hewison J 1999 Experiencing cancer. Open University Press, Buckingham

Seegenschmiedt M 1998 Interdisciplinary documentation of treatment side effects in oncology. Strahlenther Onkol 174:25–29

Serlin R, Mendoza T, Nakamura Y et al 1995 When is cancer pain mild, moderate or severe? Reading pain severity by its interference with function. Pain 61:277–284

Tan L, Jones B, Gee A et al 1997 An audit of the treatment of carcinoma of the uterine cervix using external beam radiotherapy and a single line sources brachytherapy technique. British Journal of Radiology 70:1259–1269

Tishelman C, Degner L, Mueller B 2000 Measuring symptom distress in patients with lung cancer. Cancer Nursing 23:82–90

Trotti A, Byhardt R, Stetz J 2000 Common toxicity criteria: version 2. An improved reference guide for grading the acute effects of cancer treatment: impact on radiotherapy. International Journal of Radiation Oncology, Biology, Physics 47:13–47

Tully M, Cantrill J 2000 The validity of the modified patient generated index – a quantitative and qualitative approach. Quality of Life Research 9:509–520

Van Dam F 1986 Quality of life: methodological aspects. Bulletin of Cancer 73:607–613

Waldron D, O'Boyle C, Kearney M et al 1999 Quality-of-life measurement in advanced cancer: assessing the individual. Journal of Clinical Oncology 17:3603–3611

Ward S, Goldberg N, McCauley V et al 1993 Patient-related barriers to management of cancer pain. Pain 52:319–324

Waxler N 1980 The social labelling perspective on illness and medical practice. In: Eisenberg L, Kleinmman A (eds) The relevance of social science for medicine. D Reidel, Dordrecht, p 283–306

Wells E M 1995 The impact of radiotherapy to the head and neck: a qualitative study of patients after completion of treatment. Centre for Cancer and Palliative Care Studies. Institute of Cancer Research, London, p 1–76

Young J, Maher E 1992 The role of a radiographer counsellor in a large centre for cancer treatment: a discussion paper based on an audit of the work of a radiographer counsellor. Clinical Oncology 4:232–235

Appendix 6.1 Radiation morbidity scoring criteria: acute radiation side effects

Site tissue	0	1	2	3	4
Skin	No change over baseline	Follicular, faint or dull erythema; epilation; dry desquamation; decreased sweating	Tender or bright erythema, patchy moist desquamation; moderate oedema	Confluent, moist desquamation other than skin-folds, pitting oedema	Ulceration, haemorrhage, necrosis
Mucous membrane	No change over baseline	Injection; may experience mild pain not requiring analgesic	Patchy mucositis that may produce an inflammatory serosanguineous discharge; may experience moderate pain requiring analgesia	Confluent fibrinous mucositis; may include severe pain requiring narcotic	Ulceration, haemorrhage or necrosis
Eye	No change	Mild conjunctivitis with or without scleral injection; increased tearing	Moderate conjunctivitis with or without keratitis requiring steroids and/or antibiotics; dry eye requiring artificial tears; iritis with photophobia	Severe keratitis with corneal ulceration; objective decrease in visual acuity or in visual fields; acute glaucoma; panophthalmitis	Loss of vision (unilateral or bilateral)
Ear	No change over baseline	Mild external otitis with erythema, pruritus, secondary to dry desquamation not requiring medication. Audiogram unchanged from baseline	Moderate external otitis requiring topical medication; serous otitis medius; hypoacusis on testing only	Severe external otitis with discharge or moist desquamation; symptomatic hypoacusis; tinnitus, not drug-related	Deafness
Salivary gland	No change over baseline	Mild mouth dryness; slightly thickened saliva; may have slightly altered taste such as metallic taste; these changes are not reflected in alteration in baseline feeding behaviour, such as increased use of liquids with meals	Moderate to complete dryness; thick, sticky saliva; markedly altered taste		Acute salivary gland necrosis

Appendix 6.1 (Continued) Radiation morbidity scoring criteria: acute radiation side effects

Site tissue	0	1	2	3	4
Pharynx and Oesophagus	No change over baseline	Mild dysphagia or odynophagia; may require topical anaesthetic or nonnarcotic analgesics; may require soft diet	Moderate dysphagia or odynophagia; may require narcotic analgesics; may require puréed or liquid diet	Severe dysphagia or odynophagia with dehydration or weight loss (> 15% from pre-treatment baseline) requiring nasogastric feeding tube, intravenous fluids or hyperalimentation	Complete obstruction, ulceration, perforation, fistula
Larynx	No change over baseline	Mild or intermittent hoarseness; cough not requiring antitussive; erythema of mucosa	Persistent hoarseness but able to vocalise; referred ear pain, sore throat, patchy fibrinous exudate or mild arytenoid oedema not requiring narcotic; cough requiring antitussive	Whispered speech, throat pain or referred ear pain requiring narcotic; confluent fibrinous exudate, marked arytenoid oedema	Marked dyspnoea, stridor or a hemoptysis with tracheostomy or intubation necessary
Upper gastrointestinal tract	No change	Anorexia with ≤ 5% weight loss from pre-treatment baseline; nausea not requiring antiemetics; abdominal discomfort not requiring parasympatholytic drugs or analgesics	Anorexia with ≤ 15% weight loss from pre-treatment baseline; nausea and/or vomiting requiring antiemetics; abdominal pain requiring analgesics	Anorexia with > 15% weight loss from pre-treatment baseline or requiring nasogastric tube or parenteral support. Nausea and/or vomiting requiring tube or parenteral support; abdominal pain, severe despite medication; a haematemesis or melena; abdominal distension (flat-plate radiograph demonstrates bowel loops)	Ileus subacute or acute obstruction, perforation, gastrointestinal bleeding requiring transfusion; abdominal pain requiring tube decompression or bowel diversion

Continued

Appendix 6.1   (Continued) Radiation morbidity scoring criteria: acute radiation side effects

Site tissue	0	1	2	3	4
Lower gastrointestinal tract, including pelvis	No change	Increased frequency or change in quality of bowel habits not requiring medication; rectal discomfort not requiring analgesics	Diarrhoea requiring parasympatholytic drugs (e.g. Lomotil); mucus discharge not necessitating sanitary pads; rectal or abdominal pain requiring analgesics	Diarrhoea requiring parenteral support; severe mucus or blood discharge necessitating sanitary pads; abdominal distension (flat-plate radiograph demonstrates distended bowel loops)	Acute or subacute obstruction, fistula or perforation; gastrointestinal bleeding requiring transfusion; abdominal pain or tenesmus requiring tube decompression or bowel diversion
Lung	No change	Mild symptoms of dry cough or dyspnoea on exertion	Persistent cough requiring narcotic, antitussive agents; dyspnoea with minimal effort but not at rest	Severe cough unresponsive to narcotic antitussive agent or dyspnoea at rest; clinical or radiological evidence of acute pneumonitis; intermittent oxygen or steroids may be required	Severe respiratory insufficiency; continuous oxygen of assisted ventilation
Genitourinary	No change	Frequency of urination or nocturia twice pretreatment habit; dysuria, urgency not requiring medication	Frequency of urination or nocturia that is less frequent than every hour. Dysuria, urgency, bladder spasm requiring local anaesthetic (e.g. phenazopyridine (Pyridium))	Frequency with urgency and nocturia hourly or more frequently; dysuria, pelvis pain or bladder spasm requiring regular, frequent narcotic; gross hamaturia with; without clot passage	Haematuria requiring transfusion; acute bladder obstruction not secondary to clot passage, ulceration or necrosis
Heart	No change over baseline	Asymptomatic but objective evidence of electrocardiogram changes or pericardial abnormalities without evidence of other heart disease	Symptomatic with electrocardiogram changes and radiological findings of congestive heart failure or pericardial disease; no specific treatment required	Congestive heart failure, angina pectoris, pericardial disease responding to therapy	Congestive heart failure, angina pectoris, pericardial disease, arrhythmias not responsive to non-surgical measures

Continued

Appendix 6.1 (Continued) Radiation morbidity scoring criteria: acute radiation side effects

Site tissue	0	1	2	3	4
Central nervous system	No change	Fully functional status (i.e. able to work) with minor neurological findings; no medication needed	Neurological findings present sufficient to require home care; nursing assistance may be required; medications, including steroids; antiseizure agents may be required	Neurological findings requiring hospitalisation for initial management	Serious neurological impairment that includes paralysis, coma or seizures. Three per week despite medication; hospitalisation required
Haematological White blood cells ($\times 1000$)	≥ 4.0	$3.0 \leq 4.0$	$2.0 \leq 3.0$	$1.0 \leq 2.0$	< 1.0
Platelets ($\times 1000$)	>100	$75 \leq 100$	$50 \leq 75$	$25 \leq 50$	< 25 or spontaneous bleeding
Neutrophils ($\times 1000$)	≥ 1.9	$1.5 \leq 1.9$	$1.0 \leq 1.5$	$0.5 \leq 1.0$	< 0.5 or sepsis
Haemoglobin GM%	>11	$11-9.5$	$<9.5-7.5$	$<7.5-5.0$	
Haematocrit	≥ 32	$28 \leq 32$	<28	Packed cell infusion	

7

Fatigue and radiotherapy

Sara Faithfull

INTRODUCTION

Fatigue is now recognised as a common symptom and side effect of cancer treatment; however, its occurrence and impact in radiotherapy patients have, to a great extent, remained hidden and unrecorded. Consequently it is a symptom which nurses and therapy radiographers often feel ill equipped to manage. The evidence base available provides little insight into the aetiology of radiation-induced fatigue and does not explain why treatment of certain radiotherapy sites seems to cause greater levels of fatigue.

Fatigue can seriously affect quality of life and can hinder an individual's self-care ability, rehabilitation and recovery from radiotherapy treatment. The incidence of fatigue in patients being treated with radiotherapy has been reported to range from 75% to 100% and the degree to which it is experienced varies throughout the treatment trajectory (King et al 1985, Kubricht 1984, Nail 1993). It is, however, difficult to distinguish the fatigue experienced as a side-effect of radiotherapy from that which may pre-exist as a consequence of the disease process itself or the effect of adjuvant treatment. Fatigue is characterised by patients as a feeling of overwhelming exhaustion and lack of energy, often resulting in difficulty concentrating and emotional distress or low mood. It appears to be closely associated with other symptoms, producing a combination of physiological, behavioural, mental and emotional manifestations. Cancer-related fatigue as a result of radiotherapy is therefore a complex multifactorial symptom with physical and psychological components.

AETIOLOGY

Relatively little is known about the mechanisms of radiation-induced fatigue. The systemic effects of radiotherapy may be related to the accumulation of metabolites as a result of normal tissue damage, giving rise to the experience of fatigue (Glaus 1998). Alternative theories suggest that the body's increasing requirements for molecular and cellular repair may induce fatigue by putting more demands on scarce resources (Beach et al 2001). Greenberg and colleagues (1992), for example, found that cytokine and interleukin-1 levels rose in men undergoing radiotherapy for prostate cancer, mirrored by an increase in levels of fatigue. However, no other studies have identified immunological changes of this nature (Morant 1996).

Fatigue has also been linked with physiological disorders such as cachexia (Watanabe & Bruera 1996) anorexia (Gleeson & Spencer 1995) and biochemical abnormalities (Morant et al 1993). With advanced cancer a wide range of physiological changes can result in fatigue (Moore & Hayes 2001) (Table 7.1). Many patients with advanced cancer also have palliative radiotherapy and the connection between fatigue as a result of treatment and these underlying physiological changes is unclear. Nutritional problems have also been linked with fatigue, and these commonly occur during radiotherapy, especially in patients with head and neck cancer. However Kobashi-Schoot (1985) failed to detect any correlation between fatigue and gastrointestinal symptoms, and Beach et al (2001) found no relationship between fatigue severity and nutritional problems in patients with lung cancer. Many of the associated physiological disorders identified as causal factors of fatigue are not supported by evidence.

Fatigue has also been linked with psychological disorders such as depression, although the mechanism for this has not been identified (Smets et al 1996). Early studies of psychological morbidity suggest that between 30 and 40% of individuals with cancer experience moderate anxiety during the course of their therapy (Derogatis et al 1983). Many studies have identified the emotional and physical distress associated with radiotherapy (Christman 1990, Forester et al 1985b), but the proportion of people who experience depression is largely unknown. Fatigue in itself may be a cause for depression, or it may be that it is a component of a complex syndrome of physical and emotional distress. Blesch et al (1991), investigating emotional distress in patients with lung and breast cancer, found a relationship between fatigue and negative mood. Smets and colleagues (1998a)

Table 7.1 Physiological problems which may be associated with fatigue

Physiological disorders	Associated problems/causes
Decreased oxygen-carrying capacity of the circulation	Existing heart disease
	Lung cancer
	Anaemia
Metabolic disorders	Metastases in the liver
Hypokalaemia	Dehydration
Hypophosphataemia	Diarrhoea
Hypocalcaemia	Renal damage
Hypomagnesaemia	Hyperthyroidism
	Effects of medication
Nutritional disorders	Malnutrition
Anorexia	Mucositis, xerostomia
Cachexia	Gastrointestinal symptoms
Endocrine and hormonal disturbances	Diabetes
	Low testosterone levels
Disruption of central nervous functions	Brain tumours
	Toxicity from cytotoxic treatment
Immunological disorders	Neutropenia as a result of cancer treatment

also found significant associations between postradiotherapy fatigue, psychological distress and depression. Visser & Smets (1998) in exploring correlations between quality of life and fatigue, found that there was not a strong relationship with depression and stress. Sustained symptoms of fatigue after treatment can have a continued negative effect on emotions. Fobair et al (1986), describing treatment effects in survivors of Hodgkin's disease, found that if energy levels had not returned to normal after therapy, patients were more likely to be depressed. Evidence also increasingly links the experience of fatigue with other cancer symptoms such as pain, nausea and breathlessness (Blesch et al 1991, Stone et al 1998). The aetiology of cancer fatigue is thus very complex and the multitude of treatment factors and associated conditions makes teasing out the exact causal mechanisms a challenge for future researchers.

PATTERN OF FATIGUE SYMPTOMS

Haylock & Hart (1979) first highlighted the changing pattern of radiation-induced fatigue, describing it as increasing and waning in a weekly pattern over the course of radiotherapy. Fatigue may be cumulative, increasing during the course of radiotherapy and being most severe during the last week of treatment (Fieler 1997, Graydon et al 1995, Irvine et al 1998). This suggests a linear relationship between dose and fatigue (Barrere et al 1993), but there have been differing reports in the literature (Table 7.2). In a detailed study of women with breast cancer, Greenberg et al (1992) did not detect the same weekly rise but found that fatigue decreased over the 3 weeks following radiotherapy (Table 7.2). Further studies in other patient populations have also highlighted that fatigue is not consistent with this linear trajectory. Faithfull & Brada (1998) found that patients who had received cranial radiotherapy experienced several episodes of fatigue in the course of recovering from radiotherapy treatment. The persistence of fatigue after completion of therapy is clearly shown in Eardley's work (1986), which identified that two-thirds of patients who had undergone radiotherapy to the head and neck still felt tired and weak 6–8 weeks after radiotherapy had been completed. King et al (1985) also found that 14–39% of patients were still experiencing fatigue 3 months after radiotherapy treatment. The literature reports conflicting descriptions of the pattern of fatigue in different treatment groups and sites of radiotherapy. This may be as a result of the way fatigue has been assessed, as many of the studies have used cross-sectional techniques, which provide only a snapshot of the patient's symptoms.

FACTORS AFFECTING THE PATTERN OF FATIGUE

Although small studies have looked at fatigue in site-specific groups, larger studies tend to assess fatigue levels in mixed-treatment groups, thus making it difficult to extrapolate whether patients with different cancers experience fatigue differently. Several studies do appear to illustrate that those patients with lung cancer experience particularly high levels of fatigue (Larson et al 1993, Piper & Dodd 1991). Hickok and colleagues (1996) found that fatigue and problems with pain were the most frequently reported side effects of patients undergoing radiation for

Table 7.2 Evidence from studies describing fatigue as a result of radiotherapy

Author	Site of treatment	Pattern of fatigue	Comment
Greenberg et al (1992)	Women with early-stage breast cancer ($n = 15$)	Fatigue levels decreased during the first and second week of radiotherapy, rose to a peak at the fourth week then gradually fell	Fatigue continued to be a problem following completion of treatment
Greenberg et al (1993)	Men receiving radiation for localised prostate cancer ($n = 15$)	Fatigue levels continued to rise throughout treatment	The peak of fatigue levels was the fourth week of radiotherapy treatment
Graydon et al (1995)	Women with breast cancer ($n = 53$)	Women reported increases in fatigue scores as treatment progressed	Higher fatigue scores were correlated with increased symptom distress and decreased physical functioning
Hickok et al (1996)	Lung cancer patients ($n = 50$)	Fatigue was experienced within 3 weeks of starting radiotherapy	Fatigue was experienced by 78% of patients at some point during therapy
Fieler (1997)	Patients receiving high-dose-rate brachytherapy ($n = 9$ bronchial, $n = 18$ gynaecological)	Fatigue increased over course of treatment	Patients experienced a wide range of symptoms, from fatigue to urinary frequency and shortness of breath
Irvine et al (1998)	Women with breast cancer ($n = 76$)	Fatigue significantly increased over the course of radiotherapy treatment	Fatigue was highest during the last week of treatment and returned to pre-treatment levels by 3 months
Faithfull & Brada (1998)	Cranial radiotherapy ($n = 19$)	A linear decrease in fatigue was not seen after treatment but there was a rise and fall in fatigue symptoms	Fatigue was correlated with somnolence. Fatigue symptoms were also linked with feelings of a lack of concentration, drowsiness and lethargy
Smets et al (1998a)	Patients with different cancers and sites of radiotherapy treatment ($n = 250$)	Fatigue scores increased over treatment	40% of all patients reported fatigue. In comparison to pre-treatment scores, 44% found fatigue levels were increased. Nine months after radiotherapy, fatigue levels were no different from the general population
Lovely et al (1999)	Cranial radiotherapy ($n = 60$)	Fatigue significantly increased over the course of radiotherapy	Increases in fatigue were associated with decreases in quality of life

lung cancer. Fatigue developed during the first 3 weeks of treatment in 78% of patients and was closely correlated with the onset of pain; however, those patients who had received chemotherapy or had surgery prior to radiotherapy had a lower incidence of fatigue. Blesch et al (1991) also found that lung cancer patients had higher fatigue levels at the start of treatment compared to women being treated with radiotherapy for breast cancer. It appears that men having pelvic treatment may experience a lower incidence of fatigue than women with genitourinary disease. Nail (1993) describes how intracavitary treatment for gynaecological disease significantly adds to the extent of fatigue symptoms. In breast cancer treatment, the addition of chemotherapy and surgery complicates the pattern and incidence of the symptom. Fatigue is also a very debilitating consequence of cranial irradiation for brain tumours and seems to be closely related to somnolence syndrome, which is reported to occur 2 and 6 weeks from the end of therapy (Faithfull & Brada 1998). The impact of such fatigue on quality of life is substantial (Davies et al 1996). Other factors such as gender, adjuvant treatment and age may also influence the pattern of fatigue in patients undergoing radiotherapy; however, few of these correlates have been proven.

PREDICTIVE FACTORS

Although fatigue is expected as an inevitable side effect of radiotherapy treatment, no specific predictive factors have been identified in the literature. It is thought that fatigue, like other side effects, relates to the cell type, degree of normal tissue damage, treatment site and volume and dose of radiotherapy (Table 7.3). However, given its multifaceted nature, and close association with other emotional and physical symptoms, the explanation is likely to be considerably more complex. The literature suggests that the incidence and severity of fatigue are also affected by adjuvant therapy, chemotherapy or surgery (either concurrently or prior to radiotherapy treatment), neutropenia (Molassiotis & Chan 2000) and symptom distress (Irvine et al 1998).

Evidence for the increase in fatigue with combined-modality treatment is shown in several studies. Woo et al (1998) found that women receiving combination

Table 7.3 Factors that may influence the occurrence of fatigue

Adjuvant therapy
   Chemotherapy
   Recent surgery
   Hormone therapy
Age
Frailty
Pre-treatment fatigue levels
Site of radiotherapy
Dosage of treatment
Fractionation regime
Advanced disease
Extensive physical symptoms
Pain

therapies had the highest fatigue scores and those receiving radiotherapy alone had the lowest fatigue scores. Fobair and colleagues (1986) surveyed 403 patients receiving a variety of adjuvant treatments, and found that 90% of patients reported that treatment had an effect on their energy levels. For 37% this did not improve once treatment was completed.

There have been conflicting accounts in the literature as to whether age is a predictive factor for fatigue occurrence. Kobashi-Schoot (1985) found that there was no correlation between fatigue and age of the patient. However, in Fobair's study, the younger patients (< 34 years) fared best and felt recovered within 12 months, while older patients took longer to recover. In a study of patients with prostate cancer, those men who were older than 75 were 11 times more likely to experience elevated fatigue levels than their younger counterparts (Faithfull 2000). Woo et al (1998), however, found the opposite, in that younger women with breast cancer had more severe fatigue. This may have been associated with the fact that more aggressive treatment regimes were given to younger women.

Although few studies account for this, chronological age may not be particularly meaningful in itself; differences in fatigue levels may be much more closely linked to the combination of treatments used and the patient's 'frailty'. This is a concept explored by Corner (1993), who suggests that chronological age may influence treatment decisions and hence the extent of therapy but that physical condition, comorbidity and dependence vary tremendously among older people. Pre-treatment fatigue is also an important factor in that it may explain differences in incidence for different diseases and sites of therapy. Smets and colleagues (1998a) in a study of 250 patients undergoing radiotherapy found that pre-treatment fatigue levels were the best predictor for fatigue intensity. Factors identified were the degree of functional disability and impaired quality of sleep prior to treatment, which explained as much as 38% of the variance in fatigue levels during radiotherapy. There is also evidence that patients experience fatigue prior to having their cancer diagnosed (Piper & Dodd 1991). Cox and colleagues (1987) found in a study of men and women without cancer that 20% of men and 30% of women complain of fatigue. It is therefore unclear how cancer-related fatigue differs from these more normal occurrences of fatigue.

THE IMPACT OF FATIGUE

Oberst and colleagues (1991) reported that fatigue was considered by patients to be one of the most difficult of cancer symptoms. In a study of distress associated with radiotherapy, Munro et al (1994) asked 72 patients to prioritise which symptoms or feelings were most troublesome during treatment. Fatigue was ranked second to worries about the success of therapy, but above other physical symptoms such as pain. A study by Smets et al (1998a) highlighted that fatigue after radiotherapy was listed by 46% of patients as one of the three most troublesome and distressing symptoms. The persistence of fatigue symptoms following radiotherapy particularly influenced their quality of life. Thirty-four per cent of patients had worse levels of fatigue than they had anticipated 9 months after radiotherapy was completed (Smets et al 1998b). In a large telephone survey of USA cancer patients, Vogelzang and colleagues (1997) reported that fatigue, more than pain, adversely affected patients' daily activities (61% vs 19%). Although the experience of fatigue during radiotherapy is, for many patients, expected, the long duration and severity of fatigue symptoms experienced after radiotherapy can have a substantial impact on quality of life (Fieler 1997).

It appears that the impact of fatigue is not directly proportional to its occurrence or severity. This has been demonstrated by Krishnasamy's work, which found that high fatigue scores were not necessarily associated with high levels of distress (Krishnasamy 1997). These findings highlight the importance of recognising the subjective nature and personal experience of fatigue, including physical limitations, feelings of exhaustion and subsequent distress. Krishnasamy (2001) emphasises the significance of fatigue for the individual and family, pointing out that the expression of fatigue is largely determined by the meaning attributed to it. Patients may feel that fatigue is related to healing or that it represents the advancing cancer.

Fatigue is a complex and shifting symptom and its impact on patients' lives changes according to beliefs and circumstances (Richardson & Ream 1998). Listening to patients' accounts of their experiences is vital, if clinicians and researchers are to understand the words that patients use to describe different aspects of fatigue. This is important not only for understanding the impact of fatigue, and its effect on quality of life, but also in the development of assessment tools.

Many patients experience the impact of radiation fatigue as a sense of loss, not just in terms of physical strength but also in motivation and ability to think as well as to engage in social activity (Fig. 7.1). The uncertainty of the symptom and its effects can lead to emotional distress and despair.

The feeling of cancer-related fatigue is described by Magnusson et al (1999) as a sense of both physical and mental loss:

The mere thought of getting out of bed can be too much ... When my legs are tired I haven't got any strength and then I easily stagger and fall ... you can't concentrate; when my wife asks what I've been reading, I don't know, I can't remember ... You feel like a block of concrete, there's this heaviness in your body and this tired feeling that makes you feel sleepy... you feel hundreds of pounds heavier ... I've always loved to go dancing but now I haven't got any strength left, that's sad, it's almost the worst part of it. There's so much you have to give up because you know you can't do it, you haven't got any strength left.

Every day many of us may experience fatigue as a result of exertion, but we tend to use strategies to restore our energy, for example rest or sleep. However, in cancer-related fatigue, these self-care strategies are often ineffective (Davies et al 1996), resulting not only in loss of activity (Ream & Richardson 1997) but also in a sense of loss of control (Krishnasamy 1997).

The effect on physical activity is not just about functional ability but relates to an overriding feeling of exhaustion. Ferrell et al (1996) conceptualises fatigue as affecting physical, psychological, social and spiritual well-being and illustrates these domains with qualitative narratives to define how cancer patients experience fatigue:

My level of energy affects my quality of life. I'm generally energetic, so anything that affects my energy levels affects my life ... The fatigue issue, call it wet cement. It is wet

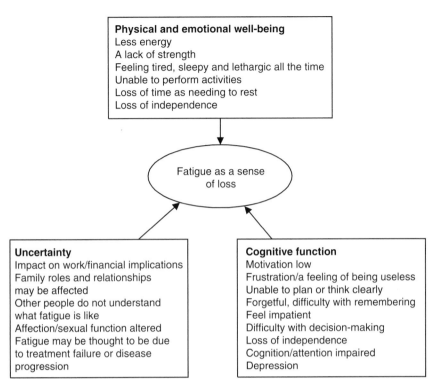

Figure 7.1 The impact of radiation-induced fatigue.

cement. [it's] very different from, 'I've worked hard and I'm really tired'. Big difference. Until you've experienced that, if you're standing up you want to lie down, If you're sitting down, you want to lie down. You feel like something is pushing you down. It's not exhaustion. I've never had fatigue like this. Its not work fatigue or emotional fatigue. It's very different. It's incredible. It's like rubber knees. All of a sudden everything's fine. And you just start sinking. You're like rubber knees. There's nothing to hold you up.

(Ferrell et al 1996, p. 1543).

This feeling leads to inactivity and isolation:

I have felt like I had lead boots … I just didn't want to do anything! I didn't feel I could do anything which was the worst thing.

Some patients describe this feeling as lethargy.

I felt lethargic. There were things which I had to think of doing, wanted to do and I just couldn't muster myself to do them you know

(Faithfull 1991, p. 943).

Patients also describe the impact of fatigue on cognitive abilities.

I mean physically. I knew I could walk across the kitchen and get myself a biscuit! But to get a biscuit! I would rather sit in a chair and think about it.

Lack of mental concentration subsequently reduces motivation, making all but the simplest of physical tasks difficult to achieve.

It felt like every day was a great effort and that just moving and doing anything was exceedingly hard, but not physically. It was more mentally than physically hard

(Faithfull 1991, p. 943).

There is little evidence in the literature of the social impact of radiation-induced fatigue. The daily journey to the radiotherapy centre over the course of treatment can also contribute to fatigue levels. Curt et al (2000) found that fatigue had economic consequences in that 75% of patients in their survey had changed employment as a result of their fatigue. Qualitative data are scarce and focus on individual experiences, but relatives often describe the dependence of those who are experiencing fatigue and the difficulty of caring for patients when motivation is low and morale is affected (Jensen & Given 1993).

MANAGEMENT STRATEGIES

One of the limitations to the recognition of fatigue in the past has been the lack of systematic assessment of the symptom. The basis of adequate management of fatigue has to be comprehensive assessment. Clearly fatigue is a multidimensional symptom influenced by a variety of factors, thus it must be considered alongside a wider assessment of other symptoms such as pain and psychological morbidity. Substantial progress has been made in the development of a framework to measure the intensity (strength or severity), timing (duration and frequency), level of perceived distress and quality of fatigue.

There has been an exponential growth in fatigue research in recent years and much of this work has centred on the definition and validation of instruments and tools, although many of these are used in a wide range of patient groups (Meek et al 2000). Qualitative research exploring patients' descriptions has contributed greatly to our ability to assess the subjective nature of fatigue.

Many quality-of-life and research tools include measurement of fatigue as a single symptom, or subscale, including the European Organisation for Research and Treatment of Cancer quality-of-life questionnaire (EORTC QLQ C30) and the Rotterdam Symptom Checklist (RSCL) (Stone et al 1998). Specific instruments have also been published, such as the fatigue assessment questionnaire (Glaus 1998) and the multidimensional fatigue inventory (Smets et al 1996). These two tools are very similar, which suggests confidence in their validity (Richardson & Ream 1998). Assessing fatigue for the purposes of research, however, is different from assessing fatigue in a clinical setting, as the aims are more diverse in research and are likely to require more lengthy assessment (Holley 2000). Mendoza et al (1999) describe a brief fatigue inventory which assesses fatigue as a single dimension and is straightforward and quick enough to use in busy areas such as radiotherapy treatment and follow-up clinics (Fig. 7.2). Whether a simple sliding scale (0–10) or a more detailed tool is used, it is important to assess baseline fatigue levels prior to treatment so that changes in fatigue over time can be monitored. Appropriate physical assessment is also important. The close association of fatigue with other symptoms such as pain and breathlessness and depression, highlights the need for consistent evaluation of changes in symptoms and toxicity (see Ch. 6). Additionally, checking biochemical and nutritional parameters should form part of comprehensive fatigue assessment. Anaemia is often not the cause of fatigue symptoms, but it would be imprudent not to check the patient's haemoglobin, given that radiotherapy treatment fields may well incorporate substantial areas of bone marrow production, thus affecting the synthesis of red blood cells. Equally, electrolyte imbalances such as low magnesium levels, uraemia or hypocalcaemia may cause symptoms similar to those experienced as part of fatigue, and it is important that these are corrected.

The need to improve the assessment of fatigue in routine clinical practice is clear. Evidence suggests that fatigue is infrequently reported in medical records and the treatment options or strategies for fatigue management are rarely discussed. The survey of Vogelzang et al (1997) found that fewer than 50% of cancer patients discussed treatment options for fatigue with their oncologist and only 27% of them were recommended any treatment. Patients felt there was little that could be done about fatigue and that it was a symptom to be endured. In the UK, a multicentre survey by Stone et al (2001) also found that fatigue was reported to affect 58% of patients 'somewhat or very much', although in 52% of cases it had never been reported to the hospital doctor. Only 14% of patients had received treatment or advice about the management of fatigue (Stone et al 2000).

The evaluation of interventions to reduce fatigue has been an area of rapid research growth in the past 5 years. There is still relatively little evidence for specific interventions to alleviate fatigue symptoms, as few have been adequately tested in cancer patients (Richardson 1995). However, some basic strategies are clear. Studies have highlighted that patients are surprised by the severity and effects of fatigue (Eardley 1986, Faithfull 1991). Forewarning patients of fatigue and providing information on strategies that may be helpful can provide some relief and prevent the anxiety of unexpected symptoms. Allowing patients to talk about their fatigue helps to make the symptom more tangible and may reduce the uncertainty of its occurrence and associated distress (Krishnasamy 1997). Identifying when patients experience fatigue through keeping diaries can help to reduce wasteful activity, and assists with interventions such as activity pacing and goal-setting. Energy conservation focuses on setting priorities, valuing rest time, delegating tasks and identifying important activities (Krishnasamy 2001).

Increasing activity rather than resting has been a major focus of intervention research. Exercise has been promoted to reduce fatigue in women with breast cancer since the beginning of the 1990s (Winningham 1991). Mock et al (1997) specifically explore how exercise influences fatigue in women receiving breast radiotherapy. This randomised study used a self-paced, incremental 20–30-min walk (four to five times a week). The researchers found that women in the walking

Brief fatigue inventory
Patient no.:
Date:
Throughout our lives most of us have times when we feel very tired or fatigued.

Have you felt unusually tired or fatigued in the last week? Yes ☐ No☐

---

1. Please rate your fatigue (weariness, tiredness) by circling the one number that best describes your fatigue right *now*

       0　1　2　3　4　5　6　7　8　9　10
No fatigue   As bad as you can imagine

2. Please rate your fatigue (weariness, tiredness) by circling the one number that best describes your usual level of fatigue during the past 24 hours

       0　1　2　3　4　5　6　7　8　9　10
No fatigue   As bad as you can imagine

3. Please rate your fatigue (weariness, tiredness) by circling the one number that best describes your worst level of fatigue during the past 24 hours

       0　1　2　3　4　5　6　7　8　9　10
No fatigue   As bad as you can imagine

4. Circle the one number that describes how, during the past 24 hours, fatigue has interfered with your:

A General Activity

       0　1　2　3　4　5　6　7　8　9　10
Does not interfere   Completely interferes

B Mood

       0　1　2　3　4　5　6　7　8　9　10
Does not interfere   Completely interferes

C Walking ability

       0　1　2　3　4　5　6　7　8　9　10
Does not interfere   Completely interferes

D Normal work (includes both work outside the home and daily chores)

       0　1　2　3　4　5　6　7　8　9　10
Does not interfere   Completely interferes

E Relations with other people

       0　1　2　3　4　5　6　7　8　9　10
Does not interfere   Completely interferes

F Enjoyment of life

       0　1　2　3　4　5　6　7　8　9　10
Does not interfere   Completely interferes

Figure 7.2 The rapid assessment of fatigue severity in cancer patients. (Reproduced with permission from Mendoza et al 1999.)

programme had better physical functioning, lower symptom intensity and lower fatigue levels than those in the control group. Exercise also improved sleep and reduced anxiety. Sarna & Conde (2001) in a pilot study found that fatigue decreased in patients who increased their activity during radiotherapy. Although exercise has demonstrated benefits, most of the patients in these studies had early-stage disease and were relatively well prior to start of treatment. It is less easy to see how patients with more extensive disease or debilitating symptoms could undertake these levels of exercise.

Healthcare professionals often recommend rest as a strategy to reduce fatigue. In a study to explore which strategies were most effective in relieving cancer treatment fatigue (chemotherapy $n = 45$, radiotherapy $n = 54$) Graydon and colleagues (1995) report that sleep and exercise were found by patients to be the most effective strategies in reducing fatigue. Most patients who are fatigued naturally tend to rest, nap or sleep (Pearce & Richardson 1994), which may lead to more night-time waking and increased fatigue levels (Berger & Farr 1999). These are passive strategies, and frequently fail to alleviate the fatigue associated with cancer-related fatigue.

Stress management techniques can also help reduce the anxiety associated with fatigue symptoms. Interventions aimed at reducing emotional distress may be an effective way of decreasing feelings of fatigue. Cimprich (1993) found that 'attention fatigue' or difficulty in thinking and concentration could be improved by focusing on recreational activities for 20–30 min three times per week. Compared to a control group, the intervention group demonstrated significant improvements in concentration and mental agility. Forester et al (1985a) investigated the effect of psychotherapy on patients undergoing radiotherapy and found that patients receiving the intervention were significantly less fatigued than those in the control group. Trijsburg and colleagues (1992) evaluated 22 research studies exploring the value of psychological treatment for patients with cancer. They found that counselling tailored to an individual's need reduced not only distress but also fatigue. However, it must be recognised that the provision of psychotherapy or counselling to all patients would require significant time and resources, and Watson (1983) suggests that psychological intervention should be targeted at those most at risk. More work is therefore needed to identify which patients would most benefit from this type of intervention and which fatigue symptoms are most affected. The wide range of scores achieved for the different interventions between individuals suggests that fatigue management techniques need to be individually tailored and that patients should be advised to try different interventions to find what works best for them. Interventions to manage cancer-related fatigue are described on a continuum from passive to active (Fig. 7.3). The more successful interventions appear to be those that require more physical effort; however these are relatively untested in patients undergoing radiotherapy. The multidimensional aspects of fatigue suggest that more holistic approaches that combine a variety of complementary strategies may be the way forward to managing this complex symptom (Ream & Richardson 1999). Comprehensive assessment is therefore crucial to identifying an individual's needs and this may require the help of all members of the multidisciplinary team.

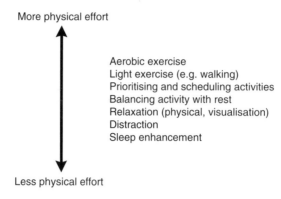

More physical effort

Aerobic exercise
Light exercise (e.g. walking)
Prioritising and scheduling activities
Balancing activity with rest
Relaxation (physical, visualisation)
Distraction
Sleep enhancement

Less physical effort

Figure 7.3 Self-care strategies advocated for the relief of fatigue. (Reproduced with permission from Ream & Richardson 1999.)

RECOMMENDATIONS FOR CLINICAL PRACTICE

• Assess fatigue levels prior to commencement of treatment in order to establish a baseline. Pre-existing fatigue may be due to previous treatment or related to the experience of the disease.

• Regular assessment is fundamental. Check for possible physical, biochemical and psychological causes of fatigue, e.g. electrolyte imbalance or anaemia and psychological morbidity such as depression.

• Encourage patients who are experiencing difficulties with fatigue to maintain a daily diary recording fatigue levels and the relationship to activity. This helps to clarify when fatigue is at its worst during the day or treatment week and hence enhances the ability to control activities or plan ahead.

• Utilise a fatigue assessment tool or ensure that fatigue is included routinely in your current assessment strategy or evaluation of radiation-induced symptoms.

• Forewarn patients of the likely occurrence of fatigue during and after radiotherapy.

• Provide information on the experience and pattern of fatigue symptoms.

• Assess an individual's self-care strategies and how effective these are in managing fatigue during radiotherapy treatment.

• Suggest a combination of strategies, for example, goal-setting and prioritising activity so as to reduce unnecessary energy loss. Although resting may help some people with fatigue, in others it may make the symptom worse. Refer to the occupational therapist if there is a need for help with activities or home aids.

• If the patient is able, encourage daily activity, suggesting 30 min brisk walking at least three to four times per week. For those not so able to exercise at that level, help them to assess and plan what they would be capable of doing. Referral to the physiotherapist may be appropriate.

• Explore the impact of fatigue and the emotions that are causing distress. Refer for counselling if patient has anxiety or depression.

CONCLUSION

The multiple factors involved in fatigue and the lack of knowledge of causative mechanisms point to a need to recognise the complexity of this symptom and the need to introduce a package of different interventions to alleviate radiotherapy induced fatigue. Symptoms may be interrelated and, as a result, may precipitate and impact on each other, increasing fatigue severity. Above all, the individual experience of fatigue must be acknowledged. There may not be one solution to the problem of fatigue, but as research in this area grows, some strategies do now exist for intervention and support. It is vital that we incorporate this new knowledge into our everyday practice.

AREAS FOR FURTHER RESEARCH

- Investigation of the pattern and incidence of fatigue in different treatment sites so that it is possible to forewarn patients of potential levels of fatigue for different therapies
- Explore how fatigue and radiation-induced symptoms interact
- Design and evaluate interventions for individuals undergoing radiotherapy that can be tailored to meet an individual's needs
- Testing more activity interventions on wider patient populations, for example, those with more debilitating or advanced disease
- Utilise existing validated tools for fatigue assessment
- Understanding how to help carers to facilitate those living with fatigue symptoms.

FURTHER INFORMATION

Cancerfatigue.org
http://www.cancerfatigue.org

MD Anderson Cancer Centre: Cancer-Related Fatigue

Beth Israel Medical Centre

http://www.mdanderson.org/news/fatigue.html

http://www.stoppain.org/services_staff/featuredprogs.html fatigue

University of Iowa Cancer centre: cancer-related fatigue
http://www.vh.org/Patients/IHB/Cancer/CancerFatigue.html

http://www.cancernet.co.uk

REFERENCES

Barrere C, Trotta P, Foster J 1993 The experience of fatigue in women undergoing radiation therapy for early stage breast cancer. Oncology Nursing Forum 20:311
Beach P, Siebeneck B, Buderer N et al 2001 Relationship between fatigue and nutritional status in patients receiving radiation therapy to treat lung cancer. Oncology Nursing Forum 28:1027–1031

Berger A, Farr L 1999 The influence of daytime activity and nightime restlessness on cancer-related fatigue. Oncology Nursing Forum 26:1663–1671

Blesch K, Paice J, Wickham R et al 1991 Correlates of fatigue in people with lung and breast cancer. Oncology Nursing Forum 18:81–87

Christman N 1990 Uncertainty and adjustment during radiotherapy. Nursing Research 39:17–20

Cimprich B 1993 Development of an intervention to restore attention in cancer patients. Cancer Nursing 16:82–92

Corner J 1993 Some reflections on frailty in elderly patients with cancer. European Journal of Cancer Care 2:5–9

Cox B, Blaxter M, Buckle A 1987 The health and lifestyle survey. Health Promotion Research Trust, London

Curt G, Breitbart W, Cella D et al 2000 Impact of cancer-related fatigue on the lives of patients: new findings from the fatigue coalition. Oncologist 5:353–360

Davies E, Clarke C, Hopkins A 1996 Malignant cerebral glioma-1: survival, disability, and morbidity after radiotherapy. British Medical Journal 313:1507–1512

Derogatis L, Morrow G, Fetting J et al 1983 The prevalence of psychiatric disorder among cancer patients. Journal of the American Medical Association 249:751–757

Eardley A 1986 Expectations of recovery. Nursing Times April 23:53–54

Faithfull S 1991 Patients' experiences following cranial radiotherapy: a study of the somnolence syndrome. Journal of Advanced Nursing 16:939–946

Faithfull S 2000 Supportive care in radiotherapy: evaluating the potential contribution of nursing: Institute of Cancer Research. London University, London, p 294

Faithfull S, Brada M 1998 Somnolence syndrome in adults following cranial irradiation for primary brain tumours. Clinical Oncology (Royal College of Radiologists) 10:250–254

Ferrell B, Grant M, Dean G et al 1996 'Bone tired': the experience of fatigue and its impact on quality of life. Oncology Nursing Forum 23:1539–1547

Fieler V 1997 Side effects and quality of life in patients receiving high dose rate brachytherapy. Oncology Nursing Forum 24:543–553

Fobair P, Hoppe R, Bloom J et al 1986 Psychosocial problems among survivors of Hodgkin's disease. Journal of Clinical Oncology 4:805–814

Forester B M, Kornfield D, Fleiss J 1985a Psychotherapy during radiation: effects on emotional and physical distress. American Journal of Psychiatry 142:22–27

Forester B M, Kornfield D, Fleiss J 1985b Psychiatric aspects of radiotherapy. American Journal of Psychiatry 142:22–27

Glaus A 1998 Fatigue in patients with cancer: analysis and assessment, vol. 145. Recent results in cancer research. Springer-Verlag, Berlin

Gleeson C, Spencer D 1995 Blood transfusion and its benefits in palliative care. Palliative Medicine 9:307–313

Graydon J, Bubela N, Irvine D et al 1995 Fatigue-reducing strategies used by patients receiving treatment for cancer. Cancer Nursing 18:23–28

Greenberg D, Sawicka J, Eisenthal S et al 1992 Fatigue syndrome due to localised radiotherapy. Journal of Pain and Symptom Management 7:38–45

Greenberg D, Gray J, Mannix C et al 1993 Treatment related fatigue and serum interleukin-1 levels in patients during external beam radiation for prostate cancer. Journal of Pain and Symptom Management 8:196–200

Haylock P, Hart L 1979 Fatigue in patients receiving localised radiation. Cancer Nursing 2:461–467

Hickok J, Morrow G, McDonald S et al 1996 Frequency and correlates of fatigue in lung cancer patients receiving radiation therapy: implications for management. Journal of Pain and Symptom Management 11:370–377

Holley S 2000 Evaluating patient distress from cancer-related fatigue: an instrument development study. Oncology Nursing Forum 27:1425–1431

Irvine D, Vincent L, Graydon J et al 1998 Fatigue in women with breast cancer receiving radiotherapy. Cancer Nursing 21:127–135

Jensen S, Given B 1993 Fatigue affecting family caregivers of cancer patients. Supportive Care in Cancer Care 1:321–325

King K, Nail L, Kreamer K et al 1985 Patients' descriptions of the experience of receiving radiation therapy. Oncology Nursing Forum 12:55–61

Kobashi-Schoot J 1985 Assessment of malaise in cancer patients treated with radiotherapy. Cancer Nursing 8:306–313

Krishnasamy M 1997 Exploring the nature and impact of fatigue in advanced cancer. International Journal of Palliative Nursing 3:126–131

Krishnasamy M 2001 Fatigue. In: Corner J, Bailey C (eds) Cancer nursing: care in context. Blackwell Science, Oxford, p 358–365

Kubricht D 1984 Therapeutic self-care demands expressed by outpatients receiving external radiation therapy. Cancer Nursing 1:43–52

Larson P, Lindsey A, Dodd M et al 1993 Influence of age on problems experienced by patients with lung cancer undergoing radiation therapy. Oncology Nursing Forum 20:473–480

Lovely M, Miaskowski C, Dodd M 1999 Relationship between fatigue and quality of life in patients with glioblastoma multiformae. Oncology Nursing Forum 26:921–925

Magnusson K, Moller A, Ekman T, Wallgren A 1999 A qualitative study to explore the experience of fatigue in cancer patients. European Journal of Cancer Care 8:224–232

Meek P, Nail L, Barsvick A et al 2000 Psychometric testing of fatigue instruments for use with cancer patients. Nursing Research 49:181–189

Mendoza T, Shelley Wang X, Cleeland C et al 1999 The rapid assessment of fatigue severity in cancer patients. Cancer 85:1186–1196

Mock V, Hassey-Dow K, Meares C et al 1997 Effects of exercise on fatigue, physical functioning, and emotional distress during radiation therapy for breast cancer. Oncology Nursing Forum 24:991–999

Molassiotis A, Chan C 2000 The association of fatigue with febrile neutropenia in patients receiving radiotherapy. European Journal of Oncology Nursing 4:249–251

Moore G, Hayes C 2001 Maintenance of comfort (fatigue and pain). In: Watkins-Bruner D, Moore-Higgs G, Haas M (eds) Outcomes in radiation therapy: multidisciplinary management. Jones and Bartlett, Massachusetts, p 459–492

Morant R 1996 Asthenia: an important symptom in cancer patients. Cancer Review 22:117–221

Morant R, Stiefel F, Berchtold W et al 1993 Preliminary results of a study assessing asthenia and related psychological and biological phenomena in patients with advanced cancer. Support Care Cancer 1:101–107

Munro A, Biruls R, Griffin A et al 1994 Distress associated with radiotherapy for malignant disease: a quantitative analysis based on patients' perceptions. British Journal of Cancer 60:370–374

Nail L 1993 Coping with intracavity radiation treatment for gynaecological cancer. Cancer Practice 1:218–224

Oberst M, Hughes S, Chang A, McCubbin M 1991 Self care burden, stress appraisal and mood among persons receiving radiotherapy. Cancer Nursing 14:71–78

Pearce S, Richardson A 1994 Fatigue and cancer: a phenomenological study. Journal of Cancer Nursing 3:381–382

Piper B, Dodd M 1991 Self initiated fatigue interventions and their perceived effectiveness. Oncology Nursing Forum 18:39

Ream E, Richardson A 1997 Fatigue in patients with cancer and chronic obstructive airways disease: a phenomenological enquiry. International Journal of Nursing Studies 34:44–53

Ream E, Richardson A 1999 From theory to practice: designing interventions to reduce fatigue in patients with cancer. Oncology Nursing Forum 26:1295–1303

Richardson A 1995 Fatigue in cancer patients: a review of the literature. European Journal of Cancer Care 4:20–32

Richardson A, Ream E 1998 Recent progress in understanding cancer-related fatigue. International Journal of Palliative Nursing 4:192–198

Sarna L, Conde F 2001 Physical activity and fatigue during radiation therapy: a pilot study using actigraph monitors. Oncology Nursing Forum 28:1043–1046

Smets E, Garssen B, Cull A, de Haes J 1996 Application of the multidimensional fatigue inventory (MFI-20) in cancer patients receiving radiotherapy. British Journal of Cancer 73:241–245

Smets E, Visser M, Willems-Groot A et al 1998a Fatigue and radiotherapy: (A) experience in patients undergoing treatment. British Journal of Cancer 78:899–906

Smets E, Visser M, Willems-Groot A et al 1998b Fatigue and radiotherapy: (B) experience in past 9 months following treatment. British Journal of Cancer 78:907–912

Stone P, Richardson A, Hardy J 1998 Fatigue in patients with cancer. European Journal of Cancer 34:1670–1676

Stone P, Richardson A, Ream E et al 2000 Cancer related fatigue: inevitable, unimportant and untreatable? Results of a multi-centre patient survey. Annals of Oncology 11:971–975

Stone P, Ream E, Richardson A et al 2001 Cancer-related fatigue – a difference of opinion? Results of a multicentre survey of healthcare professionals, patients and caregivers. Annals of Oncology 8:971–975

Trijsburg R, van Knippenberg F, Rijpma S 1992 Effects of psychological treatment on cancer patients: a critical review. Psychosomatic Medicine 54:489–517

Visser M, Smets E 1998 Fatigue, depression and quality of life in cancer patients: how are they related? Support Care Cancer 6:101–108

Vogelzang N, Breitbart W, Cella D et al 1997 Patient, caregiver, and oncologist perceptions of cancer-related fatigue: results of a tripart assessment survey. Seminars in Haematology 34:4–12

Watanabe S, Bruera E 1996 Anorexia and cachexia, asthenia and lethargy. Hematological, Oncology Clinics of North America 10:189–206

Watson M 1983 Psychosocial intervention with cancer patients: a review. Psychological Medicine 13:839–846

Winningham M 1991 Walking program for people with cancer: getting started. Cancer Nursing 14:270–276

Woo B, Dibble S, Piper B et al 1998 Differences in fatigue by treatment methods in women with breast cancer. Oncology Nursing Forum 25:915–920

8

Radiation skin reactions

Mary Wells   Sheila MacBride

INTRODUCTION

Radiation skin reactions are, to some extent, an inevitable consequence of radical radiotherapy, particularly where skinfolds are present. Although the widespread use of linear accelerators has reduced the severity of skin reactions through more sophisticated skin-sparing techniques, the increased use of concomitant chemotherapy and high-dose radiotherapy means that skin reactions can still be a significant problem for patients. There are surprisingly few data describing the patient's experience of skin reactions, and much conflicting evidence exists as to how skin reactions should be prevented, minimised and managed. Practice across UK radiotherapy departments reveals considerable inconsistency and a lack of evidence on which to base skin management decisions.

THE AETIOLOGY OF RADIATION SKIN REACTIONS

Although radiation skin reactions cannot be understood without an appreciation of the radiobiological effects of radiotherapy treatment, it is also important to consider the way in which healthy skin regenerates. The skin is composed of two main layers: the epidermis (superficial layer) and the dermis (deep layer), as shown in Figure 8.1.

Sitton (1992) describes the process in which skin homeostasis is normally achieved. As superficial cells are shed through normal desquamation, new cells are formed in the basal layer of the epidermis, and these continually replace those that are lost. The dermis, which contains blood vessels, glands, nerves and hair follicles, provides the supportive structure required for the epidermis to renew. Repopulation of the entire epidermis takes approximately 4 weeks, although this process can be shorter during times of healing.

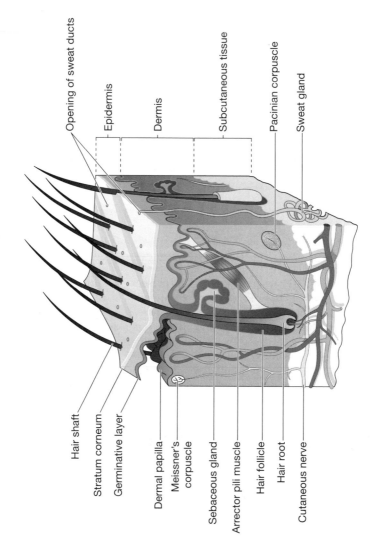

Figure 8.1 The skin, showing the main structures in the dermis. (Reproduced with permission from Waugh & Grant 2001.)

In general, the basal layer of the epidermis proliferates rapidly, so it is particularly sensitive to radiotherapy (see Ch. 5). Ionising radiation essentially damages the mitotic ability of clonogenic or stem cells within the basal layer, thus preventing the process of repopulation and weakening the integrity of the skin. Radical radiotherapy repeatedly impairs cell division within the basal layer, and so the degree to which a skin reaction develops is dependent on the survival of actively proliferating basal cells in the epidermis. Moist desquamation occurs when clonogenic cells in the basal layer are sterilised, thus rendering cells unable to repopulate in time to replace the damaged tissue. Consequently, the epidermis becomes broken (Glean et al 2001, Hopewell 1990).

Archambeau et al (1995) found that basal cell loss began once the radiation dose reached 20–25 Gy, and that maximum depletion of basal cells occurred when the patient had received a dose of 50 Gy. In practice, this means that skin reactions tend to become visible around the second to third week of radical radiotherapy, reaching a peak at the end or within 1 week of completion of treatment (Arimoto et al 1989, Ratliff 1990). Interestingly, Archambeau et al (1995) found that by the time higher doses of up to 60 Gy had been absorbed, repopulation of basal cells had occurred, so that levels were similar to those existing prior to radiotherapy.

The majority of skin reactions will have healed within 4 weeks of completion of treatment (Rezvani et al 1991). Small areas of moist desquamation tend to heal from the basal layer, whereas large areas of broken epidermis require cells to migrate from the surrounding epidermis (Hopewell 1990). Healing becomes visible as islands of epidermal cells expand and reform in central and peripheral regions of the desquamation (Cox et al 1986). Initially, this reformed skin may be hyperpigmented, due to stimulation or destruction of melanocytes as a result of exposure to radiation (Cox et al 1986, Ratliff 1990).

Skin reactions can range from mild erythema, through dry desquamation (dry, flaky or scaly skin) to confluent moist desquamation, where blistering, peeling and sloughing of the skin occur. The most severe stage of necrosis is rarely seen nowadays. At any one time, it is possible to see a combination of erythema, dry and moist desquamation within a single treatment field. Although relatively short lived, skin reactions are uncomfortable and itchy, can be painful and are sometimes dose-limiting (Campbell & Illingworth 1992, Munro et al 1989). The symptom distress associated with radiation skin reactions is particularly poorly researched.

INCIDENCE OF RADIATION SKIN REACTIONS

It is difficult to estimate the true incidence of skin reactions, given that most departments do not systematically record their occurrence or severity. A survey carried out in the early 1990s reported that more than 80% of UK radiotherapy departments frequently saw skin reactions, although these were not usually severe (Barkham 1993). The research literature supports an approximate incidence of erythematous reactions in 80–90% of patients, and a relatively low incidence of moist desquamation at around 10–15%. However, as most incidence figures are drawn from populations of patients involved in clinical trials, it is difficult to assess how much these figures are affected by the products or techniques under evaluation. One recent descriptive study of patients receiving radiotherapy to the breast reported that only 4–8% of women had no reaction at all, but fewer than 10% had moist desquamation by the completion of treatment (Porock & Kristjanson 1999). Clinical experience confirms that skin irritation and discomfort are common in patients being treated radically, and that moist desquamation reactions can be extremely difficult to manage, as well as being distressing and painful for the patient.

ASSESSMENT OF RADIATION SKIN REACTIONS

The many systems for categorising radiation skin reactions have been neatly summarised by Noble-Adams (1999a). Most include four or five stages, ranging from mild erythema to necrosis, and these form the basis of many assessment tools. The Radiation Therapy Oncology Group/European Organisation for Research and Treatment of Cancer. (RTOG/EORTC) score (Table 8.1) is probably the most widely used in practice and research. This score makes a useful distinction between faint erythema and tender, bright erythema, as well as between patchy and confluent moist desquamation. One limitation of the RTOG scoring system is that dry desquamation and faint erythema are scored equally, although they may not be equal in severity from the patient's point of view. Radiotherapy to the brain or head and neck can produce severe dry desquamation, in which thick scales develop on the scalp or neck, described by some patients as like 'crocodile skin'. The appearance of faint erythema is completely different, yet the RTOG score attributes the same score to both reactions. Similarly, an equal score is given to bright erythema and patchy moist desquamation. Because of this, many researchers have modified the four criteria to create a subdivision of score 2, thus allowing for a distinction to be made between the two (Porock et al 1998, Westbury et al 2000).

An additional limitation of the RTOG is that the scoring system only measures the appearance of the skin from the point of view of the clinician, thus giving no indication of how the patient feels. Weekly skin assessments performed by patients and clinicians have demonstrated a consistent tendency for healthcare providers to underrate the severity of skin reactions when compared with patients (Williams et al 1996). The Radiation-Induced Skin Reaction Assessment Scale (RISRAS) developed by Noble-Adams (1999b) addresses this problem. This scale,

Table 8.1 RTOG/EORTC acute radiation scoring criteria – skin

0	1	2	3	4
No change over baseline	Follicular, faint or dull erythema; epilation;dry desquamation; decreased sweating	Tender or bright erythema, patchy moist desquamation; moderate oedema	Confluent, moist desquamation other than skinfolds, pitting oedema	Ulceration, haemorrhage, necrosis

RTOG, Radiation Therapy Oncology Group; EORTC, European Organisation for Research and Treatment of Cancer.
Reproduced with permission from Cox et al (1995).

designed for weekly use, incorporates a patient-rated symptom scale and a health-care professional assessment scale (see Fig. 8.2 for the latest version).

One of the advantages of this scale is that it allows an accurate estimate of the *area* of skin affected. It also recognises that the severity of the skin reaction within a treatment area is not uniform, i.e. a patient may have a very small area of moist desquamation and a large area of bright erythema or dry desquamation. Noble-Adams (1999c) evaluated the RISRAS by asking 19 experts to assess a series of clinical photographs using the tool. Although there were some outlying responses, the overall interrater reliability coefficient was fairly high, at 0.70.

In clinical practice, the use of assessment tools such as the RISRAS are a vital component of supportive care. Systematic weekly assessment would provide excellent data on the experience of patients and the development of skin reactions, as well as guide the management of symptoms and wound healing. In clinical research, however, such tools are open to criticism because of their lack of objectivity.

Over the past few years, a variety of 'objective' skin measurement techniques have been reported in the literature. Probably the most clinically applicable technique is that of reflectance spectrophotometry, used for a number of years in dermatology settings and now gaining interest as a reliable method of measuring erythema in irradiated skin (Denham et al 1995, Simonen et al 1998). It is believed to measure the blood content of the dermal microvasculature and, as such, is sensitive to the vasodilatory effects thought to occur as a result of epithelial cell death during radiotherapy.

The erythema meter, used to take such measurements, is a compact (but expensive) piece of equipment. A probe is held against the patient's skin for a few seconds, and an average of 100 repeated measures of erythema is generated in a matter of seconds. The degree of erythema in different areas of the treatment field can be measured, and 'control' measures can also be taken outside the field. The meter is able to detect subclinical erythema and is thus considerably more sensitive than the naked eye. Studies that use reflectance spectrophotometry demonstrate that invisible but measurable erythematous reactions occur at very low doses of radiation (Simonen et al 1998), perhaps explaining why some patients appear to experience skin discomfort at an earlier stage than is thought to be related to their radiotherapy. Recent experience of using the erythema meter in a clinical research setting suggests that there are some practical difficulties associated with the technique, although the trial is still in progress, so data have not yet been analysed (MacMillan et al personal communication).

Other measurement techniques include ultrasound (Warszawski et al 1998) and dielectric constant measurements (Nuutinen et al 1998). The latter technique is based on the hypothesis that radiation damage produces a change in free and bound water molecules within the skin; the dielectric constant is related to the tissue water content of the skin. Although these techniques may provide vital objective data, they are unlikely to be adopted for everyday clinical use.

RISK FACTORS FOR RADIATION SKIN REACTIONS

A number of factors appear to influence the severity, onset and duration of radiation skin reactions. In general, moist areas of the body or those that contain skinfolds are more likely to be affected, for example, under the breast, axilla, head

Patient symptom scale

Symptoms	Not at all	A little	Quite a bit	Very much
Do you have any tenderness, discomfort or pain of your skin in the treatment area?	1	2	3	4
Does your skin in the treatment area itch?	1	2	3	4
Do you have a burning sensation of your skin in the treatment area?	1	2	3	4
To what extent has your skin reaction and your symptoms affected your day-to-day activities	1	2	3	4

Health care professional scale
Record of treatment details included here (dose, fractions, etc.)

	0	1	2	3	4
Erythema (E)	0 (normal skin)	1 (dusky pink)	2 (dull red)	3 (brilliant red)	4 (deep red-purple)
Dry desquamation (DD)	0 (normal skin)	1 (<25%)	2 (>25–50%)	3 (>50–75%)	4 (>75–100%)
Moist desquamation (MD)	0 (normal skin)	1.5 (<25%)	3.0 (>25–50%)	4.5 (>50–75%)	6.0 (>75–100%)
Necrosis (N)	0 (normal skin)	2.5 (<25%)	5.0 (>25–50%)	7.5 (>50–75%)	10 (>75–100%)

Ongoing assessment scale

Date	No.	E	DD	MD	N	Pain	Itch	Burn	Activities	Total

Treatments:

Instructions for use
1. Assess the patient as often as you feel is appropriate.
2. Rate erythema by recording the degree of colour change.
3. Rate dry desquamation, moist desquamation and necrosis by evaluating the proportion (%) of the treatment area affected by that particular reaction.
4. Record your gradings on the ongoing assessment scale.
5. Ask the patient to fill out the patient symptom scale and record the scores on the ongoing assessment scale.
6. Total the scores.

Figure 8.2 The Radiation-Induced Skin Reaction Assessment Scale (RISRAS). (Courtesy of R. Noble-Adams.)

and neck, perineum and groins (Crane 1993, Dische et al 1989, Farley 1991, O'Rourke 1987). Intrinsic factors may also play a part, including the baseline characteristics of the patient in terms of general skin condition, nutritional status, age, general health, comorbid disease and ethnicity (Blackmar 1997, Porock & Kristjanson 1999, Sitton 1992). Extrinsic factors, including the dose, energy and fractionation regime (i.e. those *prescribed* by the radiotherapist), also affect the degree of skin reaction experienced. Although the skin-sparing effect of modern linear accelerators ensures that the maximum dose of radiotherapy is reached *below* the basal layer of the skin, certain treatment techniques will increase the likelihood of the skin receiving a dose sufficient to cause a visible reaction. These include:

- the application of skin bolus (tissue-equivalent material such as wax) which is used to 'build up' the skin to ensure that a higher dose is administered to a particular area, e.g. a scar
- the use of tangential fields in breast cancer treatment. These are radiation fields which include an area of sloping skin, so that higher doses are likely to be received by skin within the 'thinner' area
- the use of parallel opposed fields where the two skin surfaces are proximal, e.g. in the treatment of laryngeal tumours
- the use of electrons, which are less penetrating than megavoltage irradiation. Sitton (1997) explains that, whilst linear accelerators deliver about 20–30% of the radiation dose to the skin, electron beam energies can deliver between 85 and 98%.

The increasing use of chemoradiotherapy also affects the severity of skin reactions experienced. The main principle of chemoradiotherapy is that the two treatments work synergistically so as to improve overall response. The other side of the coin is that radiation side effects tend to be exacerbated by the addition of chemotherapy (O'Rourke 1987, See et al 1998). Increased skin sensitivity following chemotherapy is also seen: indeed, a recall phenomenon may occur when adjuvant chemotherapy is given after completion of radical radiotherapy (Ratliff 1990, Sitton 1992). In these cases, an area of skin demarcated by the radiation field turns red and can become itchy several months after the end of radiotherapy. Cytotoxics commonly associated with an increased potential for skin reactions are dactinomycin, doxorubicin, methotrexate, 5-fluorouracil, hydroxyurea and bleomycin (O'Rourke 1987, Sitton 1992). Newer drugs such as paclitaxel have also been reported to induce 'radiation recall' (Phillips et al 1995).

However, even within a group of similar patients treated with an identical radiotherapy regime, considerable variation in skin toxicity can be seen. The nutritional status and frailty of the patient are certainly known to influence wound healing. Additionally, it has always been claimed that skin reactions could be induced or exacerbated by the application of perfumed products or substances containing metal elements (for instance, creams containing zinc or silver). A small number of studies have examined prognostic factors in patients with breast cancer, but there is no evidence to explain the nature and pattern of skin reactions in other treatment groups.

Porock et al (1998) investigated potential predictive factors for radiation skin reactions in 126 patients with breast cancer, using a conceptual framework developed from previous research, clinical knowledge and experience. A modified RTOG score and a visual analogue scale were used to measure degree of skin reaction and pain experienced at weekly intervals during radiotherapy. All women taking part in the study received a dose of 45 Gy over 5 weeks, followed by a 20 Gy electron boost to the lumpectomy scar over 2 further weeks. Patients most commonly reached a maximum RTOG score of 1 (indicating faint or dull erythema), but at the 5-week time point, between 25 and 50% of patients had developed tender or bright erythema or moist desquamation. Those areas of the breast most likely to develop severe skin reactions were the axilla, inframammary fold and sternum. Univariate and logistic regression analysis revealed that a number of variables appeared to be predictive of severe skin reactions (defined as RTOG ≥ 2). Figure 8.3 illustrates the conceptual framework of predictors of radiation skin reactions used as a basis for the study.

The predictive factors identified by Porock et al (1998) illustrate the point that a group of patients receiving very similar radiotherapy treatment may experience very different side effects. The results of the study confirm a dose–response relationship, in that patients who had received higher doses (of 45 Gy) were more likely to have a severe skin reaction in the upper quadrants of the breast, where the majority of breast cancers are located. Other interesting predictors of skin reaction were also revealed.

Weight and bra size

The authors suggest that heavier patients with large breasts are more prone to developing skin reactions because they require a greater radiation dose to the skin,

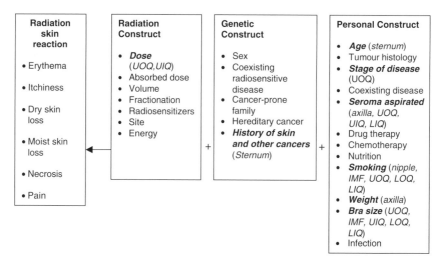

Figure 8.3 Conceptual framework of predictors of radiation skin reactions. UOQ, upper outer quadrant; UIQ, upper inner quadrant; LIQ, lower inner quadrant; LOQ, lower outer quadrant; IMF, intramammary fold. Italics show variables predictive of severe skin reactions. Specific treatment sites for which these variables were predictive are given in parenthesis. (Adapted with permission from Porock et al 1998.)

and because their potential to heal may be compromised by reduced vascularity in adipose tissue. Additionally, such patients are more likely to experience friction and moisture in the axilla and inframammary fold, where more severe skin reactions are seen.

Smoking

The significance of smoking as a highly predictive variable relates to the reduced ability of cells to reoxygenate during radiotherapy, as well as the adverse effects of nicotine on wound healing, in particular, cutaneous vasoconstriction.

Seroma aspiration

Interestingly, those patients who had required aspiration of a seroma following their breast surgery appeared to be more likely to develop a severe skin reaction. Porock et al hypothesise that damage to the lymphatic system was more likely in these patients, and that this would compromise wound healing during radiotherapy.

Stage

Porock et al patients with larger tumours (stage II) had probably experienced more trauma to surrounding tissues during surgery, and thus might have a reduced potential for wound healing.

History of skin cancer

The authors suggest that this predictor was related to previous exposure to or greater sensitivity to ultraviolet radiation (particularly as this study was carried out in Australia), although they are unable to explain why this factor was not predictive in all sites of the breast. It is possible that patients who had sunbathed in a bikini or bathing costume were more likely to have exposed their sternum than other areas of their breast, but this can only be speculation.

Age

It was found, unexpectedly, that increased age actually predicted for less severe skin reactions around the sternum. As increasing age generally results in an impaired ability to heal, the authors offer an alternative explanation for this finding. They suggest that the older patients were less likely to have received chemotherapy, and that this might have affected the degree of skin reaction they experienced.

Although the work of Porock et al (1998) requires further testing; it provides those working in radiotherapy with crucial evidence on which to base the assessment and prediction of skin reactions, so that care can be planned appropriately.

PATTERN OF ERYTHEMA

Observations made more than 60 years ago demonstrated that some patients experience a transient 'primary erythema' of the skin within hours of radiotherapy. Data from a recent study (Simonen et al 1998) suggest that the development of erythema *may* occur in two phases: the first peak is within 10 days of treatment, and the second is approximately 20 days into treatment. The findings of Simonen et al suggest that a clear dose–response relationship may not exist and that two different inflammatory responses are produced. It appears that the first occurs as a result of the direct release of substances known to cause vasodilation (such as prostaglandins). Doses as low as 1.5 Gy may be enough to produce this effect. The corresponding 'dip' in erythema is caused by the development of refractoriness to further erythematous stimuli, and possibly by an active vasoconstrictive process. This dip is followed by a second inflammatory response occurring as a result of mediators released in response to epithelial cell death.

This second inflammatory response appears to intensify as treatment progresses. Several studies support the fact that radiation skin reactions peak towards the end of radiotherapy, usually between 5 and 6 weeks (King et al 1985, Porock et al 1998, Westbury et al 2000). In King et al's study (1985) more than 80% of patients receiving chest or head and neck irradiation reported skin irritation by the last week of treatment, and this was the most common symptom experienced at this stage.

There are very few qualitative data available in the literature to describe the experience of skin reactions. Patients do, however, experience considerable distress as a result of skin damage, as these quotes illustrate.

Didn't just get redder, it erupted … it was one great big scabby thing … like it had been burnt … you see these people on television who've been burnt, you know that's all cracked, it was like that

> (patient with cancer of the larynx who developed a skin reaction after treatment was completed).

I stripped off a load of skin here, I can't feel this at all anyway and I hadn't realised it had got stripped off – it was all bleeding and raw

> (patient describing what had happened as a result of washing and shaving his radiotherapy site following a parotidectomy, which had left him with superficial numbness of his cheek and jaw).

My breast is so uncomfortable and painful. I am doing everything I should and it is not improving. The doctor warned it could be like this but I didn't expect it to be so bad. I don't think having radiotherapy was such a good idea.

Had very little sleep owing to pain from the burn on the side of my breast.

Didn't go to church because I didn't want people looking surreptitiously at my burns

> (Wells 1995, 1998).

WASHING

The freedom and ability to wash as and when you wish is a basic human need. Evidence now confirms that gentle washing during treatment does no harm, yet recent surveys have shown that some radiotherapy departments still advise patients not to wash their treatment sites for the duration of radiotherapy, or have restricted washing policies (Glean et al 2001, Lavery 1995). The idea of being unable to wash your face and neck, armpit or perineum for up to 6 weeks is at best uncomfortable and at worst positively unhygienic. Not washing may in fact promote skin infection as well as cause distress and reduce social acceptability. Three randomised trials have assessed the effect of washing on skin reactions, and all have concluded that washing is *not* associated with more severe skin reactions and that refraining from washing may in fact be detrimental (Campbell & Illingworth 1992, Roy et al 2001, Westbury et al 2000).

Campbell & Illingworth (1992) found no statistically significant differences in severity of skin reactions between those who washed with water alone and those who washed with soap, but did demonstrate that skin reactions were worse when patients were not allowed to wash at all. Westbury et al (2000) examined the role of hair washing for patients undergoing radical doses of radiotherapy for brain tumours, and concluded that the group who were randomised to no hair washing had marginally more severe symptoms 6 weeks into treatment. Unlike the previous trial, this study did attempt to measure symptom distress, finding that patients were upset by not being able to wash their hair, although the severity of symptoms was not significantly affected. The study by Roy et al (2001) found that symptoms improved in the group who were allowed to wash, and that they were also significantly less likely to develop moist desquamation. All three studies highlight the difficulties of ensuring patient compliance with professional advice, suggesting that personal experience and beliefs may have a significant influence on washing behaviour during radiotherapy. These findings reinforce the importance of patient education, supported by written information materials.

MANAGEMENT OF SKIN REACTIONS

Erythema

Surveys demonstrate that the management of skin reactions across the UK is inconsistent, and that even within hospitals and departments, practice can vary (Boot-Vickers 1999, Glean et al 2001, Lavery 1995, Thomas 1992). It is also true to say that the evidence base for practice is particularly scarce. There are relatively few published protocols and guidelines for the management of skin reactions, although many departments have developed their own and some consensus is slowly being achieved. Four recent protocols (Boot-Vickers 1999, Campbell & Lane 1996, Glean et al 2001, Mallett et al 1999) advocate a simple skin care regime, including the following advice:

- gentle washing, using mild unperfumed soap (or shampoo) and warm water
- avoidance of friction by patting the skin dry with a soft towel, and wearing loose cotton clothing

- use of a simple moisturiser, e.g. aqueous cream, either throughout treatment or when erythema develops
- avoidance of perfumed skin products, deodorants and make-up
- use of an electric razor instead of wet shaving
- protecting the skin from wind, sun and extreme temperatures
- 1% hydrocortisone cream for itchy areas

Only one author provides the sensible advice that patients with intact skin may swim during radiotherapy, provided the skin is rinsed afterwards and aqueous cream applied (Boot-Vickers 1999).

In clinical practice, there is probably a reasonable consensus about the use of simple moisturisers to relieve skin discomfort and erythema. Recently published work tends to advocate the application of creams or lotions from the first day of radiotherapy, but this is not yet routine practice in most departments, where such agents are usually reserved for symptom relief once erythematous reactions are manifest or, indeed, only when the prescribed therapy is complete. Some departments still advocate the use of powders such as talcum or cornstarch (Farley 1991), although these may in fact dry the skin and produce worse reactions as a result of the build-up effect and the blocking of sweat glands or hair follicles. Certainly, by the time the skin cracks or breaks down, powders tend to collect in messy clumps and are thought to establish a medium for fungal infections, serving no other useful purpose.

Although steroid creams such as hydrocortisone 1% may be useful to treat itching, they may also mask superficial infection and should therefore be used with caution. Lavery (1995) pointed out that there were no data to illustrate that steroid creams effectively reduce progression to moist desquamation. Similarly, there is no evidence base for the use of antibacterial creams such as Terra-Cortril ointment (hydrocortisone and tetracycline), nor is there any theoretical benefit for such creams in the absence of proven infection. However, a small study published by Simonen et al (1998) found that topical steroids do appear to reduce erythematous reactions. Hydrocortisone 1% cream appeared to modify the inflammatory response occurring during the second peak of erythema, whereas indomethacin 1% spray had no effect. Interestingly, both topical agents had been discontinued before the second peak of erythema occurred, suggesting that hydrocortisone may have a delayed effect.

In recent years, a number of research studies have investigated the application of topical agents such as ascorbic acid, or moisturising creams with active ingredients, such as sucralfate, hyaluronic acid, aloe vera gel and starch-containing creams (Table 8.2). It may be that simple emollients such as aqueous cream are just as effective as those with active ingredients, but again, little evidence exists to support this theory.

Two products have recently aroused interest, due to their potential to stimulate cell activity and growth: sucralfate and hyaluronic acid. Sucralfate has mainly been used in the treatment of gastric ulcers. It is an aluminium salt that adheres to proteins within the ulcers, thus providing a barrier to further breakdown (Delaney et al 1997). It also appears to stimulate cell growth by increasing prostaglandins and epidermal growth factor, enhancing epithelial circulation and acting as an anti-inflammatory agent (Maiche et al 1994). A number of studies have suggested

Table 8.2 Summary of research studies investigating the prevention or management of radiation-induced erythema (in chronological order)

Skin care approach evaluated	Authors	Method/strength of evidence (no. of evaluable patients/site of treatment)	Results	Endpoints/clinical outcomes
Chamomile and almond oil	Maiche et al (1991)	Physician-blinded RCT (50/breast). Chamomile cream and almond oil randomly applied above or below scar	No significant differences between areas above or below scar. Skin changes appeared later in chamomile group. Patients preferred consistency and application of chamomile cream	Four-point score for skin reaction; pain; itching
Washing	Campbell & Illingworth (1992)	RCT (99/breast or chest wall). Water alone vs soap and water vs no washing	Washing (with or without soap) diminished erythema and itching compared with no washing	RTOG scores. Itch; pain; compliance
Bioshield foam	Dini et al (1993)	Prospective evaluation (38 women with mixed sites). Bioshield only	Disappearance of symptoms (58%), improvement (37%)	Visual analogue scales, observer-rated four-point scale
Topical ascorbic acid	Halperin et al (1993)	Blinded RCT (65/brain). Ascorbic acid solution vs placebo	No benefit associated with topical ascorbic acid	Five-point skin and hair loss scales
Sucralfate cream	Maiche et al (1994)	Double-blind RCT (50/breast or chest wall). Sucralfate vs base cream	Mild reactions appeared later in sucralfate group (statistically significant at 5 weeks) Itching improved in sucralfate group	Five-point rating scale. Prevention of erythema; rate of recovery; patient preference (including cosmetic properties)
Silicone-coated polyamide net Mepitel	Adamietz et al (1995)	Prospective evaluation (21/mixed group)	No significant effects on skin reaction, but well tolerated Increased radiation dose detected under dressing, but no associated increase in skin reaction	Radiation dose measurement at skin surface Skin reaction under dressing rated on six-point scale

Continued

Table 8.2 (Continued) Summary of research studies investigating the prevention or management of radiation-induced erythema (in chronological order)

Skin care approach evaluated	Authors	Method/strength of evidence (no. of evaluable patients/site of treatment)	Results	Endpoints/clinical outcomes
Bepanthen cream	Lokkevik et al (1996)	RCT (79/breast or larynx) cream vs no cream	No benefits to using cream	Scoring criteria based on RTOG
Aloe vera gel	Williams et al (1996)	2 RCTs (breast and chest wall) double-blind; aloe vera gel vs placebo (194); aloe vera gel vs no treatment (108)	No difference between groups. Some patients experienced an allergic reaction to aloe vera	Toxicity score (patient and physician). Maximum reported severity of erythema, time to occurrence of severe erythema; duration of severe erythema
Sucralfate cream	Delaney et al (1997)	RCT (39/head and neck, breast, other) Sucralfate cream vs base cream	No significant differences	Time to healing; area of moist desquamation; pain relief; adverse effect
Superskin liquid polymer skin sealant	Goebel & Hazuka (1997)	Prospective non-comparative evaluation (54/breast, head and neck)	31% developed patchy moist desquamation (4% confluent) 65% developed redness with itching or tenderness. 'Apparent' delay in time to skin toxicity	Daily symptom record Five-point weekly score for erythema; desquamation; ulceration; pigmentation; sensitivity to touch; epilation
Hyaluronic acid cream	Liguori et al (1997)	RCT (134/breast, head and neck, pelvis) Hyaluronic acid vs placebo	Significantly less severe reactions in hyaluronic acid group between treatment weeks 3 and 8. Improved healing time in intervention group	Six-point skin toxicity score. Healing time
Usual skin care regime	Meegan & Haycocks (1997)	Prospective comparative study using consecutive samples (156/breast). Group A (92) warm water only. Group B (64) usual skin care	No significant differences	Four-point skin toxicity score. Discomfort; use of analgesics; interference with normal activities

Intervention	Study	Details	Results	Outcome measures
Homeopathy (belladonna 7 cH and X-ray 15 cH)	Balzarini et al (2000)	Double-blind RCT (66/breast) Homeopathy vs placebo	No significant differences, although total severity score suggested benefits with homeopathic treatment	Skin colour; heat; oedema; pigmentation; frequency and severity of skin reaction
Biafine wound dressing emulsion	Fisher et al (2000)	RCT (172/breast) Biafine vs best supportive care (usually aloe vera or aquaphor)	No statistically significant differences, although may reduce postradiation toxicity in large-breasted women	Prevention of skin toxicity. RTOG/EORTC + Oncology Nursing Society criteria; quality of life; patient satisfaction
Hair washing	Westbury et al (2000)	RCT (109/brain). No hair washing vs normal hair washing	No significant differences	RTOG (modified) Distress; frequency of hair washing; pain; itching
Aloe vera gel	Olsen et al (2001)	Blinded RCT (73/chest, head and neck, pelvis) Soap and aloe vera gel vs soap alone	Skin reactions later in aloe vera group, once cumulative radiotherapy dose > 27 Gy	Time to first observed skin change RTOG Skin change variables including age, ethnicity, skin type, texture, itch
Washing	Roy et al (2001)	RCT (99/breast) Washing with soap vs no washing	Significantly less moist desquamation in washing group and trend towards decreased symptoms	RTOG scores Pain; itching; burning

RCT, randomised controlled trial; RTOG, Radiation Therapy Oncology Group; EORTC, European Organisation for Research and Treatment of Cancer.

that sucralfate may reduce radiation mucositis in the gut, and these are discussed in Chapter 9 and 10. Two randomised studies have investigated the effect of sucralfate cream in the prevention and management of radiation skin reactions (Maiche et al 1994, Delaney et al 1997). Maiche et al's study of 50 patients receiving electron beam therapy to the chest wall following mastectomy found that grade 2 skin reactions (dark, painful erythema) were significantly less common ($P = 0.05$) in the areas treated with sucralfate, and that skin reactions also recovered more quickly. A smaller study assessed the effect of sucralfate on moist desquamative reactions (Delaney et al 1997). No significant differences in discomfort or skin healing were detected, although the small sample size may partially explain the lack of statistical significance. Unfortunately, neither of the studies assessed patient comfort in any detail, nor did they address the question of whether the placebo cream was more effective than applying no cream. At present, sucralfate cream is not commercially available in the UK.

Only one study has assessed the role of hyaluronic acid cream on the development of skin reactions (Liguori et al 1997). This natural polymer is found in the dermis, where it plays a key role in the healing process by stimulating fibrin, granulocyte and macrocyte activity, and inducing proliferation of fibroblasts. Liguori et al randomised 134 patients with breast, head and neck and pelvic cancers to receive hyaluronic acid cream or placebo cream to their treatment site from the first day of therapy. The placebo group suffered more severe erythema, more moist reactions and slower healing times than the hyaluronic acid group. Statistically significant differences in severity of reactions were consistently found between week 3 and week 8 of treatment. This study provides promising evidence that hyaluronic acid may improve healing in established skin reactions as well as prevent reactions happening in the first place. However, other than a physician's assessment of tolerability of the creams, this study also fails to assess the patients' perceptions of their skin reaction and its associated distress. Hyaluronic acid cream is not currently commercially available in the UK.

Moist desquamation and wound care

It is difficult to estimate with any confidence the number of individuals who will experience moist desquamation, as this information is rarely collected systematically. The risk of developing a moist skin reaction increases as higher doses are absorbed, and other factors referred to in the section on risk factors, above, also play a part. Patients undergoing concomitant chemotherapy are also more likely to experience moist desquamation (O'Rourke 1987), as are those whose treatment affects areas where skinfolds rub together. Recent studies indicate that between 2 and 10% of patients (Fisher et al 2000, Porock & Kristjanson 1999) develop confluent moist‹ desquamation during treatment. However, clinical experience shows that a number of patients develop moist reactions once treatment is over, and it is quite possible that we are not aware of the full extent of the problem.

The management of moist desquamation poses a particular challenge, not least because reactions often develop in awkward areas such as the axilla, neck and perineum, where dressings cannot easily be applied. The evidence to support the use of wound care products for moist desquamative reactions is scarce, and this remains an area of considerable controversy (Barkham 1993, Glean et al 2001, Lavery 1995). In their review of the literature, Glean et al (2001) found that, between 1979 and 1999, only eight randomised controlled trials evaluating skin products were reported.

Old-fashioned methods of drying the skin were shown to be popular with around 60% of departments surveyed by Thomas (1992). Many practitioners still favour the exposure of skin reactions to the air, using cool hairdryers or even oxygen as a means of keeping the skin dry. The application of antiseptic agents intended to dry the skin also remains relatively common, in particular the use of povidone-iodine spray, proflavine lotion (Thomas 1992), and gentian violet (Mak et al 2000). Lavery's survey (1995) reported that 63% of radiotherapy centres were still using gentian violet, despite the fact that it had been withdrawn from clinical use because of its carcinogenic properties. Other centres continue to advocate the use of combination creams containing steroid and antibiotic agents, or the application of antiseptic creams such as Flamazine, used in the treatment of burns (Atkinson 1998, Cameron 1997). However, research into the care of general wounds has long since demonstrated that the application of antiseptics to wounds confers little advantage to irrigation with saline, due to the transient nature of the antiseptic contact, the inability to effect a reduction in bacterial count and the increased risk of sensitivity reactions (Lavery 1995, Thomas 1992). There is also controversy over the use of creams that contain metallic ions (e.g. Flamazine), due to the potential for scatter of the radiation beam during treatment. This may however, present a purely theoretical concern (Thomas 1992).

Simple dressings alone, such as non-adherent layers or tulles, are not recommended, due to the pain and trauma caused at dressing changes (Glean et al 2001). Latterly there has been increasing interest in the use of dressings such as hydrocolloids, hydrogels and alginates, which provide the ideal moist wound-healing environment. These dressings have been widely researched in burns care and their role and function ascertained (Atkinson 1998). The evidence base for the management of first-degree burns with epidermal damage is much more robust, and healthcare professionals working in radiotherapy could learn a great deal from this literature (Atkinson 1998, Lavery 1995).

Thomas (1992) found a general lack of knowledge of wound care and suggested that healthcare professionals fail to appreciate the benefits of new products coming on to the market, despite these being based on the latest scientific evidence. Staff working in radiotherapy have certainly been slow to accept the virtues of moist wound-healing theory. However, considerably more research is required to demonstrate the effectiveness of newer wound care products for moist desquamation reactions. It is important that clinical trials comprehensively address issues of healing, patient comfort, pain reduction, prevention of infection and minimal trauma to wounds on dressing removal. Dressings must be readily conformable to awkward areas, able to absorb varying amounts of serous leakage associated with epidermal damage without macerating surrounding skin, and must be removed without disturbing granulation. In the radiotherapy setting, hydrogels appear to have much to offer due to their easy application, conformability, rehydration and cooling properties (Williams 1997). Most do, however, require secondary dressings and a means of holding them in place that does not compromise skin integrity. Although flexible netting tubes (such as Netelast) are a versatile means of securing

Table 8.3   Summary of research studies investigating the management of established skin reactions or moist desquamation

Skin care approach evaluated	Authors	Method/strength of evidence (no. of evaluable patients/site of treatment)	Results	Endpoints/clinical outcomes
Tegaderm	Shell et al (1986)	Pilot RCT (21/breast)	Trend towards faster healing time, reduction in discomfort	Time to healing; rate of healing/efficacy; discomfort
DuoDERM	Margolin et al (1990)	Non-comparative evaluation (20/breast, mixed group)	No wound infections. Mean healing time 12 days 83% of patients reported their comfort to be excellent or good	Infection; wound, oral and skin surface temperature; patient satisfaction with comfort, adhesion, containment of gel and aesthetic acceptability
Second Skin hydrogel dressing Gentian violet	Pickering & Warland (1991)	Prospective evaluation (19/breast) Patients alternately assigned to one or other treatment	60% complete relief of symptoms (Second Skin) vs 33% (gentian) Time to healing 4–6 days (mean 4.6) in Second Skin group and 5–22 days (mean 11) in gentian group	Relief of symptoms (pain, irritation, movement restriction, sleep disturbance, duration); time to healing; infection
Vigilon/Second Skin	Crane (1993)	Prospective evaluation, case study (4/breast)	Reduced pain and discomfort with hydrogel dressing	Comfort
Sucralfate cream	Delaney et al (1997)	RCT (39/head and neck, breast, other) Sucralfate cream vs base cream	No significant differences	Time to healing; area of moist desquamation; pain relief; adverse effects. Daily symptom record
Hydrocortisone and neomycin ointment DuoDERM dressing (control gel formula)	Chen et al (1997)	RCT (105/nasopharynx) steroid ointment vs normal saline vs gel dressing (DuoDERM)	Reduced healing time in steroid ointment group (21–28 days) and gel dressing group (7–14 days) vs normal saline (30–35 days). Only 15% in both groups satisfied with pain relief (cf. 95% in gel dressing group). Fewer local infections in gel group	Healing time; bacterial growth; pain relief

Dermofilm dressing	See et al (1998)	Prospective evaluation (50/breast, head and neck, pelvis, other)	98% gained significant symptom relief. Healing time medians between 11 and 16 days	RTOG score. Size of wound; healing. Diary of symptoms
Various dressings and topical agents	Porock & Kristjanson (1999)	Prospective descriptive study (126/breast)	Bepanthen cream found to be soothing but sticky and staining; fixomull (Mefix) improved comfort, pain and itching	RTOG (modified). Pain
Gentian violet Hydrocolloid dressing	Mak et al (2000)	Prospective RCT (39 patients; 60 wounds/nasopharynx)	No significant differences in healing. Wound size significantly smaller in gentian group; trend towards higher pain severity in hydrocolloid group; better comfort and aesthetic acceptance in hydrocolloid group	Wound size; pain, infection; time to healing: patient satisfaction

RCT, randomised controlled trial, RTOG, Radiation Therapy Oncology Group.

dressings, they can feel tight and hot to wear and are not tolerated by all patients. Other products use the body temperature to encourage adherence, e.g. Tielle, and these may be of value if they can be removed with little or no trauma, using water or saline. One interesting approach to wound care contradicts the generally accepted rule that no adhesive dressings or tape should be applied to skin within a treatment area. Porock & Kristjanson (1999) report the successful use of dressing tape such as Mefix applied to skinfold areas and left in place to *prevent* friction during treatment. Another early study (Shell et al 1986) found that adhesive moisture vapour-permeable dressings (Tegaderm) were effective at reducing healing time, and could be removed easily with the aid of baby oil.

Surveys have repeatedly shown that different departments apply conflicting and even contradictory principles to their wound care practice (Glean et al 2001, Lavery 1995, Thomas 1992). The paucity of evidence inevitably contributes to this problem. Table 8.3 summarises research studies that have been conducted on wound care products and techniques designed to manage established or moist skin reactions.

It is important that future research studies also consider the potential for dressings to *prevent* moist desquamation from occurring, for instance the use of hydrogels in brisk erythema/dry desquamation (Crane 1993), or Mefix tape to minimise friction where skin surfaces touch (Porock & Kristjanson 1999). A vital consideration is the cost-effectiveness of dressings, as modern products are often more expensive than their traditional counterparts. Their use in non-radiotherapy settings is usually justified on the basis of their remaining in place for several days, but moist desquamation reactions often require once- or twice-daily dressing changes to ensure adequate cleansing and comfort. Although this may be costly, sceptics of new dressings should be reminded that the application of unproven preparations may be just as cost-ineffective (Lavery 1995).

The latest guidelines issued by the College of Radiographers (2001) recommend hydrocolloid dressings for light to moderately exuding wounds such as patchy moist desquamation. These are both flexible and comfortable, providing a slight cushioning effect. However, most are adhesive, thus limiting the opportunity for regular skin assessment, and some are relatively thick, which could theoretically introduce a 'bolus' effect. Two studies have evaluated such dressings, but do report some practical problems associated with their use. Margolin et al (1990) found that occlusive hydrocolloid dressings appeared to reduce healing time, but were also prone to leakage – a problem often experienced with the use of these dressings in skinfold areas such as groins and buttocks. Mak et al (2000) compared the effects of a hydrocolloid dressing with gentian violet on the healing of moist desquamation wounds. The study failed to achieve statistical significance in terms of healing times, but found that wound sizes were significantly larger in the hydrocolloid group. At first glance, this appears to be a negative finding, but it may just reflect the fact that moist wound-healing products tend to promote the debridement of damaged tissue as well as the granulation of new tissue. This phenomenon also appears to occur with hydrogels, and it is important that healthcare professionals are not dissuaded from their use because of a transient increase in wound size. Mak et al's study provided a clear indication that patients found the hydrocolloid to be more comfortable and aesthetically pleasing. In contrast, those who received gentian violet commented on the skin remaining tight and dry, a feature they disliked.

The recent guidelines (College of Radiographers 2001) recommend alginate sheets for confluent moist desquamation. Their rationale is that these dressings not only convert to a hydrophilic gel on contact with the wound, lending them conformity in difficult areas, but they also encourage granulation and have haemostatic properties, which can be an advantage in areas of exposed skin. One relevant practical issue is that dressings will usually need to be removed for radiotherapy treatment, to reduce the possibility that the additional 'volume' of the dressing provides a 'bolus' effect and thus increases the dose to the skin. Thilmann et al (1996) used thermoluminescence dosimetry techniques to determine the dose increase to skin during radiotherapy with electrons and high-energy photons. Dressings tested included a silicone-coated wound dressing made of polyamide, a silk acetate dressing, a self-adhesive hydrocolloid dressing and an alginate wound dressing. These authors concluded that the use of dressings during electron therapy does not significantly increase the dose administered to skin. However, they recommend that, when using high-energy photons, only 'extremely thin' dressings are permissible, and then only when there is no 'aggravated skin reaction' (p. 181). They also emphasise the need to ensure that the dressing is accounted for in calculating the applied dose. It is also important to be aware that some products, such as silver-impregnated charcoal, contain metallic ions, which may be associated with radiation scatter.

Although the development of moist desquamation may prompt radiotherapy staff to consider the suspension or early completion of radiotherapy, it is not desirable to allow gaps in treatment, due to the potential for these to affect outcome (Hendry et al 1996). If the use of a comfortable, pain-relieving dressing can enable treatment to continue, all disciplines should work together to ensure that compliance is achieved.

One aspect of care which is not covered by the recent guidelines is that of the systemic management of symptoms associated with radiation skin reactions. Although comfortable dressings can largely relieve these symptoms, some patients experience significant pain, itching or infection which cannot be adequately managed by topical agents. It is important that the patient's need for pain management is assessed, and appropriate analgesia prescribed and evaluated. Non-steroidal anti-inflammatory drugs can often be extremely effective, and can also relieve the discomfort associated with itching and swelling around the skin reaction. Antihistamine tablets can be useful in the management of severe itching, although caution must be taken in relation to the drowsiness these can produce. If infection is suspected, appropriate wound swabs should be taken, so as to establish whether antibiotic or antifungal therapy is required. Timely management of infection can rapidly reduce the discomfort and intensity of a severe skin reaction.

CONCLUSION

Radiation skin reactions remain a significant problem for patients undergoing radical treatment. Wide variations in practice continue to exist, and there is patently a need for more research into skin and wound care products both to prevent and manage skin reactions.

Existing variations in practice suggest that the use of protocols and guidelines has much to offer, if we are to improve consistency in care (Boot-Vickers 1999,

Campbell & Lane 1996, Mallett et al 1999). A two-pronged approach that combines the conduct of research studies to enhance the evidence base with the translation of research findings into practice through protocols and guidelines has to be the way forward.

Patient information is of course an essential component of care. It is crucial that healthcare professionals work together to ensure that a consistent approach to skin care is adopted in their treatment centre. Patients must be adequately informed about the risks of skin breakdown, the self-care strategies they can employ to minimise problems and the potential for skin reactions to worsen once treatment is over. While it remains difficult to predict exactly who will develop moist desquamation, some groups are clearly identifiable as being at increased risk, and experienced healthcare professionals can often judge who is liable to further skin breakdown. If adequate end-of-treatment assessment takes place, patients whose skin is at risk can be referred to community staff and appropriate wound care planned. Skin reactions can be a particularly distressing side effect of treatment, not just because of the pain and discomfort, but also because of the 'unsightly' and 'dirty' nature of these reactions, and the disruption that is caused to daily lives. It is vital that we not only take on board new evidence of wound-healing principles, but also that we listen and respond to the symptom distress caused by radiation skin reactions.

SUMMARY OF KEY CLINICAL POINTS

- Radiation-induced skin reactions are a common side effect of radical treatment, and may become more so as further combined chemoradiotherapy regimes are introduced.
- Radiation skin reactions are a cause of considerable distress and discomfort to patients and are also difficult to manage.
- Damage to the basal layer occurs at doses of around 20–25 Gy or approximately 10 days into radical treatment.
- A number of risk factors exist, including intrinsic and extrinsic factors, which may predispose a patient to developing a skin reaction.
- Skin reactions tend to peak towards the end of treatment, and frequently worsen after treatment is completed.
- There are limited data available on the patient's experience of skin reactions and associated symptoms.
- The management of skin reactions has, until recently, been ritualistic and preference-led, rather than based on current wound-healing evidence.
- Consistent patient information is vital, as are the commitment and collaboration of the multidisciplinary team in radiotherapy.
- Systematic regular assessment of skin reactions is important, and a number of useful tools exist to guide this assessment.
- Washing the skin with or without soap during treatment has been proven not to be detrimental.
- Moisturising creams and those with active ingredients may prevent the onset and severity of erythema, but more research is needed in this area.
- Moist wound-healing methods are gaining support in the management of moist desquamation, but more evidence of their effectiveness is required.

- Most existing research studies are small and have evaluated a range of obscure products not readily available in the UK.

Recent published guidelines provide a sound basis for evidence-based supportive care. Whilst definitive evidence for and against certain dressings and skin products is still unavailable, the management of radiation skin reactions should be guided by the optimisation of patient comfort.

REFERENCES

Adamietz I A, Mose S, Harberl A et al 1995 Effect of self-adhesive, silicone-coated polyamide net dressing on irradiated human skin radiation. Oncology Investigations 2:277–285

Archambeau J O, Pezner R, Wasserman T 1995 Pathophysiology of irradiated skin and breast. International Journal of Radiation Oncology, Biology, Physics 31(5):1171–1185

Arimoto T, Maruhashi N, Takada Y et al 1989 Acute skin reactions observed in fractionated proton irradiation. Radiation Medicine 7(1):23–27

Atkinson A 1998 Nursing burn wounds on general wards. Nursing Standard 12(41):58–67

Balzarini A, Felisi E, Martini A et al 2000 Efficacy of homeopathic treatment of skin reactions during radiotherapy for breast cancer: a randomised, double-blind clinical trial. British Homeopathic Journal 89:8–12

Barkham A 1993 Radiotherapy skin reactions. Professional Nurse 8(11):732–736

Blackmar A 1997 Radiation-induced skin alterations. Medical Surgical Nursing 6(3):172–175

Boot-Vickers M 1999 Skin care for patients receiving radiotherapy. Professional Nurse 14(10):706–708

Cameron S 1997 Changes in burn patient care. British Journal of Theatre Nursing 7(5):5–7

Campbell I R, Illingworth M H 1992 Can patients wash during radiotherapy to the breast or chest wall? A randomized controlled trial. Clinical Oncology (Royal College of Radiolgists) 4: 78–82

Campbell J, Lane C 1996 Developing a skin-care protocol in radiotherapy. Professional Nurse 12(2):105–108

Chen Y, Tsang N, Tseng C et al 1997 Control gel formula dressing in the care of acute skin damage by radiation therapy in head and neck cancer patients. European Journal of Cancer 33 (suppl. 8) Abstract 1357 (ECCO9)

College of Radiographers 2001 Summary of intervention for acute radiotherapy induced skin reactions in cancer patients: a clinical guideline. College of Radiographers, London

Cox J D, Byhardt R W, Wilson F et al 1986 Complications of radiation therapy and factors in their prevention. World Journal of Surgery 10: 171–188

Cox J D, Stetz J, Pajak T F 1995 Toxicity criteria of the Radiation Therapy Oncology Group (RTOG) and the European Organization for Research and Treatment of Cancer (EORTC). International Journal of Radiation Oncology, Biology, Physics 31(5):1341–1346

Crane J 1993 Extending the role of a new hydrogel. Journal of Tissue Viability 3(3):98–99

Delaney G, Fisher R, Hook C et al 1997 Sucralfate cream in the management of moist desquamation during radiotherapy. Australasian Radiology 41:270–275

Denham J W, Hamilton C S, Simpson S A et al 1995 Factors influencing the degree of erythematous skin reactions in humans. Radiotherapy and Oncology 36:107–120

Dini D, Macchia R, Gozza A et al 1993 Management of acute radiodermatitis: pharmacological or nonpharmacological remedies. Cancer Nursing 16(5):366–370

Dische S, Warburton M F, Jones D et al 1989 The recording of morbidity related to radiotherapy. Radiotherapy and Oncology 16:103–108

Farley K M 1991 Cornstarch as a treatment for dry desquamation. Oncology Nursing Forum 18(1):134

Fisher J, Scott C, Stevens R et al 2000 Randomized phase III study comparing best supportive care to Biafine as a prophylactic agent for radiation-induced skin toxicity for women undergoing breast irradiation: Radiation Therapy Oncology Group (RTOG) 97–113. International Journal of Radiation Oncology, Biology, Physics 48(5):1307–1310

Glean E, Edwards S, Faithfull S et al 2001 Intervention for acute radiotherapy induced skin reactions in cancer patients: the development of a clinical guideline recommended for use by the college of radiographers. Journal of Radiotherapy in Practice 2:75–84

Goebel R H, Hazuka M B 1997 Prevention of radiation-induced dermatitis by Superskin, a polymer adhesive skin sealant. Medlogic, Colorado (unpublished report; personal communication)

Halperin E C, Gasper L, George S et al 1993 A double-blind, randomized, prospective trial to evaluate topical vitamin C solution for the prevention of radiation dermatitis. International Journal of Radiation Oncology, Biology, Physics 26:413–416

Hendry J H, Bentzen S M, Dale R G et al 1996 A modelled comparison of the effects of using different ways to compensate for missed treatment days in radiotherapy. Clinical Oncology (Royal College of Radiologists) 8(5):297–307

Hopewell J W 1990 The skin: its structure and response to ionizing radiation. International Journal of Radiation Biology 57(4):751–773

King K, Nail L, Kreamer K et al 1985 Patients' descriptions of the experience of receiving radiation therapy. Oncology Nursing Forum 12:55–61

Lavery B A 1995 Skin care during radiotherapy: a survey of UK practice. Clinical Oncology (Royal College of Radiologists) 7:184–187

Liguori V, Guillemin C, Pesce G F et al 1997 Double-blind, randomized study comparing hyaluronic acid cream to placebo in patients treated with radiotherapy. Radiotherapy and Oncology 42:155–161

Lokkevik E, Skovlund E, Reitan J et al 1996 Skin treatment with Bepanthen cream versus no cream during radiotherapy. Acta Oncologica 35(8):1021–1026

Maiche A, Gröhn P, Mäki-Hokkonen H 1991 Effect of chamomile cream and almond ointment on acute radiation skin reaction. Acta Oncologica 30(3):395–396

Maiche A, Isokangas O, Grohn P 1994 Skin protection by sucralfate cream during electron beam therapy. Acta Oncologica 33(2):201–203

Mak S S, Molassiotis A, Wan W et al 2000 The effects of hydrocolloid dressing and gentian violet on radiation-induced moist desquamation wound healing. Cancer Nursing 23(3):220–229

Mallett J, Mulholland J, Laverty D et al 1999 An integrated approach to wound management. International Journal of Palliative Nursing 5(3):124–132

Margolin S G, Breneman J C, Denman D L et al 1990 Management of radiation-induced moist skin desquamation using hydrocolloid dressing. Cancer Nursing 13(2):71–80

Meegan M A, Haycocks T R 1997 An investigation into the management of acute skin reactions from tangential breast irradiation. Canadian Journal of Medical Radiation Technology 28(4):169–178

Munro A J, Biruls R, Griffin A V et al 1989 Distress associated with radiotherapy for malignant disease: a quantitative analysis based on patient perceptions. British Journal of Cancer 60:370–374

Noble-Adams R 1999a Radiation-induced reactions 1: an examination of the phenomenon. British Journal of Nursing 8(17):1134–1140

Noble-Adams R 1999b Radiation-induced reactions 2: development of a measurement tool. British Journal of Nursing 8(18):1208–1211

Noble-Adams R 1999c Radiation-induced reactions 3; evaluating the RISRAS. British Journal of Nursing 8(19):1305–1312

Nuutinen J, Lahtinen T, Turunen M et al 1998 A dielectric method for measuring early and late reactions in irradiated human skin. Radiotherapy and Oncology 47:249–254

Olsen D L, Raub W, Bradley C et al 2001 The effect of aloe-vera gel/mild soap versus mild soap alone in preventing skin reactions in patients undergoing radiation therapy. Oncology Nursing Forum 28(3):543–547

O'Rourke M E 1987 Enhanced cutaneous effects in combined modality therapy. Oncology Nursing Forum 14(6):31–35

Phillips K A, Urch M, Bishop J F 1995 Radiation-recall dermatitis in a patient treated with paclitaxel [letter]. Journal of Clinical Oncology 13:305

Pickering D G, Warland S (1992) The management of desquamative radiation skin reactions. The Dressing Times 5(1)

Porock D, Kristjanson L 1999 Skin reactions during radiotherapy for breast cancer: the use and impact of topical agents and dressings. European Journal of Cancer Care 8:143–153

Porock D, Kristjanson L, Nikoletti S et al 1998 Predicting the severity of radiation skin reactions in women with breast cancer. Oncology Nursing Forum 25(6):1019–1029

Ratliff C 1990 Impaired skin integrity related to radiation therapy. Journal of Enterostomal Therapy 17(5):193–198

Rezvani M, Alcock C J, Fowler J F et al 1991 Normal tissue reactions in the British Institute of Radiology study of 3 fractions per week versus 5 fractions per week in the treatment of carcinoma of the laryngo-pharynx by radiotherapy. British Journal of Radiology 64:1122–1133

Roy I, Fortin A, Larochelle M 2001 The impact of skin washing with water and soap during breast irradiation: a randomised study. Radiotherapy and Oncology 58:333–339

See A, Wright S, Denham J W 1998 A pilot study of Dermofilm in acute radiation-induced desquamative skin reactions. Clinical Oncology (Royal College of Radiologists) 10:182–185

Shell J A, Stanutz F, Grimm J 1986 Comparison of moisture vapour permeable (MVP) dressings to conventional dressings for management of radiation skin reactions. Oncology Nursing Forum 13(1):11–16

Simonen P, Hamilton C, Ferguson S et al 1998 Do inflammatory processes contribute to radiation-induced erythema observed in the skin of humans? Radiotherapy and Oncology: Journal of the European Society for Therapeutic Radiology and Oncology 46(1):73–82

Sitton E 1992 Early and late radiation-induced skin alterations. Part 1; mechanisms of skin changes. Oncology Nursing Forum 19(5):801–807

Sitton E 1997 Managing side effects of skin changes and fatigue. In: Dow K H, Bucholtz J D, Iwamoto R (eds) Nursing care in radiation oncology, 2nd edn. W B Saunders, Philadelphia, p 79–100

Thilmann C, Adamietz I A, Mose S et al 1996 Increase of surface dose using wound dressings during percutaneous radiotherapy with photons and electrons. Radiotherapy and Oncology 40:181–184

Thomas S 1992 Current practices in the management of fungating lesions and radiation damaged skin. Surgical Materials Testing Laboratory, Bridgend

Warszawski A, Röttinger E M, Vogel R et al 1998 20 MHz ultrasonic imaging for quantitative assessment and documentation of early and late postradiation skin reactions in breast cancer patients. Radiotherapy and Oncology 47(3):241–247

Waugh A, Grant A 2001 Ross and Wilson anatomy and physiology in health and illness, 9th edn. Churchill Livingstone, Edinburgh

Wells M 1995 The impact of radiotherapy to the head and neck: a qualitative study of patients after completion of treatment. MSc Cancer Care thesis. Centre for Cancer and Palliative Care Studies, Institute of Cancer Research, London

Wells M 1998 The hidden experience of radiotherapy to the head and neck: a qualitative study of patients after completion of treatment. Journal of Advanced Nursing 28(4):840–848

Westbury C, Hines F, Hawkes E et al 2000 Advice on hair and scalp care during cranial radiotherapy: a prospective randomized trial. Radiotherapy and Oncology 54:109–116

Williams C 1997 The role of Sterigel hydrogel wound dressing in wound debridement British Journal of Nursing 6(9):494–496

Williams M S, Burk M, Loprinzi C L 1996 Phase III double-blind evaluation of an aloe-vera gel as a prophylactic agent for radiation-induced skin toxicity. International Journal of Radiation Oncology, Biology, Physics 36(2):345–349

9

Pain and breathing problems

Mary Wells

INTRODUCTION

This chapter looks at the symptoms of pain and breathing difficulties, which may not be specifically linked to one particular site of radiotherapy, yet affect a significant proportion of patients with advanced cancer, and may also be produced as a side-effect of radiotherapy treatment. Although these two symptoms are distinct from each other and will be considered separately, both are complex problems with emotional and physical components, and both cause considerable discomfort and distress. Patients suffering pain or breathing difficulties may be receiving radiotherapy to *relieve* their symptoms; others may have pre-existing pain and breathing problems as a result of comorbid disease or advanced cancer; and others may purely experience these symptoms as side effects of treatment. Although the distress experienced by each of these groups may be quite different, it is clear that the impact of pain and breathing difficulties can be profound, and that any supportive care strategy must address these complex problems.

PAIN

There are no studies which specifically assess the prevalence of pain in patients attending a radiotherapy department, but studies of various populations suggest that between 33% and 88% of all cancer patients experience pain (Higginson & Edmonds 2000). Miaskowski & Lee (1999) estimate that around 45% of adult oncology patients experience moderate to severe pain on a daily basis. Given that more than 50% of patients with cancer are likely to receive radiotherapy at some point during their trajectory, and that many of these are having palliative treatment, it is likely that pain will affect a significant number of patients. In addition to the discomfort and effects of cancer and its treatment, patients experience the daily disruption and distress of attending for radiotherapy and lying in treatment positions that may be both undignified and uncomfortable.

THE NATURE OF PAIN

The International Association for the Study of Pain (IASP) defines pain as 'an unpleasant sensory and emotional experience associated with actual or potential tissue damage, or described in terms of such damage' (Merskey & Bogduk 1994, p. 210). Another well-accepted definition that takes the subjective nature of pain into account is McCaffrey's (1972), which states that pain is 'whatever the experiencing person says it is, existing whenever he says it does'.

It is beyond the scope of this chapter to discuss either traditional or new theories of how pain occurs; concise reviews can be found in the *Lancet* series on pain (Besson 1999, Cervero & Laird 1999, Chapman & Gavrin 1999, Loeser & Melzack 1999). It is, however, important to acknowledge that current research disputes the notion that the experience of pain is an inevitable consequence of tissue or nerve damage, or indeed that it is proportional to the *extent* of that damage. Besson (1999, p. 1614) suggests that 'pain is not a unique consequence of impulses in specific, unidirectional hardwired lines that originate in the periphery and terminate in the central nervous system'. Instead, it is a phenomenon with anatomical, physiological and psychological components, which manifests in a number of different ways.

Loeser & Melzack (1999) state that the existence of many types of pain can be understood by the identification of four broad categories: nociception, pain perception, suffering and pain behaviours. Nociception involves the detection of tissue damage through a sensory process involving transduction (activation of receptors), transmission (from peripheral to central nervous system) and modulation (neural activity leading to control of the pain transmission pathway). Pain perception, although it can be triggered by injury or chronic disease, may however, occur *without* nociception. Unpleasant physical and psychological symptoms (including pain) may induce suffering, defined as a negative response which 'occurs when the physical or psychological integrity of the person is threatened' (Cassell 1982). Resulting pain behaviours are manifestations of the individual's response to that suffering and pain.

Pain is usually classified as either acute or chronic in nature, with nociceptive or neuropathic elements (Portenoy & Lasage 1999). Nociceptive pain syndromes are either somatic (related to persistent tissue injury in the bone, joint or muscle) or visceral (related to obstruction, infiltration or compression of visceral structures). Neuropathic pain syndromes are diverse in nature, although they all involve damage to the nervous system.

The body is usually able to restore and repair itself after transient or acute pain, both of which are often amenable to analgesia. However, the existence of chronic pain may signify an inability of the body to restore itself. Most chronic pain syndromes have a neuropathic element, and can be extremely difficult to manage, particularly with conventional analgesics. The nervous system or the individual's perception of pain may be so altered that pain relief is unachievable, and cognitive or behavioural therapy may be required in order to reduce the impact of the pain on that person's life.

Turk & Okifuji (1999) suggest that the pain experience must be viewed in terms of organic, functional and psychosocial processes, which take into account the degree of disease or injury, the suffering and disability caused by the pain, and the extent to which psychosocial factors influence pain perception and behaviour. This framework is similar to that of *total pain*, a concept supported by the World Health Organization (WHO) (1990), which combines physical, social, psychological and spiritual pain, each of which can exacerbate the patient's overall experience. It is vital that the assessment and management of pain in patients undergoing radio-therapy incorporate all these aspects. As Table 9.1 suggests, those commencing treatment may already have a wide variety of different pains related or unrelated to their cancer. All patients also bring their own personal history, with experiences both positive and negative. The nature of any past experience will profoundly influence response to an individual's current problems.

Pain as an underlying problem

To some extent, we assume that the greatest problem patients are dealing with is their cancer, but for some patients, the pain and immobility associated with chronic conditions such as arthritis or backache can interfere with daily life more profoundly than any pain associated with the cancer itself. Twycross et al's (1996) survey of 111 patients referred to a palliative care service revealed that 85% of patients had more than one pain, and more than 40% had more than four different pains. Although these patients all had advanced cancer, and therefore represent a slightly different population than those attending a radiotherapy department, the survey demonstrates that pain is rarely localised to one site. Indeed, in the survey, only about half these pains were directly attributable to cancer. Existing pain can make it extremely difficult for some patients to lie in the required position during radiotherapy, and therefore it is vital that a thorough assessment of the patient's mobility and pain is made before treatment. Radiotherapy treatment couches are usually unpadded, and if the patient is already suffering pain, the experience of treatment can be very uncomfortable. In addition, the efficacy of treatment may be compromised, as pain will increase patient movement, thus reducing set-up accuracy and increasing field size. Simple comfort measures such as the use of cushions and foam supports can make a huge difference, but it may also be necessary to ensure that adequate analgesia is given prior to the patient's treat-ment. Otherwise, the treatment itself may be less effective, as well as exacerbating pre-existing problems.

Table 9.1 summarises the types of pain which may exist for patients *prior* to commencing cancer treatment, therefore compromising their ability to cope with radiotherapy. Some diseases, such as rheumatoid arthritis, systemic lupus erythe-matosus and other collagen vascular diseases, are also associated with greater radiation toxicity (Morris & Powell 1997), and thus may influence pain during radiotherapy. Pains that occur as a result of radiotherapy will be dealt with later in the chapter.

Table 9.1 Main causes of underlying discomfort and pain in patients undergoing radiotherapy

Underlying cause	Type of pain	Pain problem during radiotherapy
Comorbid disease, e.g. arthritis	Chronic, can be a combination of nociceptive (soft-tissue or bone damage) and neuropathic pains	Difficulty climbing on and off treatment couch, discomfort and pain maintaining treatment position
Metastatic bone disease	Acute or chronic, can be a combination of nociceptive (bone destruction) and neuropathic pains	As above N.B.: possible pain flare soon after treatment
Tumour infiltration of soft tissues or nerves	Acute or chronic, neuropathic or visceral pain as a result of pressure or damage	Discomfort and pain lying in or maintaining treatment position
Brain tumour or metastases causing increased intracranial pressure	Most likely to be acute nociceptive or neuropathic (or combination)	Headache, visual disturbances, nausea and vomiting causing discomfort during treatment, and difficulty maintaining treatment position, particularly if immobilised
Recent surgery	Not strictly acute pain if surgery is recent, but not necessarily chronic	Reduced mobility and stiffness, particularly in maintaining treatment position, e.g. arm stiffness after axillary clearance surgery
Previous surgical damage	Chronic, largely neuropathic pain as a result of nerve damage	Difficulty lying in treatment position and discomfort or pain during treatment
Lymphoedema resulting from previous surgery	Chronic, probably a combination of nociceptive and neuropathic pains	Heavy, swollen, painful and uncomfortable limbs or tissues causing difficulty mobilising and discomfort and pain during treatment
Total pain	Likely to be chronic, combining physical and psychological pain, overwhelming in nature	Fear, anxiety and depression, discomfort and burden of pain, resulting in potential difficulty in all aspects of the treatment experience

Patients attending for adjuvant radiotherapy may already be affected by pain resulting from their primary treatment. An area that has been particularly neglected in the literature is the incidence and complexity of chronic postsurgical pain: pain lasting 2 months or more after surgery (Macrae & Davies 1999). Breast cancer surgery appears to be associated with numbness, phantom breast pains, dysaesthesiae (a sensation of cold water trickling down the arm), paraesthesiae, senstivity, arm weakness, swelling and scar pain – all of which may accompany the patient through radiotherapy treatment. The side effects of radiotherapy are then super-imposed or may exacerbate existing discomfort. In addition, clinical experience informs us that patients who have poor arm mobility after axillary clearance surgery often have difficulty raising their arm into the desired treatment position. Physiotherapy and regular arm exercises after surgery can greatly reduce the discomfort associated with radiotherapy to the breast.

Studies suggest that chronic pain is more common if patients receive radio-therapy and/or chemotherapy as well as surgery, and that radiotherapy exacerbates pain in those who have already undergone surgery. Rathmell et al (1991), for example, assessed quality of life in 96 patients who had completed treatment for advanced head and neck cancer, and found that those who received radio-therapy and surgery (39 patients) experienced pain more frequently than those who received radiotherapy alone (54 patients). Whale et al (2001) also found that patients who received both therapies experienced more troublesome pain between 6 and 12 months after treatment. Neck dissection and damage to the eleventh cranial nerve can cause particular problems.

Conflicting evidence exists on the incidence of pain in patients who receive post-operative radiotherapy to the breast. A retrospective study of 408 women between 1 and 6 years post-mastectomy found no clear association between increased pain and radiotherapy, although nearly half these women (particularly those under 50 years old) reported post-mastectomy pain syndrome (Smith et al 1999). Whelan et al (2000) prospectively examined quality of life in patients with breast cancer who had been randomised to receive post-operative radiotherapy ($n = 416$) or surgery alone (wide local excision and axillary clearance; $n = 421$). Whereas quality of life steadily increased in the surgery group, the radiotherapy group experienced deterioration in physical symptoms, fatigue and increased inconvenience during the first weeks of radiotherapy. Six months after randomisation (between 4 and 5 months post-radiotherapy), a third of patients in the radio-therapy group were troubled by breast pain compared with only a fifth of surgery patients. Twice as many patients in the radiotherapy group also experienced skin irritation within 2 months of completing radiotherapy.

Pain as a consequence of radiotherapy

Surprisingly little is written on the subject of pain and radiotherapy, except in the context of managing metastatic bone pain. The fact that radiotherapy may *cause* pain and discomfort is given little attention, and it is clear that patients undergoing radiotherapy do not always report the discomfort and pain associated with treatment. As one patient said:

> ... *you don't like asking for things because you think it's silly ... you feel it's minimal, you know, it's only feeling sick, or a slight headache, so what, or you feel tired, so what, they're only minimal things ... the radiotherapy's dealing with cancer, cancer's the big thing, having a headache, not sleeping, they're minor things so you don't want to say anything about that*

(Wells 1995).

Pain during radiotherapy does not follow a standard pattern. Although the side effects of radiotherapy can be to some extent predicted, the experience of the individual cannot. Pain associated with the acute effects of radiation generally peaks towards the end of treatment and resolves within a few weeks after treatment. The time course is, however, unpredictable. Emotional and psychosocial factors may strongly influence the experience of pain, and other symptoms such as fatigue can add to and exacerbate pain sensations. The expectations of loved ones and healthcare professionals, the experiences of other patients and the perceptions and expectations of individuals can alter their ability to express pain and discomfort. As Wall (1999; 31) states: 'Pure pain is never detected as an isolated sensation. Pain is always accompanied by emotion and meaning so that each pain is unique to the individual'. Pain in patients with cancer is loaded with meaning.

Some patients are surprised that during the actual radiation exposure, they experience no pain or unusual sensation. Cassileth et al (1980) found that more than 50% expected such discomfort. Others, however, can be surprised by the severity of pain and discomfort associated with the side effects of radiotherapy. Table 9.2 illustrates the main causes of pain and discomfort experienced as a direct result of radiotherapy, and refers to chapters in which these side effects are discussed in more detail.

Table 9.2 Main causes of discomfort and pain as a direct result of radiotherapy

Site of treatment	Nature of discomfort or pain
Any site, particularly where skinfolds are present	Itching, burning and pain as a result of erythema or desquamation of the skin (see Ch. 8)
Any site	Discomfort and indignity of treatment positions, particularly lying prone or with areas of skin and body exposed (see Ch. 17). Potential increase in toxicity for those suffering from rheumatoid arthritis, systemic lupus erythematosus and other collagen vascular diseases
Head and neck	Acute pain as a result of mucositis and dysphagia. Discomfort of xerostomia and taste changes (see Ch. 10). Musculoskeletal and neuralgic pains also occur. Late effects, including osteoradionecrosis, cause severe pain (see Ch. 19)
Chest, i.e. lung, breast or oesophagus	Acute pain as a result of oesophagitis and difficulty swallowing (see Ch. 10). Breast swelling and discomfort in breast patients (see Ch. 15). Brachial plexus damage secondary to radiotherapy to the axilla, causing nerve pain (see Ch. 14). Late effects, such as radiation pneumonitis, fibrosis and pleuritic pain from radiation-induced changes to pleura in lung patients (see this chapter and Ch.19)
Upper abdomen	Pain and discomfort associated with abdominal cramps, nausea and vomiting (see Ch. 13)
Pelvis	Pain and discomfort of abdominal cramps, urgency of elimination, diarrhoea, cystitis, tenesmus, proctitis, vaginal dryness, impotence (see Chs 12, 13 and 16). Plexopathy secondary to groin irradiation causing nerve pain (see Ch. 14)

Specific pain problems in patients undergoing radiotherapy

Radiotherapy to the head and neck is known to cause severe side effects and these problems have been specifically investigated (Epstein & Stewart 1993, Janjan et al 1992, Whale et al 2001). Epstein & Stewart (1993) used a detailed pain questionnaire to assess pain in 34 patients with oropharyngeal cancer during radiotherapy, and found that 82% of patients experienced some pain prior to commencing treatment. By the middle of radiotherapy, 100% patients were experiencing pain, 71% of whom had 'distressing' or 'horrible' pain, and around half of whom had continuous pain. At the end of treatment, 73% had 'distressing' or 'horrible' pain, although 1 month later the severity and incidence of pain had decreased, leaving 18% with 'distressing' pain, and 41% with mild pain. Epstein & Stewart found that the medications used did not appear to eliminate pain, and that this was partly explained by a reluctance to prescribe strong analgesics. They also make the important point that radiation-induced mucositis is not always the primary cause of pain during radiotherapy, and that patients also experience musculoskeletal and neuralgic pains. In addition, they highlight the fact that the significance of pain in the head and neck is magnified because of the impact it has on psychosocial interaction.

In order to build a picture of the pain experienced by individuals undergoing radiotherapy, it is necessary to look carefully at symptom assessments performed on patients taking part in clinical trials or other studies of radiotherapy. Quality-of-life assessments generally incorporate pain as a quality-of-life indicator, but pain is just one of many symptoms which have been investigated. The literature demonstrates that a proportion of patients experience pain prior to radiotherapy treatment, and that some pains improve and others deteriorate during radiotherapy. Munro & Potter's (1996) study of symptom distress in 110 radiotherapy patients found that breast patients experienced an improvement in arm numbness during radiotherapy, but an increase in 'breast pain', 'pain' and 'heaviness of the breast' as time went on. Patients with lung cancer experienced an improvement in their pain, and those with head and neck cancer had a steady rise in the pain they experienced on swallowing. Wengstrom et al's (2000) study of the experience of breast cancer treatment confirmed that a proportion of patients commence treatment in pain (20%) and that this increases to 49% at the end of treatment, with 8% experiencing severe or intolerable pain. Miaskowski & Lee (1999) found that other symptoms, such as fatigue, tended to intensify the experience of pain.

Studies suggest that patients who experience severe pain in the acute postoperative period are more likely to experience chronic pain lasting months or years (Macrae & Davies 1999). Further research is required in order to establish the relationship between acute pain as a result of radiotherapy side effects, and chronic pain or discomfort which persists beyond the treatment phase. We also have a great deal to learn about the incidence, nature and management of pains which appear to be related to late nerve damage, tissue fibrosis and necrosis. The particular problems of neural plexus injury are covered in Chapter 14.

The problem of recognising pain

The literature suggests that pain is inadequately recognised in patients attending radiotherapy and oncology departments. The attitudes and approach of staff may play a part here. A large study of 1308 patients with metastatic cancer who were attending oncology outpatient clinics revealed that 67% of patients had pain, and 62% of these rated their pain as substantial (Cleeland et al 1994). However, nearly half the patients in pain were receiving inadequate analgesia for the severity of pain experienced, and this was more likely to be the case in women, older people, ethnic minorities, apparently well patients and those whose pain was attributed to non-malignant causes.

Recent studies suggest that the assessment and management of pain are still poor. Rogers & Todd (2000) present a qualitative analysis of 74 outpatient consultations between cancer patients and their doctors, over half of which included some discussion of pain. Taped accounts demonstrate that doctors in this study tended not to address the impact of the pain on patients' lives and only pursued patients' accounts of pain when they perceived the pain as 'treatable'. The authors concluded that doctors use a variety of communication tactics to identify the 'right kind' of pain and avoid talking about problems that they do not perceive as amenable to cancer therapy.

Cleeland et al (2000) surveyed a group of US radiation oncology physicians and found that less than half the sample felt that they had been well trained in the management of cancer pain. A total of 77% believed that inadequate pain assessment prevented good pain management, and that patient and staff reluctance to use opioids was a significant barrier to pain management. When asked to comment on a case scenario of a patient with severe pain from metastatic cancer, only half stated that they would use a morphine-class analgesic. Nearly a quarter of physicians said that they would only prescribe morphine if the patient's prognosis was less than 6 months. Given that the sample was self-selected, and may represent a group already sympathetic to the issue of pain management, the authors suggest that, in reality, reluctance to use opioids may be more widespread than the survey suggests. Certainly, a recent survey of doctors and nurses in a general surgical unit in Scotland confirmed that staff are fearful of prescribing strong analgesics for patients at early stages of their diagnosis (Wells et al 2001). Another American study demonstrated that, even when quantitative pain assessments were performed and documented in patients' notes prior to outpatient consultations, nearly half the sample of 520 patients had no analgesia prescribed, despite recording significant pain scores (Rhodes et al 2001).

It is difficult to establish from the literature the nature and extent of pain experienced by radiotherapy patients, as most studies use relatively crude measurement techniques which cannot adequately capture the complexity of pain and its impact on daily life. Even studies that specifically investigate the efficacy of radiotherapy for bone pain use narrow endpoints, with the emphasis too often on the doctor's rather than the patient's perspective (Dawson et al 1999). However, a recent survey suggests that approximately one-third of patients currently being treated with radiotherapy have significant pain, and that 23% of *all* those attending an oncology outpatient clinic record pain scores of at least four out of 10 on a numerical rating scale (Rhodes et al 2001).

PAIN ASSESSMENT AND MANAGEMENT

Effective pain management is dependent on a thorough assessment of the patient's experience of pain, including the type, duration, severity and manifestations of the symptom, as well as its physical, psychosocial, spiritual and functional components. Patients should be given the opportunity to express, in language and terms with which they are familiar, problems related to their pain. An accurate and detailed history of the pain(s) must be taken, including an account of all factors that aggravate or alleviate the pain(s) as well as their duration, timing, severity, quality and type (Scottish Intercollegiate Guidelines Network 2000). An analgesic record is also important, as is a consideration of possible aetiological factors, including pains unrelated to cancer and its treatment as well as those that can be attributed to the cancer experience. The assessment of the patient's beliefs, anxieties, mood, culture and reactions to pain is a vital component of this process.

Pain is an exceptionally complex symptom and, provided they are used appropriately, the use of standardised assessment tools is helpful. Body charts and simple visual analogue scales or numerical/Likert rating scales are useful for serial assessments, but tools should also measure the intensity of pain, relief of pain, psychological distress and functional impairment associated with the symptom (Scottish Intercollegiate Guidelines Network 2000).

The management of pain using radiotherapy

The usefulness of radiotherapy for relieving bone pain is well established. Techniques include single-field administration, hemibody irradiation or radioisotopes. Two principal mechanisms are invoked to explain how radiotherapy relieves pain (Mercadante 1997):

1. The cytotoxic effect of radiotherapy on normal bone cells inhibits the release of chemical mediators of pain, such as prostaglandins. This effect explains the fact that some patients get rapid relief, often within 24 h of their treatment.
2. The cytotoxic effect of radiotherapy on abnormal (i.e. cancer) cells prevents any further bone destruction, reduces the size of the tumour and enables resorption of bone to take place. This effect explains the pain relief achieved between 2 and 8 weeks after radiotherapy.

McQuay et al (1997) reviewed 13 published trials of radiotherapy for bone pain and concluded that, overall, 42% of patients can expect at least 50% pain relief from radiotherapy, and that just under 30% achieve complete pain relief by 1 month after treatment. The review found no discernible difference between the effectiveness of different fractionation schedules. A large study conducted by the Bone Pain Trial Working Party has since confirmed that a single fraction of 8 Gy is as safe and effective as a multifraction regimen for the palliation of metastatic bone pain (Yarnold 1999) and a recent consensus statement (Hoskin et al 2001) supports this practice, although points out that areas of controversy remain. It has, for instance, recently been suggested that patients with a good prognosis and performance status may achieve greater pain relief from radical doses of radiotherapy delivered over a longer treatment period (Arcangeli et al 1998). However, not only do single fractions appear to be safe and effective, but they also reduce the distress and inconvenience associated with repeated visits to the department or prolonged admission to hospital during a time at which most patients want to be at home. Single treatments to painful bones are unlikely to produce side effects, although a sudden increase in pain 'flare' can occur soon after administration of radioisotopes or following a large single fraction of external beam radiotherapy. This usually disappears within 48 h, and may be predictive of a good clinical response to treatment.

If pain is caused by multiple bone metastases, hemibody irradiation or treatment with radioisotopes may be indicated. Evidence suggests that both these treatments reduce the number of new pain sites after radiotherapy (McQuay et al 1997), and pain relief is often rapid, but side effects are more common. Hemibody irradiation involves the administration of a single fraction of radiotherapy to the upper or lower half of the body. McQuay et al (1997) conclude that 50% of patients achieve pain relief within 48 h. If pain in both halves of the body is a problem, each half can be treated sequentially, provided there is a 4–6-week gap between the treatments. This allows time for migration of haemopoietic stem cells from unirradiated to irradiated bone marrow. Supportive care at and around the time of treatment should include antiemetics (and/or dexamethasone); antidiarrhoeals (lower hemibody); careful monitoring of fluid balance and renal function, with intravenous hydration if necessary.

The use of radioisotopes for bone pain is confined to patients with prostate cancer, who can be effectively treated with radioactive strontium, provided it is used early (Hoskin et al 2001). This has the advantage of being easy to administer and causing relatively little toxicity, as well as having the ability to reach subclinical metastases. Patients who are radioactive do, however, require particular information and psychological support to ensure that they do not feel isolated and contaminated by the experience.

Approaches to pain relief in radiotherapy

In common with the management of any cancer pain, analgesia should be administered according to the three-step analgesic ladder developed by the WHO (World Health Organization 1996) (Table 9.3). Pain management should usually commence at step 1 of the analgesic ladder, moving to steps 2 and 3 if pain persists or increases.

The Expert Working Group of the European Association for Palliative Care has now issued clear recommendations for the use of opioids in cancer pain (Hanks et al 2001) and these offer extremely helpful advice. If patient-suffering during radiotherapy is to be reduced, there is a need for a more consistent, liberal attitude towards pain relief.

Simple step 1 analgesics, such as those suggested in Table 9.3, can be extremely effective for mild to moderate pain associated with radiotherapy. Although some patients tolerate radiotherapy treatment with mild analgesia or even no pain relief, others require fairly large doses of opioids to keep pain under control. It is vital that pain assessment forms part of routine radiotherapy care, so that the individual's need for analgesia is adequately assessed, and the side effects of any analgesia are adequately managed. If the cause(s) of pain cannot be addressed effectively and quickly using straightforward measures, patients should be referred to specialist pain or palliative care teams for further assessment and management.

Recent pain guidelines (Scottish Intercollegiate Guidelines Network 2000) provide a useful overview of analgesic management, emphasising the importance

Table 9.3 The three steps of the World Health Organization analgesic ladder (WHO 1996)

Step 1 Mild pain	Step 2 Mild to moderate pain	Step 3 Moderate to severe pain
Non-opioids ± adjuvant	Opioid for mild to moderate pain ± non-opioid ± adjuvant	Opioid for moderate to severe pain ± non-opioid ± adjuvant
Drug options include paracetamol, aspirin and NSAIDs	Drug options include codeine, dihydrocodeine, dextro-propoxyphene	Drug options include morphine, diamorphine (or alternatives such as fentanyl, hydromorphone, oxycodone, methadone, phenazocine)
	N.B.: If a weak opioid is ineffective, move to step 3. Do not change to an alternative weak opioid	

NSAIDs, non-steroidal anti-inflammatory drugs.

of regular analgesia, delivered by an appropriate route, with a dose that is titrated according to the individual's needs. These comprehensive guidelines also recognise the need for careful treatment of adverse effects such as constipation, and discuss the potential for adjuvant analgesics and interventional techniques to relieve pain. Adjuvant analgesics such as non-steroidal anti-inflammatory drugs (NSAIDs) can be useful in the management of radiotherapy-related pain, which is often inflammatory in nature, although caution is required due to the potential for gastric bleeding and hepatic or renal damage. NSAIDs act by inhibiting the synthesis of prostaglandins, normally activated by the release of chemical mediators in response to inflammation. This, in turn, reduces the stimulation of nociceptors responsible for the sensation of pain. As prostaglandin synthesis appears to be increased by radiation (Tanner et al 1981), NSAIDs may directly reduce the oedema and inflammation associated with radiation damage. However, only one small randomised controlled trial appears to have specifically investigated the use of NSAIDs during radiotherapy (Soffer et al 1994). This grossly underpowered study of only 28 patients found that daily naproxen and ranitidine did not reduce the pain or dysphagia produced by radiotherapy to the oesophagus.

Non-pharmacological approaches to pain management

Convincing proof of the efficacy of non-pharmacological interventions to manage pain is lacking (Scottish Intercollegiate Guidelines Network 2000), but many patients do appear to benefit from approaches that help them to relax or be distracted from their pain. The discomfort associated with lying in the treatment position for radiotherapy may be particularly amenable to such approaches. There is increasing interest in relaxation as a method of reducing pain or helping patients to manage pain, and this is a technique that can be easily learnt by healthcare professionals working with radiotherapy patients. Other techniques include visual imagery, music, acupuncture, massage and hypnosis.

Radiotherapy techniques

Modern radiotherapy techniques have also changed the experience of pain in patients undergoing radiotherapy treatment. The techniques of continuous hyperfractionated accelerated radiotherapy (CHART) and chemoradiotherapy are essentially designed to enable the biologically effective dose of radiotherapy to the tumour to be increased so as to improve response. The price of improved survival and local control by the use of CHART and chemoradiotherapy appears to be an increase in acute side effects, and pain is no exception. It is acknowledged that acute reactions appear sooner and are more severe with CHART, but that late morbidity is reduced (Dische & Saunders 1999). One study demonstrates that pain can be a significant problem in CHART patients (Bailey et al 1998). Three weeks into treatment, 44% were experiencing moderate or 'very much' pain, in comparison with 23% who were receiving conventional radiotherapy. Similarly, 60% of CHART patients had a sore mouth or pain on swallowing, compared with 37% in the conventional group, and 43% vs 17% experienced heartburn 3 weeks into treatment. Interestingly, significantly fewer patients in the CHART group had moderate or very much pain 1 year after radiotherapy (17% compared with 34% in conventional group). These results demonstrate the importance of recognising pain severity in patients receiving different fractionation regimes, as well as adequate pain management throughout the different stages of the cancer trajectory.

The technique of conformal radiotherapy may also influence the incidence and pattern of pain experienced during treatment. As Tait et al (1997) state, the hypothesis behind conformal therapy is that the reduction in volume of normal tissue irradiated should reduce toxicity and thus improve patient tolerance, or should enable a larger dose to be given without increasing toxicity. However, the randomised controlled trial conducted by Tait et al found no significant differences in the acute reactions experienced by patients undergoing conformal or conventional radiotherapy to the pelvis.

This study of 266 patients undergoing pelvic radiotherapy also demonstrates that patients have a number of different pains which behave differently during radiotherapy treatment. For instance, pain during and after passing urine or a bowel motion tended to increase towards the end of treatment and start decreasing approximately 2 weeks after treatment, as did general discomfort in the bowels. However, the extent to which cramp-like or other abdominal pains interfered with activities of daily living was variable throughout the treatment period.

Other approaches to pain management in patients undergoing radiotherapy

A number of other approaches are thought to reduce side effects, including the pain associated with radiotherapy. Many of these are currently undergoing investigation.

Sucralfate

Conflicting evidence exists for the benefits of sucralfate in reducing pain and discomfort associated with radiotherapy. Sucralfate is an aluminium hydroxide complex of sulphated sucrose, normally used in the treatment of gastric ulcers, which works by forming a viscous barrier, protecting damaged mucosal tissues against acid and enzyme irritation. It may also act by stimulating other protective mechanisms such as growth factors, bicarbonate and mucus secretion, synthesis of endogenous prostaglandins and absorption of bile salts. Henriksson et al (1992) reported the reduction of bowel discomfort during and after radiotherapy as a result of sucralfate granules, and Sur et al (1994) found that sucralfate suspension was superior to conventional antacids in the treatment of dysphagia caused by oesophageal radiotherapy. However, other studies have shown no significant benefits from sucralfate enemas for proctitis (O'Brien et al 1997) or oral suspension for mucositis (Meredith et al 1997).

Radioprotectors

A variety of radioprotective agents have recently been tested in clinical trials, and there are indications that such agents do reduce the severity of side effects experienced as a result of radiotherapy. Amifostine (Ethyol) appears to have a protective effect against normal cells and is being promoted for its ability to reduce xerostomia in patients undergoing radiotherapy to the head and neck. Organic thiophosphates were originally identified for the potential protection they might offer to troops involved in nuclear warfare, by protecting normal cells against ionising radiation. They appear to work by free radical scavenging, direct chemical repair at sites of DNA damage and induction of the antioxidation process. Other agents currently being investigated include misoprostol, growth factors such as granulocyte colony-stimulating factor (G-CSF), angiotensin-converting enzyme (ACE) inhibitors, essential fatty acids and agents which appear to prevent or reverse radiation fibrosis, for example, superoxide dismutase and pentoxifylline. An overview of these protective agents can be found in Trotti (1997).

Hyperbaric oxygen

Hyperbaric oxygen (HBO) treatment, although not widely available, has also been used successfully in the management of radiation-induced symptoms, particularly those associated with late soft-tissue damage or necrosis (Krahn 1999). HBO may act by stimulating angiogenesis with consequent benefits for healing. One study, for example, reports that the symptoms of pain, rectal bleeding, incontinence and diarrhoea improved in nine out of 18 patients with radiation proctitis who underwent hyperbaric oxygen (HBO) treatment (Woo et al 1997). (See Chapters 14, 18 and 19 on late effects for further information.)

BREATHLESSNESS

Although the management of breathlessness may not appear to constitute a significant part of the general supportive care of patients undergoing radiotherapy, it deserves particular mention because of the distress that breathing problems can cause, and the specific lung toxicities that may occur as a result of treatment to the chest. Like pain, breathlessness and other breathing difficulties cannot be considered merely as physical symptoms. Instead, breathlessness is defined 'as a problem where there is complex interplay between physical, psychological, emotional and functional factors' (O'Driscoll et al 1999, p. 37). Like pain, breathlessness may exist as an underlying problem for the patient who is undergoing radiotherapy, and it can interfere with that patient's ability to cope with treatment. Alternatively, breathlessness may occur as a direct result of radiotherapy. Table 9.4 illustrates the range of breathing problems which can affect patients treated with radiotherapy. Radiotherapy treatment can be frightening, and patients who have no physiological reason to feel breathless can experience panic, anxiety and breathing problems, merely because of the fear and claustrophobia induced by the treatment environment.

Table 9.4 Breathing problems affecting patients undergoing radiotherapy

Site of treatment	Breathing problems	Specific symptoms requiring regular monitoring, and strategies for their management
Head and neck	Difficulty breathing due to • excessive secretions, (particularly if tracheostomy is present) • claustrophobia associated with immobilisation shell, or • airway narrowing due to oedema (see Ch. 10)	Hoarseness of voice, noisy breathing, difficult or painful breathing may indicate narrowing of airway. Regular indirect laryngoscopy is performed routinely in some centres to ensure that patency of airway is assessed. It may be sensible to record resuscitation status in the notes and treatment sheet. If symptoms are worsening, refer for immediate examination by medical staff in case airway is at risk. If secretions are excessive, refer to physiotherapy, and employ tracheal suction if tracheostomy is present
Chest	Discomfort of cough, breathlessness, secretions and underlying disease in lung patients. Tumour infiltration of chest wall or pleura	Worsening cough, secretions or breathlessness may indicate inflammation or infection, or increasing panic and anxiety. Acute onset of breathlessness and chest pain following treatment completion may indicate radiation pneumonitis. Manage symptoms accordingly (see management section of this chapter)
Any	Chest tightness, fear and restricted breathing due to pain at any site, particularly abdomen	Pain and discomfort at any site causing restricted breathing. Ensure analgesics are given prior to treatment and monitor efficacy regularly
Underlying cardiopulmonary disease	Breathlessness, difficulty lying down for treatment, excessive secretions	Degree of breathlessness, use of bronchodilators and steroid inhalers, peak flow. Encourage use of respiratory drugs prior to treatment, and assist with comfortable positioning as far as possible

Assessment of breathing difficulties

The assessment of breathing difficulties is fundamental to the achievement of comfort for patients who are undergoing radiotherapy. It is vital that all patients are assessed for their ability to lie flat: many appear to be able to breathe normally when in a sitting or standing position, but cannot manage this lying down. As treatment progresses, side effects may interfere with the patient's ability to breathe easily, either because of scant or excessive secretions in the mouth or airways, or because of local irritation, pain or inflammation in the upper airway or lungs. The psychosocial impact of undergoing radiotherapy treatment for cancer, or the experience of wearing an immobilisation device, may also produce discomfort, panic attacks and breathing difficulties.

Table 9.4 illustrates the specific breathing problems that should be monitored regularly during treatment, such as the patency of the airway in patients undergoing laryngeal radiotherapy. These problems are referred to in more detail in specific chapters. Those patients who are already suffering from breathlessness as an underlying symptom, or those who develop breathlessness during treatment, require a more comprehensive assessment. Based on extensive investigation and work with breathless patients, Corner & O'Driscoll (1999) have developed an invaluable tool to guide the assessment and management of breathlessness in the clinical setting. This tool addresses the psychological, physical, functional and practical components of breathlessness, as well as providing a basis for understanding the impact that breathlessness has on the individual's quality of life so that the symptom can be managed holistically.

Specific breathing problems occurring as a result of radiotherapy

Radiotherapy to the upper airway

The local oedema and inflammation associated with radiotherapy to the head and neck can cause particular breathing difficulties because of the complex anatomy of the upper airway. Patients receiving radiotherapy to the nasal cavity or nasopharynx may experience congestion, build-up of thick and crusty secretions and local discomfort or pain, all of which may interfere with breathing. Nebulised saline, humidification or inhaled steam can ease symptoms, as can the use of lubricating jelly on dry mucous membranes. Meticulous oral hygiene and regular mouthwashes can also help, as these patients are often unable to breathe through their nasal passages, and can develop an extremely dry and sore mouth.

Similarly, radiotherapy to the oral cavity or tongue can cause local swelling and discomfort, so that breathing is more difficult. Sensations of choking whilst eating or drinking are not uncommon. These are likely to occur because of swelling in the epiglottis, which results in poor closure of the airway on swallowing. Practical techniques such as lowering the chin when swallowing, drinking thicker liquids, and deliberately swallowing more than once may help. If patients are experiencing consistent problems, it is important to seek the advice of a speech therapist. Adequate pain control is also fundamental, as patients will be unable to swallow effectively if they are in pain.

Radiotherapy to the larynx or pharynx can cause significant local swelling resulting in compromise to the airway. Patients with large tumours may be advised to undergo elective tracheostomy prior to commencing radiotherapy, so as to avoid any unnecessary risk of airway obstruction. Although this is a relatively simple surgical procedure, it can have major implications for patients, particularly if they live alone and are reluctant or unable to manage their own care. Discharge planning for a patient with a tracheostomy can be extremely complicated, and the potential impact of such a procedure on the individual's quality of life must be carefully assessed. If radiotherapy commences soon after a tracheostomy is formed, patients may not have developed the ability to cough effectively enough to expel excessive secretions, and it is important that suction equipment is available in the treatment room and staff are able to use it. The experience of lying flat whilst immobilised in a plastic shell is uncomfortable enough without the problem of feeling drowned in secretions. Patients with tracheostomies may need particular reassurance before and during treatment.

Those patients who do not require an elective tracheostomy may still develop breathing problems during treatment, and it is vital that any difficulties, discomfort or noisy breathing are reported to the medical team and assessed rapidly by indirect laryngoscopy. If a patient does develop stridor, immediate administration of Heliox (helium and oxygen) can improve symptoms. Steroids may also help, and, very rarely, emergency tracheostomy may be required. The experience of stridor can be extremely frightening, and it is important that the environment is as relaxed and calm as possible. Relaxation and breathing techniques which reduce panic can be effectively employed if patients are experiencing acute difficulty breathing, although medical intervention may still be necessary.

Radiotherapy to the chest

Radiotherapy can be used for the effective treatment of pain and breathlessness associated with obstruction or tumour infiltration into the lungs. Little research addresses the immediate side effects of radiotherapy to the chest, but clinical experience demonstrates that existing breathing problems or chest pain can sometimes be initially exacerbated by radiotherapy. A survey of 118 patients following palliative radiotherapy to the lung found that 58.5% of patients reported symptoms during the first 24 h, most commonly chest pain (46%) and systemic symptoms such as fevers, rigors and sweating (36%) (Devereux et al 1997). Almost 70% of those who experienced symptoms stated that they were short-lived, lasting less than 2 h. However, half of those with chest pain required analgesia. No significant differences were found between the side effects experienced by patients who were given a single fraction, two fractions one week apart, or several daily fractions. The authors propose that steroids may reduce the immediate side effects of bronchial radiotherapy, and suggest that patients should be warned about the likelihood of these symptoms.

One of the most serious (and sometimes fatal) complications of radiotherapy to the chest is radiation pneumonitis (RP), which usually occurs 1–3 months after completion of treatment, although it is seen as early as 3 weeks after radiotherapy. Acute RP can develop in patients treated for breast, oesophageal or lung cancer, and it is characterised by fever, breathlessness on exertion and unproductive cough (Johansson et al 1998). A lack of uniform scoring criteria means that the true incidence of RP is difficult to determine precisely (Senan 2000). A retrospective study reported that mild RP occurred in 36% of patients with lung cancer, and severe RP in a further 13% (Inoue et al 2001). Another recent study found that RP occurred in only 20% of patients receiving definitive or adjuvant radiotherapy for lung cancer (Monson et al 1998), but that it was more likely in those who had not undergone surgical resection. Other risk factors included poor performance status, comorbid lung disease, poor pulmonary function and smoking, although conversely, another study found that smoking appeared to be protective (Johansson et al 1998). Earlier authors have also identified radiation dose, field size, prior chemotherapy, combined chemoradiotherapy and total body irradiation (TBI) as potential risk factors (Molls et al 1993).

The symptoms of RP are produced as a result of damage to epithelial cells in the alveoli, leading to loss of surfactant and alterations in alveolar surface tension. These changes impair ventilation, perfusion and gas exchange, and cause progressive fibrosis and collapse of alveolar tissue (Gift 2001). Classic radiographic changes are seen on X-ray and computed tomographic scan, where the area of haziness and opacity largely conforms to the rectangular margins of the radiation field (Sigmund et al 1993).

RP can lead to severe and chronic respiratory dysfunction as a result of the insidious development of pulmonary fibrosis. This is an irreversible situation, and it is therefore vital that acute RP is recognised and treated promptly. Further research is required to evaluate effective preventive strategies: it has been reported that amifostine may, for instance, reduce the incidence of RP (Antonadou 2002). The management of established RP largely relies on the administration of corticosteroids, although the optimum dose and timing of these drugs have not really been confirmed, and antibiotics and oxygen therapy may also be necessary (Inoue et al 2001).

The management of breathlessness

Traditionally, the management of breathlessness has relied upon the treatment of underlying causes or the employment of pharmacological interventions, with many patients receiving oxygen therapy or bronchodilators, and those with advanced disease being prescribed opiates, anxiolytics or steroids to ease their symptoms. Although these strategies can be useful in specific circumstances, they do not always improve the distress associated with breathlessness, a symptom which is heavily influenced by both emotional and physical factors. A review (Ripamonti et al 1998) provides valuable guidance on conventional approaches to the management of breathlessness, including the use of cancer therapies, pharmacological treatments and radiological interventions. However, it is the work of Jessica Corner and colleagues which has changed the way in which breathlessness is viewed and managed from a supportive care perspective (Corner et al 1995, 1996). Recognising the emotional and physical aspects of breathlessness as inseparable, Corner suggests an integrated approach to the management of the symptom,

---

Box 9.1   Essential components of the integrative model of breathlessness

- Detailed assessment of breathlessness and factors that ameliorate or exacerbate it
- Exploration of the meaning and experience of breathlessness
- Practical advice and support for patients and families
- Rebreathing training to encourage diaphragmatic breathing and improve ventilation, strength and control as well as promote a relaxed and gentle breathing pattern
- Relaxation, distraction and visualisation
- Goal-setting and advice on pacing activities so as to improve functional and social well-being and enhance coping
- Early recognition of problems requiring medical intervention

---

(Reprinted with permission from Corner et al 1995.)

which involves a combination of assessment, breathing retraining, relaxation, psychological exploration and rehabilitative strategies. The essential components of Corner's integrative model are illustrated in Box 9.1. An interactive CD-ROM provides further information on all aspects of the work (see further information section at the end of this chapter).

A multicentre study has demonstrated the efficacy of this approach (Bredin et al 1999), and many clinical nurse specialists now incorporate these strategies into their everyday work, as well as providing breathlessness clinics for comprehensive management of chronic symptoms. Breathless patients undergoing radiotherapy may benefit from referral to such clinics, particularly if their symptoms persist. Those whose breathlessness appears to be specifically related to treatment position or feelings of claustrophobia may find relaxation or visual imagery helpful. Radiographers and clinic staff are in an excellent position to learn and utilise simple relaxation schedules to make the treatment experience more tolerable for these patients. The timing of tracheal suction, oxygen therapy, nebulised drugs, analgesics and inhalers may also make a difference to the severity and distress of breathlessness experienced during treatment, and these aspects of care must be given adequate attention.

CONCLUSION

The symptoms of breathlessness and pain can be extremely debilitating, and may affect a significant number of patients undergoing radiotherapy. The basis of supportive care is founded on adequate recognition of underlying problems, assessment of relevant toxicities during treatment and acknowledgement of the emotional and functional components of these distressing symptoms. A multidisciplinary approach is essential to optimum management, as the complexity of both symptoms requires a range of perspectives and skills to address the physical, psychosocial and functional impact they may have on the individual.

This chapter has illustrated the many ways in which pain and breathlessness can cause problems for cancer patients undergoing radiotherapy. It has not been possible to provide a comprehensive review of the nature or management of these complex symptoms; much greater detail is found in most palliative care texts. For the purposes of this book, however, it is vital that staff working in radiotherapy appreciate that patients on treatment may already be coping with pain and/or breathlessness, and that, for many, undergoing treatment is an uncomfortable ordeal which exacerbates such symptoms, or produces new challenges to their management.

SUMMARY OF KEY CLINICAL POINTS

- Pain and breathlessness may exist prior to radiotherapy, either as a consequence of underlying disease or as a result of the cancer itself.
- The incidence and nature of pain in radiotherapy patients is largely under-recognised and undocumented.
- Patients who are breathless or in pain may find it difficult to comply with treatment positions. Timely medication, relaxation and comfort measures may help.
- Pain associated with radiation-induced symptoms can be severe.
- Assessment of pain and breathlessness is crucial to optimum symptom management.
- Pain and breathlessness can be managed with a combination of pharmacological and non-pharmacological measures. It is vital that the emotional and functional aspects of both symptoms are considered.
- Adequate analgesia is crucial. A proportion of patients will require opioids to relieve radiotherapy-induced symptoms.
- Palliative radiotherapy can relieve pain and discomfort, particularly if symptoms are caused by bone metastases.
- Other approaches to pain management which are currently under investigation include radioprotectors, sucralfate, and HBO therapy.
- Specific breathing problems associated with radiotherapy include airway narrowing and radiation pneumonitis.
- A holistic approach to the management of pain and breathlessness requires the input of the multidisciplinary team.

AREAS FOR FURTHER RESEARCH

- The incidence and nature of pain in the radiotherapy population
- The nature and severity of pain associated with specific radiation-induced symptoms such as oral mucositis, oesophagitis, cystitis, bowel symptoms
- The efficacy of pharmacological and non-pharmacological interventions to relieve radiation-induced pains
- The use of relaxation and breathing techniques to improve the experience of radiotherapy in patients who are breathless or in pain
- The evaluation of measures to improve difficult symptoms which interfere with breathing, such as excessive secretions, dry mouth
- The relationship between acute pain during radiotherapy and chronic or late effects.

FURTHER INFORMATION

American Pain Society
www.ampainsoc.org

International Association for the Study of Pain
www.iasp-pain.org

Evidence based health care (including Pain Research at Oxford)
www.jr2.ox.ac.uk/bandolier

Palliative Drug information
www.palliativedrugs.com

Wisconsin Cancer Pain Initiative
www.wisc.edu/wcpi

Pain Relief Foundation
www. painrelieffoundation.org.uk

Dept of Pain Medicine and Palliative Care at Beth Israel Medical Center
www.stoppain.org

Breathlessness CD ROM A breath of fresh air: An interactive guide to managing breathless-ness in patients with lung cancer. Interactive Education Unit, Institute of Cancer Research 2001. email: ieu@icr.ac.uk (freephone 0800 9177263)

REFERENCES

Antonadou D 2002 Radiotherapy or chemotherapy followed by radiotherapy with or without amifostine in locally advanced lung cancer. Seminars in Radiation Oncology 12(1):50–58

Arcangeli G, Giovinazzo G, Saracino B et al 1998 Radiation therapy in the management of symptomatic bone metastases: the effect of total dose and histology on pain relief and response duration. International Journal of Radiation Oncology, Biology, Physics 42:1119–1125

Bailey A, Parmar M, Stephens R 1998 Patient-reported short-term and long-term physical and psychologic symptoms: results of the continuous hyperfractionated accelerated radio-therapy (CHART) randomized trial in non small-cell lung cancer. CHART Steering Committee. Journal of Clinical Oncology 16:3082–3093

Besson J 1999 The neurobiology of pain. Lancet 353:1610–1615

Bredin M, Corner J, Krishnasamy M et al 1999 Multicentre randomised controlled trial of nursing intervention for breathlessness in patients with lung cancer. British Medical Journal 318:901–904

Cassell E J 1982 The nature of suffering and the goals of medicine. New England Journal of Medicine 306 (11):639–645

Cassileth B, Volckman D, Goodman R 1980 The effect of experience on radiation therapy patients' desire for information. International Journal of Radiation Oncology, Biology, Physics 6:493–496

Cervero F, Laird J 1999 Visceral pain. Lancet 353:2145–2148

Chapman C, Gavrin J 1999 Suffering: the contributions of persistent pain. Lancet 353:2233–2237

Cleeland C, Gonin R, Hatfield A K et al 1994 Pain and its treatment in outpatients with metastatic cancer. New England Journal of Medicine 300:592–596

Cleeland C, Janjan N A, Scott C B et al 2000 Management by radiotherapists: a survey of radiation therapy oncology physicians. International Journal of Radiation Oncology, Biology, Physics 47:203–208

Corner J, O'Driscoll M 1999 Development of a breathlessness assessment guide for use in palliative care. Palliative Medicine 13:375–384

Corner J, Plant H, Warner L 1995 Developing a nursing approach to managing dyspnoea in lung cancer. International Journal of Palliative Nursing 1:5–11

Corner J, Plant H, A'Hern R et al 1996 Non-pharmacological interventions for breathlessness in lung cancer. Palliative Medicine 10:299–305

Dawson R, Currow D, Stevens G et al 1999 Radiotherapy for bone metastases: a critical appraisal of outcome measures. Journal of Pain and Symptom Management 17:208–218

Devereux S, Hatton M, Macbeth F 1997 Immediate side effects of large fraction radiotherapy. Clinical Oncology (Royal College of Radiologists) 9:96–99

Dische S, Saunders M 1999 The CHART regimen and morbidity. Acta Oncologica 38:147–152

Epstein J, Stewart K 1993 Radiation therapy and pain in patients with head and neck cancer. Oral Oncology 29B:191–199

Gift A 2001 Maintenance of efficient ventilation. In: Watkins-Bruner D, Moore-Higgs G, Haas M (eds) Outcomes in radiation therapy: multidisciplinary management. Jones and Bartlett, Sudbury, Massachusetts, p 590–610

Hanks G, De Conno F, Cherny N et al 2001 Morphine and alternative opioids in cancer pain: the EAPC recommendations. British Journal of Cancer 84:587–593

Henriksson R, Franzen L, Littbrand B 1992 Effects of sucralfate on acute and late bowel discomfort following radiotherapy of bowel cancer. Journal of Clinical Oncology 10:969–975

Higginson I J, Edmonds P M 2000 Effectiveness and efficiency in the management of cancer pain: current dilemmas in clinical practice. In: Hillier R, Finlay I, Welsh R, Miles A (eds) The effective management of cancer pain. Aesculapius Medical Press, London

Hoskin P, Yarnold J, Roos D et al 2001 Radiotherapy for bone metastases. Clinical Oncology 13:88–90

Inoue A, Kunitoh H, Sekine I et al 2001 Radiation pneumonitis in lung cancer patients: a retrospective study of risk factors and the long-term prognosis. International Journal of Radiation Oncology, Biology, Physics 49:649–655

Janjan N, Weisman M, Pahule A 1992 Improved pain management with daily nursing intervention during radiation therapy for head and neck carcinoma. International Journal of Radiation Oncology Biology Physics 23:647–652

Johansson S, Bjermer L, Franzen L et al 1998 Effects of ongoing smoking on the development of radiation-induced pneumonitis in breast cancer and oesophagus cancer patients. Radiotherapy and Oncology 49:41–47

Krahn M 1999 Analgesic effect of hyperbaric oxygen for pain caused by cancer treatment. Journal of Palliative Care 15:53–55

Loeser J, Melzack R 1999 Pain: an overview. Lancet 353:1607–1609

Macrae W, Davies H 1999 Chronic postsurgical pain. In: Crombie I (ed.) Epidemiology of pain. IASP Press, Seattle, p 125–142

McCaffrey M 1972 Nursing management of the patient in pain. J B Lippincott, Philadelphia

McQuay H, Carroll D, Moore R 1997 Radiotherapy for painful bone metastases: a systematic review. Clinical Oncology 9:150–154

Mercadante S 1997 Malignant bone pain: pathophysiology and treatment. Pain 69:1–18

Meredith R, Salter M, Kim R et al 1997 Sucralfate for radiation mucositis: results of a double-blind randomized trial. International Journal of Radiation Oncology, Biology, Physics 37:275–279

Merskey H, Bogduk N 1994 Classification of chronic pain. International Association for the Study of Pain Press, Seattle

Miaskowski C, Lee K 1999 Pain, fatigue, and sleep disturbances in oncology outpatients receiving radiation therapy for bone metastasis: a pilot study. Journal of Pain and Symptom Management 17:320–332

Molls M, Herrmann T, Steinberg F et al 1993 Radiopathology of the lung: experimental and clinical observations. In: Bruggmoses G, Frommhold H, Wannenmacher M (eds) Recent results in cancer research, vol. 130. Springer-Verlag, Berlin, p 109–121

Monson J, Stark P, Reilly J et al 1998 Clinical radiation pneumonitis and radiographic changes after thoracic radiation therapy for lung carcinoma. Cancer 82:842–850

Morris M, Powell S 1997 Irradiation in the setting of collagen vascular disease: acute and late complications. Journal of Clinical Oncology 15:2728–2735

Munro A, Potter S 1996 A quantitative approach to the distress caused by symptoms in patients treated with radical radiotherapy. British Journal of Cancer 74:640–647

O'Brien P, Franklin C, Dear K et al 1997 A phase III double blind randomised study of rectal sucralfate suspension in the prevention of acute radiation proctitis. Radiotherapy and Oncology 45:117–123

O'Driscoll M, Corner J, Bailey C 1999 The experience of breathlessness in lung cancer. European Journal of Cancer Care 8:37–43

Portenoy R, Lasage P 1999 Management of cancer pain. Lancet 353:1695–1700

Rathmell A, Ash D V, Howes M et al 1991 Assessing quality of life in patients treated for advanced head and neck cancer. Clinical Oncology (Royal College of Radiologists) 3:10–16

Rhodes D, Koshy R, Waterfield W et al 2001 Feasibility of quantitative pain assessment in outpatient oncology practice. Journal of Clinical Oncology 19:501–508

Ripamonti C, Fulfaro F, Bruera E 1998 Dyspnoea in advanced cancer: incidence, causes and treatments. Cancer Treatment Reviews 24:69–80

Rogers M, Todd C J 2000 The 'right kind' of pain: talking about symptoms in outpatient oncology consultations. Palliative Medicine 14:299–307

Scottish Intercollegiate Guidelines Network 2000 Control of pain in patients with cancer. Scottish Intercollegiate Guidelines Network and Scottish Cancer Therapy Network, Edinburgh

Senan S 2000 Regarding scoring of radiation pneumonitis. International Journal of Radiation Oncology, Biology, Physics 48:609

Sigmund G, Slanina J, Hinkelbein W 1993 Diagnosis of radiation-pneumonitis. In: Bruggmoser G, Frommhold H, Wannenmacher M (eds) Recent results in cancer research, vol. 130. Springer-Verlag, Berlin, p 123–131

Smith W, Bourne D, Squair J et al 1999 A retrospective cohort study of post mastectomy pain syndrome. Pain 83:91–95

Soffer E, Mirtros F, Doornbos J et al 1994 Morphology and pathology of radiation-induced esophagitis. Digestive Diseases and Sciences 39:655–660

Sur R, Kochhar R, Singh D 1994 Oral sucralfate in acute radiation oesophagitis. Acta Oncologica 33:61–63

Tait D, Nahum A, Meyer L et al 1997 Acute toxicity in pelvic radiotherapy; a randomised trial of conformal versus conventional treatment. Radiotherapy and Oncology 42:121–136

Tanner N, Stamford I, Bennett A 1981 Plasma prostaglandin in mucositis due to radiotherapy and chemotherapy for head and neck cancer. British Journal of Cancer 43:767–771

Trotti A 1997 Toxicity antagonists in cancer therapy. Current Opinion in Oncology 9:569–578

Turk D, Okifuji A 1999 Assessment of patients' reporting of pain: an integrated perspective. Lancet 353:1784–1788

Twycross R, Harcourt J, Bergl S 1996 A survey of pain in patients with advanced cancer. Journal of Pain and Symptom Management 12:273–282

Wall P 1999 Pain. The science of suffering. Weidenfeld and Nicolson, London

Wells M 1995 The impact of radiotherapy to the head and neck: a qualitative study of patients after completion of treatment. Centre for Cancer and Palliative Care Studies. Institute of Cancer Research, London

Wells M, Dryden H, Guild P et al 2001 The knowledge and attitudes of surgical staff towards the use of opioids in cancer pain management: can the Hospital Palliative Care Team make a difference? European Journal of Cancer Care 10:201–211

Wengstrom Y, Haggmark C, Strander H et al 2000 Perceived symptoms and quality of life in women with breast cancer receiving radiation therapy. European Journal of Oncology Nursing 4:78–90

Whale Z, Lyne P, Papanikolaou P 2001 Pain experience following radical treatment for head and neck cancer. European Journal of Oncology Nursing 5:112–120

Whelan T, Levine M, Julian J et al 2000 The effects of radiation therapy on quality of life of women with breast carcinoma: results of a randomized trial. Ontario Clinical Oncology Group. Cancer 88:2260–2266

Woo T, Joseph D, Oxer H 1997 Hyperbaric oxygen treatment for radiation proctitis. International Journal of Radiation Oncology, Biology, Physics 38:619–622

World Health Organization 1990 Cancer pain relief and palliative care. World Health Organization, Geneva

World Health Organization 1996 WHO guidelines: cancer pain relief, 2nd ed. World Health Organization, Geneva

Yarnold J 1999 8 Gy single fraction radiotherapy for the treatment of metastatic skeletal pain: randomised comparison with a multifraction schedule over 12 months of patient follow-up (Bone Trial Working Party). Radiotherapy and Oncology 52:111–121

10

Oropharyngeal effects of radiotherapy

Mary Wells

INTRODUCTION

The direct oropharyngeal effects of radiotherapy only affect patients who are being treated for head and neck cancer and these represent a very small proportion of all radiotherapy patients. However, the distress associated with these side effects is significant. Several studies confirm that patients are unprepared for the severity and duration of symptoms (Eardley 1986, Wells 1998). Incidence of side effects is also high, with approximately 60% of patients receiving standard radiotherapy and more than 90% of those receiving chemoradiotherapy or alternative fractionation developing severe mucositis (Sutherland & Browman 2001). The increasing use of chemoradiotherapy to treat cancers of other sites also means that a greater proportion of patients may be experiencing similar oral effects as a result of toxicity from chemotherapy.

Oropharyngeal symptoms caused by radiotherapy can be so severe that the patient's treatment has to be stopped either prematurely or temporarily, resulting in a lower than intended dose or a gap in treatment, which may affect overall response to treatment (Hendry et al 1996). Modern techniques such as accelerated and hyperfractionated radiotherapy appear to cause more severe acute toxicity, suggesting that the management of oral symptoms is an increasingly vital part of supportive care (Allal et al 1997, Griffiths et al 1999, Skladowski et al 2000).

Studies have repeatedly shown that the commonest and most troublesome symptoms experienced by patients treated with radiotherapy to the head and neck are dry mouth and eating difficulties related to swallowing or taste changes (Epstein et al 1999b, Harrison et al 1997, Langius & Lind 1995). Such studies also reveal that pain is extremely prevalent in this patient group, and that it can persist months or years after radiotherapy (Bjordal et al 1999, Epstein et al 1999b).

AETIOLOGY

There are a number of reasons why the oropharynx is particularly vulnerable to direct and indirect damage as a result of radiotherapy. Firstly, the mucosa has a high cellular turnover rate, which increases its susceptibility to irradiation. The effects of radiotherapy on this highly vascular tissue are to induce congestion and swelling, which may alter patterns of normal blood flow to surrounding tissues. The damaged mucosa becomes vulnerable to infection and trauma, to such an extent that even everyday activities such as chewing can be potentially traumatic. In addition, direct damage to salivary glands within the radiation field depletes saliva production, resulting in the loss of protection offered by the saliva as well as the discomfort associated with dry mouth. Changes to the complex oral microflora also increase the patient's susceptibility to infection. Poor dental health, gum disease, poor general condition, poor nutritional status, smoking, alcohol, anaemia and immunosuppression (in chemotherapy patients) are all factors that contribute to the increased risk of oropharyngeal effects in this patient group. The heavy smoking and drinking habits of many patients present a particular challenge to professionals involved in supportive care.

As explained in Chapter 6, toxicities associated with radiotherapy to the head and neck may be divided into acute and late effects. Acute effects occur during and in the first few weeks or months after radiotherapy, and these include mucositis, dry mouth (xerostomia), thick tenacious saliva, difficulty swallowing (dysphagia) and taste changes or loss (dysgeusia). As a result of these effects, patients are extremely vulnerable to oral infection, and can experience considerable pain and discomfort. If the patient's neck, pharynx or larynx is being treated, all the above side effects are still likely, although the throat is the focus for symptoms. Depending on the position and size of the treatment field, the patient's airway may also be at risk of oedema, resulting in hoarseness, breathing difficulties and even stridor.

The combination of side effects can have an enormous impact on the patient's ability to carry out the most basic activities of daily living, including eating, drinking, speaking, breathing, communicating and kissing. In the short term, acute oropharyngeal effects can profoundly interfere with quality of life, and the late effects of radiotherapy can cause long-term disability and distress because of damage to the mucosa, vasculature, bone structure and muscle of the irradiated area. Late effects include mucosal fibrosis and atrophy, chronic xerostomia, dental caries, osteoradionecrosis, taste dysfunction, infection and hypothyroidism. These tend to occur several months to years after treatment and, unlike most acute effects, they are largely irreversible. However, the severity of potential late effects of radiotherapy to the head and neck can be reduced if care throughout the treatment trajectory is carefully planned with involvement from key members of the multidisciplinary team – dental hygienist, dietician, physiotherapist, speech therapist, nurse specialist and radiotherapist. Assessment *prior* to radiotherapy is crucial, but additionally, so is the contribution of the multidisciplinary team in the continuing care of the patient post-treatment, as the patient remains at risk of developing complications in the longer term. More details of the management of these complications can be found in Chapters 18 and 19.

One complicating factor is that the side effects of radiotherapy are often super-imposed on to functional difficulties resulting from surgery. Patients who have undergone laryngectomy, for example, are already coping with a fundamental change in their ability to communicate, but also experience loss in many other basic ways. As a patient's wife poignantly described:

He can't taste, he can't smell, he can't spit.

Others who have undergone surgery to the salivary glands may experience nerve damage, which results in a loss of sensation or numbness in the cheek. One patient, postparotidectomy, developed severe mucositis during radiotherapy and was causing daily trauma to his already damaged mucosa, explaining,

I couldn't taste anything and I couldn't feel anything, I was biting my tongue and lips and cheek

(Wells 1995).

THE PATTERN OF OROPHARYNGEAL TOXICITY

Relatively few studies specifically look at the pattern of toxicity during radio-therapy to the head and neck, which makes it extremely difficult to understand what symptoms cause people the most problems during treatment. Data from the large series of patients in trials of continuous hyperfractionated accelerated radio-therapy (CHART) are limited by the fact that the quality-of-life tools used do not provide detailed information on the specific problems of patients with head and neck cancer (Griffiths et al 1999). A much-quoted early study by King et al (1985) used a symptom profile to assess symptoms in 25 patients undergoing radio-therapy to the head and neck and found that, by the third week of treatment, around 70% were experiencing continuous sore throat and 'moderately bad' changes in saliva. They described their sore throat as scratchy, lumpy, dry, sore and sometimes burning. Patients reported that their salivary flow decreased during the second week of treatment, and became thicker during the third week, when swallowing also became much more difficult.

As previously stated, one of the problems faced by patients with head and neck cancer is that symptoms existing prior to radiotherapy may be poorly controlled, and are exacerbated by treatment. A large study of 500 patients with head and neck cancer (86% of whom received radiotherapy) assessed quality of life before, during and after treatment (Bjordal et al 1999). Nearly one-third had lost weight prior to treatment starting, and this proportion increased to 49% during treatment. A total of 39% had moderate or severe dry mouth and sticky saliva *prior* to radiotherapy, but once treatment was underway, 90% were affected by these symptoms. Eleven per cent had moderate to severe pain prior to treatment, and nearly a third experienced such levels of pain during radiotherapy.

The high prevalence of symptoms in head and neck cancer patients has been illustrated by several small studies. Huang et al (2000) described the symptom profile of 37 patients receiving nasopharyngeal radiotherapy, a treatment known to cause severe side effects. Most patients experienced moderate to severe dry mouth, difficulty in swallowing and sore throat from the third week of treatment. Taste changes, difficulty with mouth-opening (trismus) and hoarseness also became more severe as treatment progressed, and skin problems were experienced from week 4 onwards. Anorexia affected the majority of patients, which, combined with severe oral toxicity, resulted in an average weight loss of nearly 4 kg. As expected, those patients who received sequential chemotherapy experienced more severe oropharyngeal problems.

Munro & Potter (1996) investigated a broader range of symptoms and found some interesting trends. Prior to treatment starting, patients scored highly on anxiety, family worry, being immobilised, tiredness, dryness and hoarseness. Anxiety and family worry scores had almost disappeared by the end of treatment, but specific physical symptoms tended to be more troublesome at the end of radiotherapy. Symptoms such as pain on swallowing, inability to eat, change in taste and difficulty in swallowing were at their worst during the last week of treatment, but had begun to improve by 1 month after radiotherapy. Others, such as tiredness, persisted even weeks after the end of treatment.

A qualitative study of patients' experiences after completion of radiotherapy illustrated the severity and impact of side effects to the mouth and throat (Wells 1998). The most common physical side effects (identified by selection of symptom cards) were tiredness, sore and dry mouth or throat, difficulty swallowing and sleeping. Diaries completed by patients illustrated the day-to-day impact of symptoms on basic activities of daily living – how painful it was to eat a satsuma or even a banana, how much effort it took to eat:

> ... *everything bland like mashed potato ... you cannot describe what it's like losing your taste, that was the worst thing ... you don't feel like eating and that makes you worse because you're not getting enough nourishment so you get tired, it's a sort of vicious circle.*

Several patients described an insidious onset of symptoms, which made it difficult for them to seek help at the right time. Attempts at relieving symptoms were often ineffective, thus inhibiting the patient's faith in both the medication and the doctor. As one said,

> *It's not bad enough to tell anybody about, and when it is bad enough to tell anyone about the pills you get aren't good enough to do anything about it ... you think they should be working and if they're not working then you must be doing something wrong because the doctor knows what he's doing and he's given you these pills, they're not having any effect but they must be helping the pain because the doctor's given them to you*

(Wells 2001).

The effects of radiotherapy to the head and neck can have a major and long-lasting impact on quality of life. Two separate studies (Epstein et al 1999b, Harrison et al 1997) carried out between 1 and 5 years after radical radiotherapy have found that around 90% of patients are still experiencing moderate to severe dry mouth, and between 65 and 75% have difficulty swallowing, eating and tasting food.

ASSESSMENT OF OROPHARYNGEAL TOXICITY

Regular assessment of oropharyngeal toxicity during treatment is a vital part of any supportive care strategy. Detailed assessment, using a tool which combines subjective and objective measures, enables subtle changes to be detected and prompt action to be taken in the event of any deterioration or infection. Probably the most widely used objective scoring criteria is the Radiation Toxicity Oncology Group (RTOG) acute radiation scoring system. RTOG scales are available for the assessment of laryngeal oedema (larynx), dysphagia (pharynx/oesophagus), mucositis (mouth), skin reactions (skin) and xerostomia (salivary gland) (see Ch. 6, Appendix 6.1). There are limitations to the sensitivity of these criteria, as categories are broad, and tend to include a number of different aspects of symptoms in one score. The Oncology Nursing Society (Bruner et al 1998) has also developed scales for the assessment of common toxicities, and these have been incorporated into radiation therapy patient care records for site-specific groups. Oral assessment tools more commonly used by UK radiotherapy nurses are those devised by Eilers et al (1988) and Feber (1996), and specific tools have also been developed in the USA (Dibble et al 1996). These offer a more comprehensive and holistic guide, as they score eating and drinking, pain, speech and individual mucous membranes separately and then combine them for an overall risk score.

However, none of the above tools takes into account the patient's self-rating of their symptoms. A multidisciplinary group of oral care experts recognised the need for a simple, quantitative and accurate research tool for clinical mucositis assessment and has developed and validated such a tool for use with radiotherapy and chemotherapy patients (Sonis et al 1999). The tool contains three patient-rated questions: one assessing ability to eat, and two visual analogue scales assessing pain and ability to swallow. Measurements completed by the investigator include an erythema and ulceration score, as well as a record of analgesic use. Preliminary data show that changes in oral mucosa over time can be effectively measured using this tool, and that interrater reliability is high. The authors suggest that the objective measurements of erythema and ulceration were so highly correlated with pain and swallowing that it may not be necessary to ask patients to complete the visual analogue scales and questionnaires. However, this correlation was less significant in radiotherapy than in chemotherapy patients, indicating that the degree of mucositis observed by healthcare professionals may not reflect the degree of pain and discomfort felt by patients. This would certainly concur with clinical experience in a nurse-led on-treatment review clinic for head and neck patients, where it has been noted that levels of pain and dysphagia appear to be extremely subjective and cannot always be explained by objective scoring systems.

One of the issues which also needs to be considered is the assessment of risk factors. Studies have shown that the mucositis in chemotherapy patients is significantly associated with xerostomia and a low baseline neutrophil count (<4000 cells/mm^2) (McCarthy et al 1998). A baseline assessment of symptoms and a full blood count at the beginning of treatment may identify patients who are particularly at risk. Where the neck (and particularly larynx) is within the treatment field, it is vital that the risk assessment includes the airway. Symptoms of increasing hoarseness, heavy breathing, wheezing, snoring at night and cyanosis can indicate that the airway is restricted and should always trigger an indirect

---

Box 10.1 Statements listed in the quality-of-life – radiation therapy instrument head and neck module

---

I have pain in my mouth
I have pain in my throat
I have a normal amount of saliva
My saliva is too thick
I have trouble eating or breathing because of mucus in my mouth or throat
I can taste food normally
I am bothered by how my face and neck look
People have trouble understanding me when I speak
I am bothered by frequent or severe coughing
I can chew as well as ever
I am eating regular food
I am embarrassed to eat in public or with others
I can swallow all food without difficulty (including meat and bread)
I can swallow any type of liquid without difficulty

Reprinted from *International Journal of Radiation Oncology, Biology, Physics*, 42, Trotti A, Johnson D et al, Development of a head and neck companion module for the quality of life – radiation therapy instrument (QOL-RTI), 257–261, Copyright (1998) with permission from Elsevier Science.

laryngoscopy by an experienced doctor. Patients who continue to smoke and drink alcohol may also increase their risk of severe side effects, thus advice and support to reduce or discontinue smoking and drinking are also important.

More extensive assessment tools include those that have been developed to evaluate the quality of life of patients with head and neck cancer. Some of these are specific to radiotherapy and are highly relevant to the assessment of patients on treatment (Browman et al 1993, Rathmell et al 1991, Trotti et al 1998). Others have been designed for head and neck cancer patients in general (Hassan & Weymuller 1993, Terrell et al 1997), measure specific difficulties with eating and speech (List et al 1996) or include individual head and neck modules which can be added to generic quality-of-life measures, such as the European Organisation for Research and Treatment of Cancer quality-of-life questionnaire (EORTC QLQ-C30) and H & N module (Bjordal et al 1999), and Functional Assessment of Cancer Therapy for patients with head and neck cancer (FACT–HN) (List et al 1996). Many of these tools provide a more global assessment of quality of life, but may be too cumbersome for patients to complete on a regular basis throughout treatment. Trotti et al (1998) suggest that their 14-item scale shows excellent compliance and provides specific and complete information which can be used directly to influence clinical decisions. This instrument asks patients to rate a series of statements, listed in Box 10.1, on a scale of 0–10, from 'not at all' to 'very much so'.

COMMON OROPHARYNGEAL SIDE EFFECTS

Mucositis

Mucosal toxicity is regarded as the main dose-limiting factor in radical treatment regimes (Trotti 2000). During radiotherapy, cell damage to the basal layer of the mucous membranes results in inadequate replenishment of cells lost through inactivation or exfoliation (Symonds et al 1996). Mucositis is the resulting inflammation of mucosal tissue, usually manifested as erythema or ulceration of the oropharyngeal area, which lies within the treatment field. Significant pain is associated with mucositis, and a fair proportion of patients require opiates in order to get through treatment.

Sonis (1998) proposes a model for the development of mucositis, which also takes into account the role of cytokines, immune regulation and the oral microflora. This model includes four phases of mucositis, described in Box 10.2.

Mucositis generally does not start to become noticeable until approximately 10 Gy has been administered to the oropharnyx. Most patients will have developed a degree of mucositis by about 12 days after the start of radiotherapy, and

---

Box 10.2 Stages in the development of mucositis

Inflammatory/vascular
Soon after the administration of radiotherapy, cytokines are released from the epithelial and connective tissues within the radiation field. These cytokines, which probably include tumour necrosis factor-α and interleukin-1, cause local tissue damage and may also increase vascularity, thus enhancing the cell-killing effect of the ionising radiation
Epithelial
During this phase, the direct effect of radiotherapy on the basal epithelial layer is seen. The cytotoxic effect of ionising radiation on the rapidly dividing cells of the basal epithelium results in reduced cell renewal, cell death, atrophy and ulceration. The timing of this phase is dictated by the normal turnover rate of the basal epithelium and thus commences approximately 9–16 days after the onset of treatment. Cytokine activity continues during this phase, and any functional trauma that occurs is likely to exacerbate mucosal damage. The mucosa will appear erythematous at this stage
Ulcerative/bacterial
During this phase, full-thickness erosions occur, with denudation of the surrounding mucosa. The body's response is to form a fibrinous pseudomembrane, which appears as a whitish and opalescent layer on top of the ulcerated mucosa and can sometimes be mistaken for a candidal infection. Bacterial colonisation of the complex microflora within the mouth can stimulate further cytokine release, thus producing more severe mucositis, as well as causing secondary infection. *Candida* (thrush) and Gram-negative infections are particularly common. Unfortunately, such infections are even more likely to occur in patients who wear dentures, experience dry mouth as a result of radiotherapy or who continue to smoke and drink alcohol during treatment (Singh et al 1996)
Healing
During this phase, the process of epithelial proliferation and differentiation is renewed and the normal microflora is able to reestablish homeostasis. It is difficult to predict exactly when this will occur following radiotherapy, as the dose and fractionation schedule will influence the healing process, as will the condition of the patient. However, Singh et al (1996) report that healing usually occurs by 3 weeks after the end of treatment, as surviving epithelial cells are stimulated into dividing more rapidly as a result of radiation damage. In patients who receive concomitant chemotherapy, healing time is likely to take much longer

---

this can last for at least 6–8 weeks. A small study found that ulceration of the oral mucosa occurred at an average of 28 Gy (or 15 days into treatment) and that whitening of the mucosa was observed at around 35 Gy (or 19 days into treatment) (Dibble et al 1996). The duration of radiation-induced mucositis thus differs greatly from chemotherapy-related mucositis, which tends to last between 5 and 14 days (National Cancer Institute 2000).

The pain of mucositis can be extremely intense – patients describe the inside of their mouth or throat as feeling like it has been prodded with a red-hot poker. Patients with severe mucositis often find it difficult to open their mouths and become reluctant to speak, drink or swallow their saliva for fear of the pain and discomfort it may cause. This acute pain and discomfort are intensified by severe mucosal dryness. One patient undergoing radiotherapy to the tonsil described feeling as if he had Velcro inside his mouth and throat which was being ripped apart each time he tried to speak or swallow.

Dry mouth and throat (xerostomia)

Radiotherapy causes inflammatory, degenerative and vascular changes to the salivary glands at a cellular level, resulting in the reduction and even permanent destruction of saliva production. The severity of xerostomia depends on the amount of salivary gland tissue included within the radiation field, and is therefore likely to be most severe in patients receiving radiotherapy to the nasopharynx or salivary glands themselves. However, dry mouth and throat commonly affect patients with head and neck cancers at other sites, including the tongue, mouth, pharynx, larynx or neck. One of the most unpleasant symptoms associated with xerostomia is the problem of thick tenacious saliva.

Guchelaar et al (1997) state that a 50–60% decrease in salivary flow occurs during the first week of radiotherapy, and that this trend continues as treatment goes on. Consequently, patients experience the discomfort of an extremely dry mouth and, in addition, lose the mechanical and enzymatic protection of the saliva, thus rendering them much more prone to bacterial and fungal infection, oral trauma, tooth decay and nutritional problems (Holmes 1998). Xerostomia may cause oral tenderness, pain and burning sensations, as well as chewing, swallowing and speech difficulties and extreme sensitivity of the teeth. Saliva often becomes sticky and viscous, difficult to remove from gums and teeth, and difficult to spit out. Many patients complain of having thick, sticky mucus at the back of the throat, mouth or nose, which can cause retching, coughing, nausea and even vomiting. As a result of dry mouth or throat, speaking on the telephone can become a major ordeal, sleeping may be disrupted, and using dentures can be uncomfortable and damaging to the dry oral mucosa (Warde et al 2000).

Taste alteration

Relatively little research has been carried out into the pattern or management of taste changes that occur during radiotherapy. Many patients are already experiencing taste changes by the time treatment starts, and the radiotherapy is likely to induce changes that become progressively worse from the second week of treatment onwards. It appears that thresholds for bitter and salt are most severely affected, and sweet thresholds the least. Taste loss can occur after doses of around 20 Gy have been administered (Ripamonti et al 1998), and probably affects about 90% of patients by the end of a radical dose of 60 Gy. Fernando et al (1995) report that subjective and objective taste loss appears to be related to the volume of tongue irradiated and that, although taste loss is associated with xerostomia, it is less dependent on the degree to which the parotid glands are included within the treatment field. Although this study was small, the results support the view that taste loss occurs as a result of a direct effect on the taste buds.

Wells' (1995) qualitative study illustrated the unpleasantness of taste changes. Patients' comments included:

Still no taste and lack of appetite – food is not easy when it only has texture.

and

I fancy all these things but they taste so horrible, like a soda sort of taste.

One of the most vivid descriptions of the experience of xerostomia and loss of taste was reported by a physician treated for carcinoma of the pharynx in the 1950s, who described the sensation as 'mouth blindness' (MacCarthy-Leventhal 1959). As someone who enjoyed food and cooking, she describes the lack of understanding shown by staff about 'food' as distinct from 'diet'. She says,

Imagine having taken a large dose of atropine and then being presented with a piled-high plate of charcoal biscuits by a menacing giant who says, "Eat it up, it will do you good".

EATING DIFFICULTIES AND WEIGHT LOSS

As a result of all the above symptoms, eating difficulties are extremely prevalent in this patient group. One recent study found that 57% of patients presenting to a regional cancer centre had already lost an average of 10% of their body weight prior to commencing radiotherapy (Lees 1999). Radiotherapy-related symptoms of dry mouth, mucositis, pain, trismus, difficulty chewing, taste perception, nausea and constipation inevitably further restrict patients' ability to eat. A study of chemoradiation therapy found that patients lost 10% of their pre-treatment body weight *during* treatment (Newman et al 1998), resulting in sustained nutritional problems for many. Patients and relatives find it extremely distressing to observe this loss of weight, and a great deal of psychological, physical and nutritional support may be necessary. As one patient said:

I thought that I was going to fade away, that's the only thing that worried me, I would have hated it for people to say to me, you do look ill, you're losing weight

(Wells 1995).

PREVENTION AND MANAGEMENT OF OROPHARYNGEAL EFFECTS

MUCOSITIS

Despite a number of studies investigating the prevention and management of oral effects during radiotherapy, little consensus exists as to the best possible supportive care strategy for these patients. Surveys suggest that oral care protocols vary considerably from centre to centre (Ganley 1996, Jansma et al 1992). A wide variety of mouthwashes, both commercial and homemade, have been reported, including water, saline or salt/bicarbonate of soda, as well as more unusual rinses such as old brown ale and blueberry juice (Jansma et al 1992).

An important aim in the management of mucositis is the reduction of potential trauma to the irradiated mucous membranes. There are two main sources of potential trauma: mechanical, caused by food, drink, dentures or teeth, or even opening the mouth when mucous membranes are dry and stuck together, and bacterial, caused by abnormal microflora in the mouth which may colonise and invade an already erythematous or ulcerated mucosa.

Regular and systematic mouth care is fundamental to the prevention of mechanical or bacterial trauma. A moist, clean mucosa that is free of debris is less likely to be traumatised by the everyday functions of eating, drinking and opening the mouth, and is less susceptible to infection. The frequency of mouth care is probably more important than the mouth care agent used, therefore patients need education and support to ensure optimum self-care. A small study conducted by Shieh et al (1997) suggests that specific oral care instructions given by nurses prior to radiotherapy can delay the onset of mucositis and reduce its severity. Other studies have also shown the beneficial effects of systematic oral care protocols and nursing advice in reducing the incidence of mucositis and pain (Janjan et al 1992, Larson et al 1998).

Most oral care protocols advocate a basic policy of non-irritant, simple mouthwashes such as sterile water, 0.9% saline, sodium bicarbonate solution or a mixture of the two (Feber 1996, Ganley 1996, Shieh et al 1997). Guidelines from the National Cancer Institute (2000) recommend that a normal saline solution can be prepared by adding approximately one teaspoon of salt to 32 oz (approx. 1 litre) water, and that one to two tablespoons of sodium bicarbonate can be added if saliva is viscous. Biron et al (2000) support this approach, suggesting that, apart from the assessment and prevention of dental complications prior to therapy, the use of saline mouthwashes and the provision of adequate pain relief, all other procedures are controversial.

The care of teeth and dentures is also a vital component of basic mouth care. If the patient's teeth are in poor condition, assessment by a dentist or hygienist is essential so that dental extractions can be carried out prior to radiotherapy, in order to reduce the risk of osteoradionecrosis. Twice-daily tooth-brushing with a fluoride toothpaste and soft toothbrush is recommended throughout treatment. Some centres advocate a policy of fluoride gel applications in custom-made applications. Chlorhexidine mouthwash may be used for its antiplaque effect if tooth-brushing is too painful (Singh et al 1996), although this may need to be diluted and should only be used twice a day. In edentulous patients, it is important that dentures are brushed and rinsed after meals and soaked in an antimicrobial solution each day. If oral thrush is present, dentures must also be treated for *Candida*. Similarly, mouth gags used to shield areas of the oral mucosa from the direct effect of radiotherapy must be scrupulously cleaned and soaked in an antimicrobial solution to avoid infection. These can significantly reduce mucositis (Perch et al 1995), but are not always tolerated in patients who are already experiencing pain and ulceration from oral cancers.

Optimum pain management is central to the supportive care of patients receiving radiotherapy to the head and neck, as the pain of mucositis, the discomfort of trismus and the severity of dysphagia can have a major impact on quality of life. Regular assessment, regular mouth care and the administration of adequate and timely analgesia form the basis of good pain management. Referral to speech therapists is essential if trismus or dysphagia is particularly distressing, as specific exercises and swallowing techniques can reduce discomfort and further complications. In terms of analgesia, many patients gain excellent relief from simple gargles such as aspirin and paracetamol, but a considerable proportion of patients may require opiates towards the end of radiotherapy. Unfortunately, there is still reluctance to prescribe strong analgesics, particularly as the side effects of radiotherapy are seen to be self-limiting. However, if pain is controlled, patients are much more likely to maintain their fluid and dietary intake, and hospital admission for intravenous fluids or enteral feeding can often be prevented. It is essential that the World Health Oranization analgesic ladder is followed closely, and that adjuvant analgesics such as non-steroidal antiinflammatory drugs are considered at an early stage. Pain management approaches are discussed more fully in Chapter 9.

Avoidance of spicy foods, smoking and spirits also helps to reduce potential trauma. A high-calorie, high-protein diet is usually required for patients undergoing radiotherapy to the head and neck, and foods must be soft and bland if they are to be tolerated in an ulcerated and painful mouth. Nutritional approaches to the management of oropharyngeal effects are discussed in Chapter 11. One essential component of the treatment plan is the involvement of the dietician at an early stage (Lees 1999). Comprehensive nutritional assessment should guide the advice given, timing of referral and degree of nutritional intervention required.

The relatively unsophisticated approach to mouth care described exists because there is still a lack of evidence to support other measures. Recent reviews (Plevova 1999, Wilkes 1998) demonstrate that the effectiveness of some of the more commonly used drugs, such as chlorhexidine (Corsodyl), benzydamine (Difflam) and sucralfate suspension, is still in question. A recent metaanalysis suggests that, when data on all prophylactic agents are combined, the overall risk of severe mucositis appears to be reduced by preventive measures (Sutherland & Browman 2001). However, this benefit was only clearly seen in assessments carried out by physicians; none of the interventions appeared to reduce patients' ratings of the symptoms of oral mucositis. Sutherland & Browman (2001) propose a classification system which illustrates the three principal actions of prophylactic agents: direct cytoprotection, indirect cytoprotection and antimicrobial action. These are shown in Table 10.1.

Table 10.1   Agents used in the prophylaxis of irradiation-induced oral mucositis

Category	Mode of action	Examples
Direct cytoprotectants	Formation of a protective barrier or stimulation of the basal epithelium to increase mucosal cell regeneration (so as to exceed mucosal cell kill)	Sucralfate Misoprostol – increases blood flow, mitotic activity β-Carotene – antioxidant Hydrogen peroxide – damages mucosa so as to promote proliferation Low-energy laser treatment Silver nitrate
Indirect cytoprotectants	Modulation of the immune system or modulation of the inflammatory response	Granulocyte-macrophage colony-stimulating factor Benzydamine mouthwash Corticosteroids
Antimicrobials	Reduction of harmful bacteria present in oral flora, which may predispose to mucositis	*Broad-spectrum* Chlorhexidine mouthwash Povidone-iodine mouthwash *Narrow-spectrum* Polymyxin, tobramycin and amphotericin (PTA) lozenges

Modified with permission from Sutherland & Browman 2001.

Agents providing a protective barrier

Topical coating agents may also be helpful to protect mucous membranes from trauma. One of the most commonly used coating agents in the UK is Mucaine, which is a mixture of aluminium hydroxide, magnesium hydroxide and oxethazine. Clinical experience demonstrates that Mucaine can ease dysphagia if administered approximately 20 min before meals, but there are no studies evaluating its efficacy, and at the time of going to press, it had been withdrawn in the UK. The evidence for the use of sucralfate suspension is conflicting; some studies have shown a significant reduction in radiation-induced mucositis, but others found no difference (Carter et al 1999, Plevova 1999). However, the studies which found no difference in levels of mucositis did demonstrate that sucralfate could reduce the pain associated with mucositis (Epstein 1994, Makkonen et al 1994, Meredith et al 1997) and this in itself could be extremely useful.

One of the problems with most coating agents is their lack of adhesion to ulcerated mucous membranes. Although oral pastes such as Orabase sometimes provide relief, they are sticky, difficult to apply and do not adhere readily to painful areas. Anaesthetic gels such as Teejel or Bonjela can be applied more easily, but quickly dissolve. If the same degree of mucosal damage *inside* the mouth was seen on the skin within the radiation field, it would be possible to apply a dressing to protect that skin from trauma and infection and relieve any discomfort. No such dressing exists for the oral mucosa. However, an interesting approach to the protection of oral mucosa has been reported (Oguchi et al 1998). This study, using historical controls, examined the use of a mucosa-adhesive water-soluble film in radiation-induced oral mucositis. The film contained a topical anaesthetic (tetracaine) and antibiotics (ofloxacine, miconazole and guaizulene) in a hydroxypropyl cellulose base. It was applied to painful areas of the mouth in 25 patients with acute radiation mucositis. The severity of pain and mucositis was compared with that of 27 similar patients who received topical anaesthetics instead. Patients who applied the film had significantly less pain and less severe mucositis than those in the anaesthetic group. Systemic analgesics were necessary in nearly all patients who received topical anaesthetics and in only four of the group who applied the water-soluble film. Significantly more patients in the film group could be maintained on an oral diet. The film was easily applied by patients themselves, and was successful at coating the oral mucosa for between 30 min and 2 h at a time. The authors suggest that it could also be used as a drug delivery system for topical administration. Despite the fact that this study was limited by its small sample and historical control, it suggests that mucosa-adhesive substances may have considerable potential.

Stimulation of the basal epithelium to increase mucosal cell regeneration

Studies investigating the potential for epithelial stimulation are scarce. Most agents have been investigated in very small numbers of patients, and it is difficult to draw conclusions for practice from their results. One used silver nitrate paint on one side of the tongue in 16 patients having radiotherapy to the oral cavity, the hypothesis being that silver nitrate would stimulate the irradiated epithelium to proliferate more rapidly (Maciejewski et al 1991). Mucositis scores were significantly lower in the half of the tongue that had been painted, but no further research appears to have corroborated these interesting results. Another pilot study has evaluated oral glutamine in 17 patients with head and neck cancer; the results indicated that objective mucositis is reduced in patients randomised to glutamine suspension, and that the duration of subjective mucositis is shorter in patients with severe mucositis (Huang et al 2000). Glutamine appears to play an important role in preserving intestinal epithelium after radiotherapy and chemotherapy.

Peterson (1999) reports on the potential for misoprostol oral rinse to mitigate mucosal reactions following stem cell transplant, but further studies are required in radiotherapy patients. A small randomised trial did not support the routine use of hydrogen peroxide mouthwash (Feber 1996), and the role of antioxidants such as β-carotene remains to be determined (Peterson 1999). Nonpharmacological approaches, including the use of low-energy helium laser delivered prior to each fraction of radiotherapy, have demonstrated beneficial effects in terms of objective mucositis and pain (Bensadoun et al 1999), but these approaches obviously have considerable resource implications.

Modulation of the immune system or inflammatory response

To date, only one randomised study has looked at the effects of systemic GM-CSF on radiation-induced mucositis (Makkonen et al 2000). This study demonstrated no improvement in either mucositis or pain in the GM-CSF group, and found that most patients experienced some side effects. However, the authors are now investigating the use of GM-CSF mouth washings, which have shown some promise in small studies and do not produce side effects.

Anti-inflammatory agents have been studied more widely. Abdelaal et al (1989) claimed that regular use of a high-dose corticosteroid mouthwash in five patients undergoing radiotherapy to the parotid completely prevented discomfort and bleeding, even at the end of treatment. Jansma et al (1992) report that chamomile solution, used commonly in the Netherlands, appears to have an anti-inflammatory action and may reduce the severity of mucositis. The use of topical anaesthetics to relieve the pain of mucositis is controversial. Many patients dislike the taste and numbing effect of topical anaesthetics, and can experience stinging and pain on administration. Oguchi et al (1998) also point out the potentially dangerous effect of topical anaesthetics in suppressing gag reflexes; two of the patients in their study experienced aspiration pneumonia. Two studies have compared benzydamine mouthwash with a placebo and claim significant reduction in mucositis as well as less pain (Plevova 1999). However, another study comparing benzydamine with chlorhexidine found that benzydamine caused more discomfort and produced no difference in mucositis scores. Also, pharmaceutical recommendations are that benzydamine mouthwash (Difflam) should only be used for 7 days (Twycross et al 1998).

Antimicrobials

The evidence for broad-spectrum antimicrobials is still patchy. Adameitz et al (1998) found a statistically significant reduction in oral mucositis in 20 patients who received prophylactic povidone-iodine mouthwashes four times daily compared with 20 patients who rinsed with sterile water only. However, no assessment of pain was made, and the authors admit that the mouthwash is irritating to the mucosa. Although several small studies demonstrate that the use of chlorhexidine reduces oral mucositis in patients undergoing chemotherapy, a larger study (Dodd et al 1996) of chemotherapy found no difference. The evidence for chlorhexidine in radiotherapy patients is equally unconvincing. Two randomised trials showed no difference in mucositis as a result of using chlorhexidine (vs placebo) (Ferretti et al 1990, Spijkervet et al 1989), and a more recent study found that chlorhexidine actually aggravated mucositis, causing more discomfort than the placebo mouthwash (Foote et al 1994). Despite these findings, chlorhexidine is believed to be effective in the inhibition of plaque, and it is for this reason that it is recommended by some authors (Feber 2000) for radiotherapy patients, although in diluted form. One paper suggests that chlorhexidine should not be used at exactly the same time as either nystatin or toothpaste, as the effectiveness of each agent is reduced (Barkvoll & Attramadal 1989).

More substantial evidence exists for narrow-spectrum antimicrobials. It has been proposed that Gram-negative bacteria play a significant role in the development of oral mucositis, and several studies have investigated the application of selective decontamination by topical antibiotics. Symonds et al (1996) conducted a randomised controlled trial of 275 patients undergoing radiotherapy to the head and neck, comparing antibiotic pastilles containing polymyxin E 2 mg, tobramycin 1.8 mg and amphotericin B 10 mg with a placebo pastille. Mucositis was graded according to the area and distribution of mucosa affected, the type of pseudo-membrane and the degree of erythema. Oropharyngeal flora was sampled twice weekly, and weekly weights were recorded. Patient ratings included severity of pain and dysphagia. The pastilles were prescribed four times a day every day during radiotherapy treatment to the head and neck for a duration of 8 weeks. Compliance with the pastilles appeared to be good, and where *worst* mucositis scores were compared, significant differences were found in the area and distribution of mucositis – those in the placebo group generally had more severe mucositis. Weight loss, pain on swallowing and severity of dysphagia were also more severe in patients randomised to placebo. Oral cultures showed that the active pastilles significantly reduced the number of yeasts present in the oral microflora, but had no statistically significant impact on the number of aerobic Gram-negative bacilli found in the mouth. The authors found an association between yeast cultures and degree of mucositis, thus concluding that yeast colonisation is an important factor in the pathogenesis of irradiation mucositis.

One of the limitations of this trial was that, despite the fact that patients were stratified according to whether they received conventional radiotherapy, CHART or postoperative radiotherapy, there is no analysis of any differences in mucositis between these groups. Also, patients in both arms of the trial received additional antibacterial and antifungal agents such as chlorhexidine (if they were smokers and drinkers) and nystatin (if oral thrush was present) (McIlroy 1996). A more recent study evaluating the use of a paste containing polymyxin, tobramycin and amphotericin versus a placebo oral paste found no significant differences between mucositis scores or pain severity and duration in a group of 74 patients receiving radiotherapy to the head and neck (Wijers et al 2001). A statistically significant reduction in coliform bacteria was found in the polymyxin, tobramycin and amphotericin group, but complete eradication of Gram-negative bacteria and *Candida* was not seen. This study does not support the hypothesis that Gram-negative bacteria play a crucial role in the pathogenesis of mucositis.

DRY MOUTH

Dry mouth develops earlier and appears to be the most prevalent of oral symptoms (Huang et al 2000). Holmes' (1998) review article summarises a variety of approaches to the management of xerostomia, emphasising the important and neglected point that many common drugs can potentiate or exacerbate dry mouth, and that these should be avoided or eliminated. Case studies demonstrate that discontinuing drugs such as amitriptyline and Moduretic (amiloride 5 mg and hydrochlorothiazide 50 mg) can result in subjective and objective improvement in salivary gland function in patients already affected by radiation dryness (Leslie & Glaser 1993).

Simple comfort measures such as regular mouthwashes, frequent sips of water, carbonated drinks and petroleum jelly applied to the lips can provide temporary relief. Avoiding alcohol, tobacco, spicy and dry foods may also help, and a moist, sloppy diet is likely to be easier to tolerate. The use of saliva stimulants such as citric acid, sweets and ascorbic acid is controversial, particularly in dentate patients whose teeth can be damaged as a result of demineralisation (Davies 1997). Although salivary stimulation approaches are thought to be more effective than salivary substitutes (Holmes 1998), irradiated patients may have to rely on saliva substitutes, as the radiotherapy may have eliminated functioning salivary gland tissue. Traditional saliva substitutes such as artificial salivas, generally based on mucin or carboxymethylcellulose, are available in spray and lozenge form (Davies 1997). As Warde et al (2000) state, these are often ineffective, and patients may prefer to increase their water consumption instead.

Three recent studies have investigated the use of alternative saliva substitutes, which appear to resemble natural human saliva closely. Jellema et al (2001) compared a placebo gel with a gel based on xanthan gum (Xialine) in a cross-over trial. Although results indicated a trend towards improved speech and other senses, Xialine had no effect on dry mouth, sticky saliva and eating difficulties, and therefore appears to offer no advantage over conventional saliva substitutes.

More positive results have been obtained by two pilot studies of a new saliva substitution treatment (Oral Balance gel and Biotene mouthwash/toothpaste). These products contain hydroxypropyl methylcellulose, lactic acid, sorbitol, xylitol and methyl/propyl parabens, which mimic the antibacterial and enzyme components of normal saliva (Epstein et al 1999a). Epstein et al (1999a) conducted a double-blind crossover trial in a group of patients with persisting xerostomia following radiotherapy to the head and neck. Compared with a carboxymethyl cellulose-based gel and ordinary toothpaste, the Oral Balance system resulted in significant improvements in dry mouth and taste. Patients preferred the consistency and lubrication of the new product and found that it improved dry mouth at night. Warde et al (2000) evaluated the use of Biotene mouthwash, toothpaste and chewing gum and Oral balance saliva replacement gel in 28 patients with postirradiation xerostomia, and found similar results. More than half reported a substantial improvement in dryness, discomfort and denture wearing, and between 25% and 46% experienced substantial or major improvement in sleeping, speaking and chewing or swallowing food.

Despite these encouraging results, larger trials are needed to support the findings of these small studies. Warde et al (2000) propose that a combination of pilocarpine and Biotene should be tested in a randomised controlled trial, and they also emphasise the need to develop alternative radiotherapy techniques, which will reduce damage to salivary glands.

A number of studies have now evaluated the use of pilocarpine hydrochloride in the prevention and treatment of xerostomia, suggesting that approximately 50% of patients experience an improvement in their symptoms. However, reviews suggest that up to two-thirds of patients are affected by increased sweating, and that other side effects such as urinary frequency, headache, rhinitis and abdominal cramping may be experienced (Guchelaar et al 1997, Hawthorne & Sullivan 2000). The review by Guchelaar et al concludes that pilocarpine therapy should be the treatment of choice for radiation-induced xerostomia. However, some patients do not experience any benefit from pilocarpine, and others find the side effects too unpleasant to continue therapy (Johnstone et al 2001).

Other approaches to managing dry mouth

Recent studies indicate that radioprotectors such as amifostine (Ethyol) may markedly reduce the incidence and severity of xerostomia and mucositis (Bourhis et al 2000, Brizel et al 2000). Wasserman et al (2000) found that overall scores on a patient benefit questionnaire assessing difficulty eating and speaking, dry and sore mouth, sleep problems and use of oral comfort aids or liquids were significantly better in those patients treated with amifostine. Differences were most significant in patients with chronic or late xerostomia (up to 1 year post-treatment). Although these results are extremely promising, it is important to note the resource implications of new drugs such as amifostine. Not only are the drugs themselves expensive, but they require daily intravenous infusion up to 30 min before each fraction of radiotherapy, and thus have implications for nursing, medical and radiography staff workload.

A preliminary study suggests that acupuncture may have a significant role to play in the palliation of xerostomia in patients who are not helped by other management approaches. Johnstone et al (2001) report that 16 out of 18 patients experienced an improvement in symptoms after several sessions of acupuncture, and that effects sometimes lasted for many weeks. Half of the patients treated reported significant improvements in aspects of quality of life.

The management of viscous, sticky saliva has not been addressed by existing studies, although the prevention or alleviation of dry mouth may have an impact on the severity of this associated symptom. Patients sometimes do gain relief from the saliva replacement products already mentioned, and from the modification of dietary intake to include softer, sloppier foods. Humidified air, nebulised saline and steam inhalations also seem to help to loosen thick secretions. Anecdotal evidence suggests that home humidifiers may reduce the distress and discomfort of this difficult symptom, and that nasal douches (sniffing water through the nose from a saucer) may help to shift sticky nasal secretions, although performing this activity on a regular basis is not pleasant. Similarly, mucolytic agents such as nebulised acetylcysteine can sometimes provide relief (Twycross et al 1998) although there are no data to support their use in this particular clinical situation.

Very little research exists to guide the management of taste changes. Generally, some improvement in taste is experienced between 3 and 8 weeks after the end of radiotherapy, although problems are likely to continue in patients with severe dry mouth. Although dietary measures such as those referred to in Chapter 11 can be helpful, few other approaches have been investigated. One exception is a pilot study by Ripamonti et al (1998), who found that the administration of zinc sulphate slowed down the worsening of taste changes and accelerated the improvement of taste acuity after treatment.

CONCLUSION

The oropharyngeal effects of radiotherapy can be particularly severe, and may have a profound impact on fundamental aspects of quality of life, such as eating, drinking and communication. The most dose-limiting side-effect is mucositis, but despite considerable research, there is still little evidence that any particular pharmacological agents can prevent its development. A simple approach involving systematic assessment of the oral mucosa and relevant symptoms, frequent saline mouthwashes, adequate pain management and nutritional support provides a basis for comprehensive supportive care. The importance of holistic assessment and timely symptom management for patients receiving radiotherapy for head and neck cancer cannot be overemphasised. A multidisciplinary team approach is essential, with particular input necessary from the dietician. However, the complexity of problems experienced by these patients cannot easily be addressed in a conventional on-treatment review clinic. Further research is required to explore alternative ways of providing the support that these patients require.

SUMMARY OF KEY CLINICAL POINTS

- Oropharyngeal radiotherapy can produce severe side effects, including mucositis, dry mouth and throat, sticky saliva, taste changes and taste loss, dysphagia and pain.
- Side effects interfere profoundly with activities of daily living, particularly eating, drinking and speech.
- A variety of assessment tools exist to monitor symptoms during treatment. Subjective as well as objective assessment is important, as is a comprehensive assessment of nutritional needs.
- A multidisciplinary approach to the prevention and management of symptoms is vital.
- Although a considerable body of research has been carried out, most pharmacological approaches to the prevention and management of mucositis remain controversial.
- Agents and techniques which use the principle of increasing cell growth, such as silver nitrate and laser therapy, show some promise for the future in prevention, but more research is required.
- Oral care protocols should include regular systematic assessment, frequent use of saline mouthwashes, prompt treatment of fungal infection and adequate pain management.
- Saliva replacement products and oral pilocarpine may be helpful in the management of dry mouth.
- Anecdotal evidence suggests that humidification approaches may ease the discomfort associated with thick, sticky saliva.
- Taste changes and taste loss may be alleviated with dietary advice. Zinc supplements show some potential in reducing the duration of taste loss.
- Many patients will require support to reduce smoking and alcohol intake.

There is a need to develop alternative strategies to support patients to cope with the severity and duration of oropharyngeal effects. Nurse-led clinics may offer a more holistic and comprehensive approach to care. Further research is needed into the pattern and experience of oropharyngeal side effects and the pharmacological and non-pharmacological management of symptoms.

FURTHER INFORMATION

The Joanna Briggs Institute Best Practice: Oral Mucositis in cancer patients
www.joannabriggs.edu.au/bp5.html

Oral complications PDQ
www.cancer.gov/cancerinfo/pdq/supportivecare

Oral complications during cancer treatment
www.dent.ucla.edu/pic/members/cancer

REFERENCES

Abdelaal A, Barker D, Fergusson M M 1989 Treatment for irradiation-induced mucositis. Lancet 1(8629):97

Adamietz I, Rahn R, Bottcher H D et al 1998 Prophylaxis with povidone-iodine against induction of oral mucositis by radiochemotherapy. Support Care Cancer 6:373–377

Allal A., Bieri B, Mirabell R et al 1997 Feasibility and outcome of a progressively accelerated concomitant boost radiotherapy schedule for head and neck carcinomas. International Journal of Radiation Oncology, Biology, Physics 38(4):685–689

Barkvoll P, Attramadal A 1989 Effect of nystatin and chlorhexidine digluconate on *Candida albicans*. Oral Surgery Oral Medicine Oral Pathology 67(3):279–281

Bensadoun R, Franquin J, Ciais G et al 1999 Low-energy He/Ne laser in the prevention of radiation-induced mucositis. A multicenter phase III randomised study in patients with head and neck cancer. Support Care Cancer 7(4):244–252

Biron P, Sebban C, Gourmet R et al 2000 Research controversies in management of oral mucositis. Support Care Cancer 8:68–71

Bjordal K, Hammerlid E, Ahlner-Elmqvist M et al 1999 Quality of life in head and neck cancer patients: validation of the European Organisation for Research and Treatment of Cancer Quality of Life Questionnaire-H&N35. Journal of Clinical Oncology 17(3):1008–1019

Bourhis J, De Crevoisier R, Abdulkarim B et al 2000 A randomised study of very accelerated radiotherapy with and without Amifostine in head and neck squamous cell carcinoma. International Journal of Radiation Oncology, Biology, Physics 46(5):1105–1108

Brizel D, Wasserman T, Henke M et al 2000 Phase III randomised trial of Amifostine as a radioprotector in head and neck cancer. Journal of Clinical Oncology 18(19):3339–3345

Browman G, Levine M N, Hodson D I et al 1993 The head and neck radiotherapy questionnaire: a morbidity/quality of life instrument for clinical trials of radiation therapy in locally advanced head and neck cancer. Journal of Clinical Oncology 11(5):863–872

Bruner D, Bucholtz J D, Iwamoto R et al 1998 Manual for radiation oncology nursing practice and education. Oncology Nursing Press, Pittsburgh

Carter D, Hebert M, Smink K et al 1999 Double-blind randomized trial of sucralfate vs placebo during radical radiotherapy for head and neck cancers. Head and Neck 21(8):760–766

Davies A 1997 The management of xerostomia: a review. European Journal of Cancer Care 6:209–214

Dibble S, Shiba G, Macphail L et al 1996 MacDibbs mouth assessment. a new tool to evaluate mucositis in the radiation therapy patient. Cancer Practice 4(3):135–141

Dodd M, Larson P, Dibble S L et al 1996 Randomized clinical trial of chlorhexidine versus placebo for prevention of oral mucositis in patients receiving chemotherapy. Oncology Nursing Forum 23:921–927

Eardley A 1986 Patients and radiotherapy. 3. Patients' experiences after discharge. 4. How patients can be helped. Radiography 52(601):17–22

Eilers J, Berger A, Petersen M C 1988 Development, testing and application of the oral assessment guide. Oncology Nursing Forum 15(3):325–330

Epstein J 1994 The efficacy of sucralfate suspension in the prevention of oral mucositis due to radiation therapy. International Journal of Radiation Oncology, Biology, Physics 28:693–698

Epstein J, Emerton S, Le N D et al 1999a A double-blind crossover trial of Oral Balance gel and Biotene toothpaste versus placebo in patients with xerostomia following radiation therapy. Oral Oncology 35:132–137

Epstein J, Emerton S, Kolbinson D A et al 1999b Quality of life and oral function following radiotherapy for head and neck cancer. Head and Neck 21(1):1–11

Feber T 1996 Management of mucositis in oral irradiation. Clinical Oncology (Royal College of Radiologists) 8(2):106–111

Feber T 2000 Head and neck oncology nursing. Whurr, London

Fernando I, Patel T, Billingham L et al 1995 The effect of head and neck irradiation on taste dysfunction: a prospective study. Clinical Oncology (Royal College of Radiologists) 7:173–178

Ferretti G, Raybould T, Brown A T 1990 Chlorhexidine prophylaxis for chemotherapy and radiotherapy-induced stomatitis: a randomized double-blind trial. Oral Surgery Oral Medicine Oral Pathology 76:441–448

Foote R, Loprinzi C, Frank A R et al 1994 Randomized trial of a chlorhexidine mouthwash for alleviation of radiation-induced mucositis. Journal of Clinical Oncology 12:2630–2633

Ganley B 1996 Mouth care for the patient undergoing head and neck radiation therapy: a survey of radiation oncology nurses. Oncology Nursing Forum 23(10):1619–1623

Griffiths G, Parmar M, Bailey A J et al 1999 Physical and psychological symptoms of quality of life in the CHART randomised trial in head and neck cancer: short-term and long-term patient reported symptoms. British Journal of Cancer 81(7):1196–1205

Guchelaar H, Vermes A, Meerwaldt J H 1997 Radiation-induced xerostomia: pathophysiology, clinical course and supportive treatment. Support Care Cancer 5:281–288

Harrison L, Zelefsky M J, Pfister D G et al 1997 Detailed quality of life assessment in patients treated with primary radiotherapy for squamous cell cancer of the base of the tongue. Head and Neck 19(3):169–175

Hassan S, Weymuller J 1993 Assessment of quality of life in head and neck cancer patients. Head and Neck 15:485–496

Hawthorne M, Sullivan K 2000 Pilocarpine for radiation-induced xerostomia in head and neck cancer. International Journal of Palliative Nursing 6(5):228–232

Hendry J H, Bentzen S M, Dole R G et al 1996 A modelled comparison of the effects of using different ways to compensate for missed treatment days in radiotherapy. Clinical Oncology (Royal College of Radiologists) 8(5):297–307

Holmes S 1998 Xerostomia: aetiology and management in cancer patients. Support Care Cancer 6:348–355p

Huang H, Wilkie D, Schubert M M et al 2000 Symptom profile of nasopharyngeal cancer patients during radiation therapy. Cancer Practice 8(6):274–281

Janjan N A, Weisman M D, Pahule A 1992 Improved pain management with daily nursing intervention during radiation therapy for head and neck carcinoma. International Journal of Radiation Oncology, Biology, Physics. 23:647–652

Jansma J, Vissink A, Bouma J et al 1992 A survey of prevention and treatment regimes for oral sequelae resulting from head and neck radiotherapy used in Dutch radiotherapy institutes. International Journal of Radiation Oncology, Biology, Physics 24(2):359–367

Jellema A, Langendijk H, Bogenhenegouwen L et al 2001. The efficacy of Xialine in patients with xerostomia resulting from radiotherapy for head and neck cancer: a pilot study. Radiotherapy and Oncology 59:157–160

Johnstone P, Peng Y, May B C et al 2001 Acupuncture for pilocarpine-resistant xerostomia following radiotherapy for head and neck malignancies. International Journal of Radiation Oncology, Biology, Physics 50(2):353–357

King K, Nail L, Kreamer K et al 1985 Patients' descriptions of the experience of receiving radiotherapy. Oncology Nursing Forum 12(4):55–61

Langius A, Lind M 1995 Well-being and coping in oral and pharyngeal cancer patients. Oral Oncology 31B(4):242–249

Larson P, Miaskowski C, MacPhail L et al 1998 The PRO-SELF mouth aware program: an effective approach for reducing chemotherapy-induced mucositis. Cancer Nursing 21(4):263–268

Lees J 1999 Incidence of weight loss in head and neck cancer patients on commencing radiotherapy treatment at a regional oncology centre. European Journal of Cancer Care 8(3):133–136

Leslie M, Glaser M 1993 Impaired salivary gland function after radiotherapy compounded by commonly prescribed medications. Clinical Oncology (Royal College of Radiologists) 5:290–292

List M, D'Antonio L, Cella D F et al 1996 The Performance Status Scale for head and neck cancer patients and the functional assessment of cancer therapy-head and neck scale. Cancer 77:2294–2301

MacCarthy-Leventhal E 1959 Post-radiation mouth blindness. Lancet 19:1138–1139

Maciejewski B, Zajusz A, Pilecki B et al 1991 Acute mucositis in the stimulated oral mucosa of patients during radiotherapy for head and neck cancer. Radiotherapy and Oncology 22:7–11

McCarthy G, Awde J D, Ghandir T et al 1998 Risk factors associated with mucositis in cancer patients receiving 5-fluorouracil. Oral Oncology 34:484–490

McIlroy P 1996 Radiation mucositis: a new approach to prevention and treatment. European Journal of Cancer Care 5:153–158

Makkonen T, Bostrom P, Vilja P et al 1994 Sucralfate mouth washing in the prevention of radiation-induced mucositis: a placebo-controlled double-blind randomized study. International Journal of Radiation Oncology, Biology, Physics 30(1):177–182

Makkonen T, Minn H, Jekunen A et al 2000 Granulocyte macrophage-colony stimulating factor (GM-CSF) and sucralfate in prevention of radiation-induced mucositis: a prospective randomized study. International Journal of Radiation Oncology, Biology, Physics 46(3):525–534

Meredith R, Salter M, Kim R et al 1997 Sucralfate for radiation mucositis: results of a double-blind randomized trial. International Journal of Radiation, Oncology, Biology, Physics 37:275–279

Munro A, Potter S 1996 A quantitative approach to the distress caused by symptoms in patients treated with radical radiotherapy. British Journal of Cancer 74:640–647

National Cancer Institute 2000 Oral complications of chemotherapy and head/neck radiation (PDQ). CancerNet. Available online at: http://cancernet.nci.nih.gov

Newman L, Vieira F, Schwiezer V et al 1998 Eating and weight changes following chemoradiation therapy for advanced head and neck cancer. Archives of Otolaryngology – Head and Neck Surgery 124(5):589–592

Oguchi M, Shikama N, Sasaki S et al 1998 Mucosa-adhesive water-soluble polymer film for treatment of acute radiation-induced oral mucositis. International Journal of Radiation, Oncology, Biology, Physics 40(5):1033–1037

Perch S, Machtay M, Markiewicz D A et al 1995 Decreased acute toxicity by using midline mucosa-sparing blocks during radiation therapy for carcinoma of the oral cavity, oropharynx and nasopharynx. Radiology 197(3):863–866

Peterson D 1999 Research advances in oral mucositis. Current Opinion in Oncology 11:261–266

Plevova P 1999 Prevention and treatment of chemotherapy and radiotherapy induced oral mucositis: a review. Oral Oncology 35:453–470

Rathmell A, Ash D V, Howes M et al 1991 Assessing quality of life in patients treated for advanced head and neck cancer. Clinical Oncology Royal College of Radiologists 3:10–16

Ripamonti C, Zecca E, Brunelli C et al 1998 A randomised controlled clinical trial to evaluate the effects of zinc sulphate on cancer patients with taste alterations caused by head and neck irradiation. Cancer 82:1938–1945

Shieh S, Wang S T, Tsai S T et al 1997 Mouth care for nasopharyngeal cancer patients undergoing radiotherapy. Oral Oncology 33(1):36–41

Singh N, Scully C, Joyston-Bechal S 1996 Oral Complications of cancer therapies: prevention and management. Clinical Oncology (Royal College of Radiologists) 8:15–24

Skladowski K, Maciejewski B, Golen M et al 2000 Randomised clinical trial on 7-day continuous accelerated irradiation (CAIR) of head and neck cancer – report on 3-year tumour control and normal tissue toxicity. Radiotherapy and Oncology 55:101–110

Sonis S 1998 Mucositis as a biological process: a new hypothesis for the development of chemotherapy-induced stomatotoxicity. Oral Oncology 34:39–43

Sonis S, Eilers J P, Epstein J B et al 1999 Validation of a new scoring system for the assessment of clinical trial research of oral mucositis induced by radiation or chemotherapy. American Cancer Society 85(10):2103–2113

Spijkervet F, van Saene H, Panders A K et al 1989 Effect of chlorhexidine rinsing on the oropharyngeal ecology in patients with head and neck cancer who have irradiation mucositis. Oral Surgery Oral Medicine Oral Pathology 69:154–161

Sutherland S, Browman G 2001 Prophylaxis of oral mucositis in irradiated head and neck cancer patients: a proposed classification scheme of interventions and meta-analysis of randomised controlled trials. International Journal of Radiation Oncology, Biology, Physics 49(4):917–930

Symonds R, McIlroy P, Khorrami J et al 1996 The reduction of radiation mucositis by selective decontamination antibiotic pastilles: a placebo-controlled double-blind trial. British Journal of Cancer 74:312–317

Terrell J, Nanavati K A, Esclamado R M et al 1997 Head and neck cancer-specific quality of life. Archives of Otolaryngology Head and Neck Surgery 123:1125–1132

Trotti A 2000 Toxicity in head and neck cancer: a review of trends and issues. International Journal of Radiation Oncology, Biology, Physics 47(1):1–12

Trotti A, Johnson D J, Gwede C et al 1998 Development of a head and neck companion module for the quality of life-radiation therapy instrument (QOL-RTI). International Journal of Radiation Oncology, Biology, Physics 42(2):257–261

Twycross R, Wilcock A, Thorp S et al 1998 PCF 1 palliative care formulary. Radcliffe Medical Press, Abingdon

Warde P, Kroll B, O'Sullivan B et al 2000 A phase II study of Biotene in the treatment of postradiation xerostomia in patients with head and neck cancer. Support Care Cancer 8:230–238

Wasserman T, Mackowiak J I, Brizel D M et al 2000 Effect of Amifostine on patient assessed clinical benefit in irradiated head and neck cancer. International Journal of Radiation Oncology, Biology, Physics 48(4):1035–1039

Wells M 1995 The impact of radiotherapy to the head and neck: a qualitative study of patients after completion of treatment. MSc thesis. Centre for Cancer and Palliative Care Studies, Institute of Cancer Research, London

Wells M 1998 The hidden experience of radiotherapy to the head and neck: a qualitative study of patients after completion of treatment. Journal of Advanced Nursing 28(4):840–848

Wells M 2001 The impact of cancer. In: Corner J, Bailey C (eds) Cancer nursing: care in context. Oxford, Blackwell, p 63–85

Wijers O, Levendag P C, Harms E R E et al 2001 Mucositis reduction by selective elimination of oral flora in irradiated cancers of the head and neck: a placebo-controlled double-blind randomised study. International Journal of Radiation Oncology, Biology, Physics 50(2):343–352

Wilkes J 1998 Prevention and treatment of oral mucositis following cancer chemotherapy. Seminars in Oncology 25:538–551

11

The effects of radiotherapy on nutritional status

Jill Ireland   Mary Wells

INTRODUCTION

Food and drink have an enormous significance in our society; adequate nourishment symbolises health and well-being. For most people, mealtimes are an important daily ritual, as well as a source of enjoyment and social interaction. Any threat to nutritional status or to the fundamental activities of eating and drinking can therefore have a profound impact on the well-being of individuals and families.

Up to 85% of cancer patients are malnourished, due to a variety of complex factors which interfere with the enjoyment, intake and digestion of food (Shaw 2002). The nutritional status of patients with cancer may be compromised either as a direct result of the disease or as a consequence of treatment. High incidences of anorexia, reduced food intake and weight loss are found in cancer patients, particularly those with metastatic disease (Mercadante 1996). Those with head and neck, oesophageal, lung and gastrointestinal cancers are most at risk of nutritional problems, due to the nature and site of their disease as well as the side effects of treatments (Curtis 1991, Donnelly & Walsh 1995, Vianio & Auvinen 1996).

Not all patients undergoing radiotherapy will experience side effects that directly compromise nutrition, but all require a balanced nutritional intake in order that adequate tissue repair and growth can take place. Both general and site-specific side effects of radiotherapy can affect nutritional status; symptoms such as fatigue or anxiety often reduce the individual's desire and ability to eat and drink, and others such as mucositis, enteritis and dysphagia directly interfere with nutritional intake.

The assessment and management of nutritional problems are vital to the supportive care for patients undergoing radiotherapy. Not only does altered nutritional status affect patients and their families physically, psychologically and socially, but it may also compromise the immune system and reduce the individual's ability to withstand treatment. Around two-thirds of hospitalised cancer patients are malnourished (Wilson 2000) and because of the frequently complex aetiology of their nutritional problems their management presents a major challenge to health professionals.

AETIOLOGY OF ALTERED NUTRITIONAL STATUS

Altered nutritional status may occur as a result of pre-existing problems, the cancer itself or the side effects of treatment. Almost all patients with cancer are affected by anorexia and weight loss to some degree, and the majority develop cancer cachexia before death (Ottery 1994). Nutritional problems are usually multifactorial, and it is vital that all physical, psychological, social and functional causes are considered. Figure 11.1 illustrates the complexity of altered nutritional status, listing some of the many factors that can contribute to malnutrition in cancer before radiotherapy even starts.

CANCER-RELATED CAUSES OF ALTERED NUTRITIONAL STATUS

Anorexia and weight loss

Most patients with cancer experience anorexia (or loss of appetite) at some stage of their disease trajectory, in response to a variety of physiological, psychological and social causes. Physical symptoms such as pain, fatigue, breathlessness, nausea and altered bowel function may profoundly interfere with the patient's desire or ability to eat. The body's ability to absorb and metabolise food may be impaired, and the side effects of toxic treatment are likely to compound existing difficulties. Psychological and social factors such as depression and anxiety, reduced mobility, inadequate social support or decreased income further diminish the individual's interest in food. In addition, the effect of many commonly used medications is to suppress appetite and reduce intake.

It appears that a number of metabolic changes occur in patients with cancer. Glucose turnover is significantly increased which, in turn, drives the process of gluconeogenesis (the breakdown of fatty acids and amino acids to produce energy). Whereas this process is carefully regulated in healthy people, adaptive mechanisms do not occur in patients with cancer (Shaw 2002). Elevated blood glucose levels generally suppress the appetite (Tait 1999), and increased glucose utilisation results in an increased rate of muscle breakdown and fat mobilisation, leading to progressive weight loss (Heber et al 1986). Some studies suggest that peptides such as bombesin, which are produced by certain tumours, also have a role to play in anorexia (McNamara et al 1992).

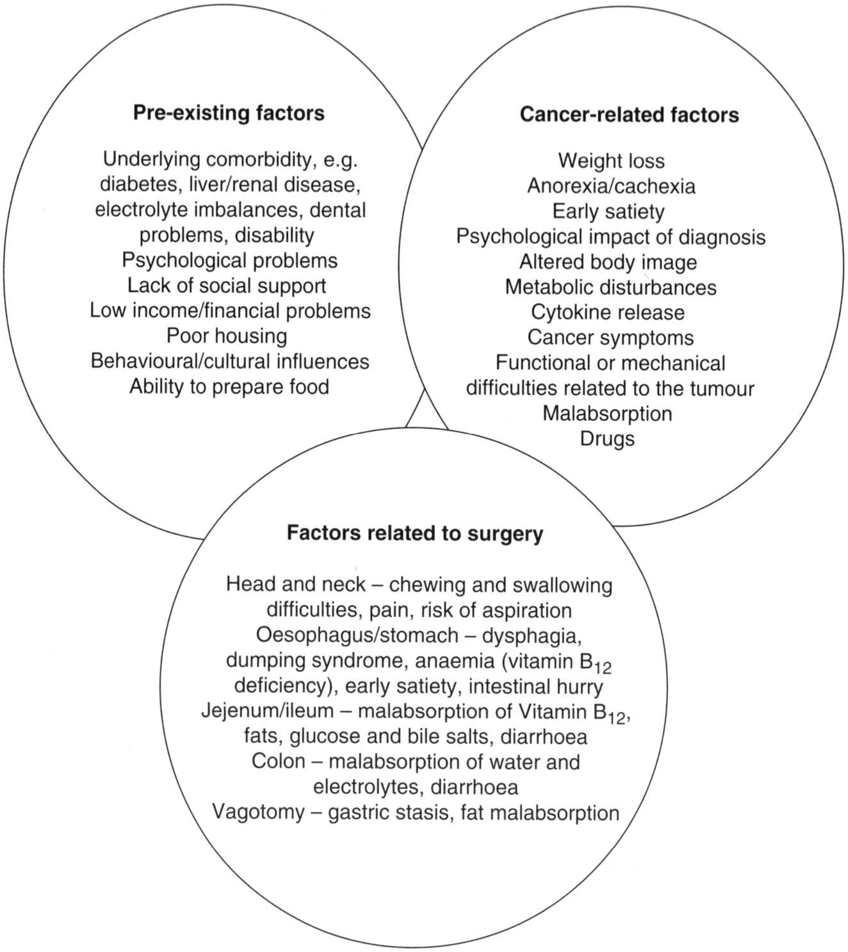

Pre-existing factors

Underlying comorbidity, e.g.
diabetes, liver/renal disease,
electrolyte imbalances, dental
problems, disability
Psychological problems
Lack of social support
Low income/financial problems
Poor housing
Behavioural/cultural influences
Ability to prepare food

Cancer-related factors

Weight loss
Anorexia/cachexia
Early satiety
Psychological impact of diagnosis
Altered body image
Metabolic disturbances
Cytokine release
Cancer symptoms
Functional or mechanical
difficulties related to the tumour
Malabsorption
Drugs

Factors related to surgery

Head and neck – chewing and swallowing
difficulties, pain, risk of aspiration
Oesophagus/stomach – dysphagia,
dumping syndrome, anaemia (vitamin B_{12}
deficiency), early satiety, intestinal hurry
Jejenum/ileum – malabsorption of Vitamin B_{12},
fats, glucose and bile salts, diarrhoea
Colon – malabsorption of water and
electrolytes, diarrhoea
Vagotomy – gastric stasis, fat malabsorption

Figure 11.1 Factors affecting nutritional status in cancer patients prior to radiotherapy.

The metabolic abnormalities directly related to tumour burden may result in early satiety – sensation of fullness after eating only a few mouthfuls of food. Large abdominal tumours or ascites can also contribute towards feelings of satiety, mainly because of the space already occupied by the cancer. Anorexia can also be caused by the release of cytokines such as tumour necrosis factor (TNF) and inter-leukin-1 (IL-1), plasma levels of which are elevated in patients with cancer. It is thought that TNF and IL-1 decrease gastric emptying, thus delaying digestion, suppressing appetite and causing satiety.

Tumour-induced anorexia is a major cause of weight loss in patients with cancer. Weight loss occurs in response to the imbalance between calorific intake and metabolic needs. When the individual's intake of protein and calories is inadequate, and there is competition for nutrients between the cancer and the host, progressive muscle wasting occurs. Body mass is persistently eroded, and organ function and strength are inevitably reduced (Wilson 2000). The larger the tumour burden, the more difficult it may be to restore the energy balance to normal (De Wys 1980).

Clinically significant weight loss is usually defined as a loss of 10% or more of prediagnosis body weight. This degree of weight loss can occur in the absence of any other specific symptoms, and is frequently the reason patients and carers first suspect that something is seriously wrong. Unfortunately, significant weight loss prior to diagnosis is a poor prognostic indicator, particularly in the case of patients with cancers of the lung and head and neck (Brookes 1985, Hespanhol et al 1995). A significant proportion of patients commencing radiotherapy have already experienced weight loss. One study of head and neck patients found that 57% had lost, on average, 10% of their original weight prior to treatment (Lees 1999).

Cachexia

The complex syndrome of cancer cachexia is not fully understood. Contributory factors include altered metabolism, reduced food intake and impaired digestion or absorption as a result of surgery, chemotherapy or radiotherapy (Shaw 2002). The catabolic state described above results in the progressive loss of lipid and protein stores, thus inducing weight loss, muscle wasting, lethargy, anorexia, taste changes, early satiety, chronic nausea and weakness (Bruera 1997). A vicious circle of symptoms can then build up, as weakness and fatigue can further diminish nutritional intake (Fig. 11.2). The altered metabolic state may also reduce cellular and humoral immunity, thus decreasing resistance to infection. Dehydration can disturb cellular metabolism through the reduction of circulatory blood volume (Naylor et al 2001) and wound healing is impaired as a result of abnormal protein metabolism and lack of essential nutrients; this has important implications for patients who experience severe radiation skin reactions.

Patients with advanced disease – particularly those with cancers of the lung, pancreas and gastrointestinal tract – are more at risk of developing cancer cachexia (Shaw 2002). Although it is not an inevitable consequence of the disease process, it is estimated that around 80% of patients with cancer will develop cachexia before they die (Bruera 1997). Not only does cachexia reduce survival and produce chronic nausea, anorexia and weakness, but it is also associated with increased complications of surgery, radiotherapy and chemotherapy. In addition, the psychological effects of cachexia may be significant. McClement & Woodgate (1997) stated that the wasted appearance of the cachectic individual is probably the most recognisable sign of serious illness, and represents a major source of concern for both patients and their families.

Psychological and social factors

Although the disease process and physical symptoms associated with cancer are primarily responsible for altered nutritional status, psychological and social factors

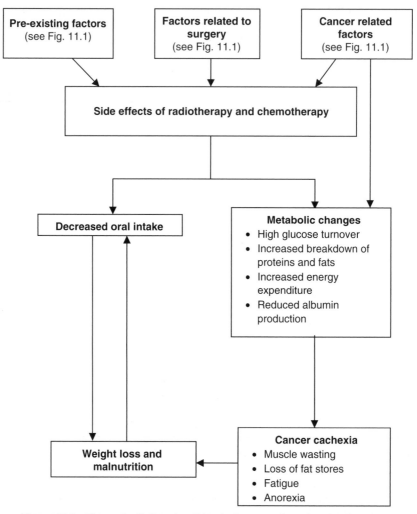

Figure 11.2   The cycle of altered nutrition in the anorexic and cachectic patient.

also play an important part. The impact of a cancer diagnosis can reduce the desire to eat, as can the uncertainty, anxiety and inconvenience associated with cancer treatment. Usual eating patterns can be upset by the timing of radiotherapy treatments and the effects of travelling to and from the hospital, and certain smells or tastes may become associated with treatment so as to cause food aversions. A small descriptive study found that 55% of patients undergoing radiotherapy had pre-existing food aversions, and 59% developed new aversions during treatment (Mattes et al 1991). Those patients obliged to eat in hospital often face unappetising preplated meals, served in an atmosphere not always conducive to an enjoyable dining experience.

For outpatients who are already coping with daily radiotherapy treatments, the physical and financial demands of purchasing, preparing and eating food may be significant. Eating special diets and additional foods recommended by well-meaning healthcare professionals may be expensive and time-consuming. Some patients may just be too tired to think about food or cook for themselves, or may be embarrassed to eat in front of loved ones because of functional problems or symptoms which interfere with acceptable table habits. As the wife of a laryngectomy patient explained,

Sometimes when he's eating, he can't help it, he makes a [imitates loud gulping sound] type of noise … he would be embarrassed if he was sitting in a restaurant, and had to drink with a straw

(Wells 1995).

Effects of the tumour or previous treatments

Mechanical and functional difficulties resulting from tumours of the head and neck or gastrointestinal tract can profoundly interfere with nutritional intake. The tumour itself may invade the oropharynx, oesophagus, stomach, bowel or peritoneum, causing compression or obstruction, which in turn limits food intake. Surgery may produce difficulties with chewing, swallowing and digestion. Resections of the oesophagus, stomach or bowel may result in malabsorption, reduced enzyme production and increased transit time. Oral prostheses or badly fitting dentures can make eating an ordeal and the risk of aspiration due to poor oral control may be increased (Shaw 2002). The toxicity associated with chemotherapy can also affect nutritional status. Drugs such as cisplatin and Adriamycin can cause severe nausea and vomiting, and others such as 5-fluorouracil can produce nausea and diarrhoea. Combination regimes are often responsible for painful oral mucositis and bone marrow depression causing increased susceptibility to oral or gut infections and unpleasant taste changes. In addition, the fatigue and emotional burden associated with chemotherapy can further reduce the desire to eat and drink.

RADIOTHERAPY-INDUCED SIDE EFFECTS CONTRIBUTING TO REDUCED NUTRITIONAL INTAKE

The side effects of radiotherapy can have a major impact on nutritional intake. Those most at risk of nutritional problems include patients who have already undergone surgery, who have already lost weight or who are having treatment to the head and neck or gastrointestinal tract. Patients with oesophageal cancer who are prescribed concomitant chemoradiotherapy also experience severe nutritional problems, due to the local and systemic effects of combining the two treatments. Both general and site-specific radiation-induced side effects can interfere with nutritional status (Table 11.1). Their assessment and management are explored in the relevant chapters indicated in Table 11.1.

Table 11.1 Radiotherapy side effects causing altered nutritional status

Site of treatment	Side effects (late effects in italics)	Relevant chapter(s)
Head and neck	Mucositis Oral infections, including Candida Xerostomia/thick saliva Taste changes or loss of taste Altered sense of smell Dysphagia Pain Difficulties with chewing Local oedema causing aspiration *Trismus* *Dental caries or loss of teeth* *Osteoradionecrosis*	Oropharyngeal effects Pain Body image Late effects
Oesophagus or chest (may include breast patients)	Mucositis (oesophagitis) Dysphagia Nausea and vomiting Anorexia *Oesophageal stenosis, strictures, fibrosis*	Oropharyngeal effects Pain Body image Enteritis Late effects
Abdomen	Nausea and vomiting Acute gastritis Malabsorption *(acute and late)* Anorexia	Enteritis Late effects
Pelvis	Nausea and vomiting Acute radiation enteritis Diarrhoea Malabsorption *(acute and late)* *Fistulae, fibrosis, stenosis* *Partial or complete obstruction* *Chronic radiation enteritis*	Enteritis Late effects
Any (general side effects)	Anorexia Nausea Fatigue Anaemia Psychological factors *Fibrosis*	Fatigue Treatment trajectory After treatment's over Late effects

THE IMPORTANCE OF NUTRITIONAL STATUS IN RADIOTHERAPY PATIENTS

The value of food

Food not only holds nutritional value, but also has unique sociological, psychological and cultural significance. Holden (1991) explored the way in which patients with advanced cancer and their primary caregivers viewed and responded to the experience of anorexia. The findings of this study revealed that loss of appetite is a source of anxiety and distress within the family, with the amount of food being eaten by the patient being used as a barometer of the patient's condition.

Patients were more likely than their carers to speak positively about their food intake. Carers expressed anger, fear, frustration and sadness when patients could not maintain usual eating patterns. One carer said:

> It is so frightening for me to see her lose weight. I knew something was drastically wrong. I blamed myself for not feeding her the right things.

Whereas patients reported other symptoms as being more significant, anorexia caused most concern to caregivers.

The author Marilyn French (1999) describes her experience of receiving radiotherapy for oesophageal cancer and highlights the impact of the nutritional problems she endured:

> My biggest problem in this period was starvation. I could not eat and could drink only water, weak tea, apple juice and aloe vera. But I was being hydrated through my IV line. When I was at home, I could occasionally get some soup down (my kids and my friends made soups for me, out of thoughtfulness and love), and I drank vegetable juices that the kids prepared. And while the kids brought me food I could keep in the hospital refrigerator and heat in the microwave, I lacked the energy to do so. Even if I got something down, it wasn't enough. I had lost about 30 pounds and smilingly told the doctors I was starving; they smiled back. Jamie bought me a pin to attach to my velour tops; it said, in great big letters, I want food! But no one suggested that I be fed through my IV line; nor did I suggest it. I was waiting for the doctors to do so. My weakness seems to have affected my brain. Maybe the doctors weren't aware that my oesophagus was ulcerated from radiation. No one was watching over my whole person. Not even me.

Given the potential impact and high incidence of nutritional problems in cancer patients, there is surprisingly little research on the experience of anorexia, weight loss, cachexia or functional difficulties with eating and drinking. Much of the research to date has explored the biological and physical impact of alterations in nutrition and effects of nutritional support. However, as McClement & Woodgate (1997) suggest, nutritional problems need to be understood within social, historical and cultural contexts. Without an appreciation of the meaning and impact of altered nutritional status on both individuals and families, we cannot effectively address the problem.

The effects of altered nutritional status may be far-reaching. Many patients are no longer able to enjoy food or become socially isolated as a result of functional difficulties with eating and drinking. They and their families may also find the visible effects of anorexia and weight loss extremely distressing to watch. In addition, the physical and psychosocial consequences of these symptoms can be considerable. Malnutrition is associated with reduced muscle strength, impaired organ function, poor wound healing, increased treatment-related morbidity and mortality, poor quality of life and reduced survival (Shaw 2002). Studies have shown that patients with weight loss are more likely to require breaks in radiotherapy due to severe treatment reactions, reduced tolerance to treatment and poor performance status (Nayel et al 1992, Shaw 2002).

ASSESSMENT OF NUTRITIONAL STATUS

Unfortunately, malnutrition is frequently underrecognised (McWhirter & Pennington 1994). Delmore (1996) argues that the 'attitude of frustrating neglect' towards nutrition in cancer patients can no longer continue. Adequate nutritional assessment is the key to early recognition and support but, in practice, few patients having radiotherapy are properly assessed. Wilson (2000) emphasises the importance of listening to patients and observing their skin, hair and nails for signs of malnutrition. Laboratory tests can also identify nutritional deficiencies, although these must be carefully interpreted as certain changes may be related to underlying malignancy rather than specific nutritional problems (Mercadante 1996). A number of nutritional screening tools have also been developed, although it is argued that none of these is ideal. However, some consensus exists as to the importance of assessing weight loss, normal and current weight, height and appetite (Mercadante 1996, Shaw 2002). In the UK, body mass index (BMI) is accepted as a basic indicator of nutritional problems, calculated by measuring height and weight (in kilograms) (Garron & Janes 1993), with a score of less than 20 indicating the need for nutritional intervention (Lees 1999). A weight loss of 10% or more is also considered clinically significant.

Ferguson et al (1999) pointed out that there are no published studies of malnutrition in outpatients undergoing radiotherapy. His team devised a malnutrition screening tool (MST), specifically for use with radiotherapy patients, and tested this against the subjective global assessment (SGA) tool, accepted as the standard by the American Dietetics Association (Brown 1999). Although Ferguson et al (1999) endorse the value of the SGA, which assesses changes in weight, dietary intake, gastrointestinal symptoms and functional capacity as well as physical examination (Detsky et al 1987), they point out that it is too time-consuming and complex to screen all patients. In contrast, the MST is a simple tool, which the authors believe can be used by medical, nursing, dietetic or administrative staff. It asks three straightforward questions, as shown in Table 11.2. When compared with the SGA, the new tool was found to be both valid and reliable, with a sensitivity of 100% and a specificity of 81%, identifying all patients who were malnourished in a population of 106 radiotherapy patients. Ferguson et al (1999) suggest that the MST can be used to screen all patients undergoing radiotherapy, thus identifying those who require more detailed nutritional assessment.

Other authors support the use of a simple assessment which is able to identify patients most at risk. Detoog (1985) formulated risk criteria, using weight loss, serum albumin, dietary changes and use of supplementary feeding, to detect patients most in need of specialist dietetic input. Delmore (1997) also suggested a 'minimal screening assessment' (present weight in relation to ideal weight, weight change and serum albumin) which would lead into a complete assessment for those patients who are malnourished. He proposed that the following parameters should be included in this complete assessment:

- Dietary history (use of a food diary, 24-h recall of dietary intake)
- Comorbid disease
- Physical examination (of body fat, muscle wasting, specific nutritional deficiencies)
- Anthropometrics (height, weight, skinfold thickness measurements)

Table 11.2   Malnutrition screening tool (MST)

Question	Score
Have you lost weight recently without trying?	
No	0
Unsure	2
Yes	See below
If yes, how much weight (kg) have you lost?	
1–5	1
6–10	2
11–15	3
>15	4
Unsure	2
Have you been eating poorly because of a decreased appetite?	
No	0
Yes	1
Total[a]	

[a]Score of 2 or more = patient at risk of malnutrition.
Reprinted from Nutrition, vol. 15, Ferguson et al Development of a valid and reliable Malnutrition Screening Tool for adult acute hospital patients, p 458–464, copyright 1999, with permission from Elsevier Science.

- Laboratory tests (serum albumin – lowered in malnourished patients, creatinine – excretion can be indicative of protein mass)
- Immune function (total lymphocyte count – reduced in malnourished patients)
- SGA.

Although they are all relevant, there are a number of limitations to assessing some of the parameters described above. Taking a full dietary history, including detailed dietary patterns and preferences, can be time consuming, but methods such as 24-h recall or food diaries completed by patients or nurses are dependent on the accuracy and commitment of the person remembering or recording the dietary intake. Regular anthropometric measures such as height and weight may be inappropriate or inaccurate for patients with very advanced disease, oedema or lymphoedema, and are only reliable if patients are weighed on the same well-calibrated machine, in the same clothing each week. Skinfold thickness measurements are dependent on the skill of the person measuring, and they are not appropriate for general clinical use. Blood tests may be helpful, but only represent part of the picture.

When making a nutritional assessment, it is important to consider all the factors highlighted in Figure 11.1. Cultural, social and financial issues must be taken into account if nutritional intervention is to be acceptable and realistic for the patient. A dietary history should, ideally, include input from individuals and their families, as it is so often the carers who are responsible for preparing food. Additionally, it is vital that comorbid disease is taken into account. The presence of irritable bowel syndrome, for example, may exacerbate bowel symptoms produced in response to pelvic radiotherapy. Smoking and drinking tend also to be associated with greater nutritional problems (Hunter 1996). A patient who drinks heavily may be used to ingesting a large percentage of his calories from alcohol, and if he cuts down significantly during radiotherapy, he may require particularly close nutritional surveillance and support. A full blood count as well as baseline urea and electrolytes (U&Es) can help to ensure that any biochemical imbalances can be monitored carefully.

A drug history should also form part of a patient's nutritional assessment. Drugs such as opioid analgesics and antidepressants can cause constipation, dry mouth, nausea and anorexia, all of which are likely to interfere with nutritional intake. Others, such as bulk laxatives, may cause altered taste sensations or feelings of satiety because of the gastric bulk produced, and medications such as non-steroidal anti-inflammatory drugs may be associated with indigestion. Complementary medicines such as mineral, herbal and vitamin supplements can compromise the effects of other medications or treatments (Brown et al 2001), thus it is important that these, too, are considered.

Following initial assessment of an individual's nutritional risk and needs, it is essential that regular reassessment takes place. Visual analogue scales may be a helpful adjunct, enabling the patient's perspective to be taken into account (Macqueen & Frost 1998). Weekly 'on-treatment' review should incorporate assessment of weight, swallowing ability, pain, nausea and vomiting, appetite, oral intake, bowel habits and other associated symptoms such as indigestion, heartburn and excessive wind. Regular blood counts (including U&Es) may be indicated, particularly in patients undergoing radiotherapy to the head and neck or gastrointestinal tract.

Specialist dietetic input

As Lees (1999) points out (p. 134) 'the actual implementation of dietetic intervention is reliant upon other members of the multi-professional team detecting nutritional status of their client group and making the appropriate referral'. If nurses and radiographers on the front line do not make an initial assessment, nutritional status can become severely compromised by the time a referral is made, thus making it much more difficult to reverse the problem and improve quality of life. Timely referral is crucial if nutritional support is to be instigated when it can still be effective. Lees (1999) suggests the following criteria for referral to the dietician:

• Unexplained or sudden unplanned fall in body weight or existing low body weight (BMI < 20)
• Impaired food intake due to dysphagia, dry/sore mouth, chewing/dental difficulties, altered taste perception, nausea and vomiting, constipation, early satiety, anorexia
• Already taking prescribed nutritional supplements or tube/parenteral feeding
• Increased nutritional requirements, e.g. due to surgery, sepsis, infection, wounds
• Already requiring therapeutic diet, e.g. diabetic
• Following a complementary/alternative diet, e.g. Bristol
• Patient or carer expresses a wish for nutritional information or dietetic consultation.

Referral for specialist dietetic advice is not likely to be helpful unless the symptoms that are interfering with nutritional intake are adequately managed. If a patient is vomiting as a result of abdominal radiotherapy, or having severe pain from oral mucositis, no amount of dietetic input is likely to improve oral intake. Identifying the cause or causes of impaired nutritional intake and reversing or alleviating those causes is therefore a fundamental first step. Although the management of specific radiation-induced symptoms is addressed in other chapters within this book, dietary advice for patients suffering from these symptoms is given below.

THE MANAGEMENT OF ALTERED NUTRITIONAL STATUS

In common with all symptoms related to radiotherapy treatment, optimum management of altered nutritional status relies on a comprehensive assessment of the patient's needs. If all the factors contributing to altered nutritional status are identified, appropriate interventions can be instigated. As already stated, symptoms that interfere with the patient's ability to maintain nutrition must be effectively managed. The provision of information and education to patients and carers is also fundamental to any management strategy. Although nurses, doctors and radiographers working in radiotherapy can identify those at risk of nutritional problems and make the initial assessment, the input of the multidisciplinary team is essential. The contribution of the dietician is self-evident, but other members of the team also have an important role to play in nutritional management. Patients with swallowing or aspiration problems should be referred to the speech therapist, and patients with practical or functional difficulties should be assessed by the occupational therapist. Some patients may find it difficult to afford food items (such as extra cream and butter) to supplement their calorie intake, and others may not have access to essential equipment such as a liquidiser. A specialist nurse or social worker may be able to arrange financial help in these circumstances.

Wilson (2000) suggests some useful guidelines on which to base nutritional management (p. 25):

- Assess current nutritional status and potential for its deterioration
- Determine calorie and protein needs in collaboration with dietician
- Monitor and maintain food intake
- Incorporate creative presentation and preparation of foods as appropriate to patient's symptoms
- Assess patient's meal habits, food preferences and socialisation when eating
- Assess lifestyle choices that affect nutritional status
- Assist with feeding as needed
- Assist in providing community support (e.g. with food shopping and preparation)
- Provide enteral or parenteral support if prescribed
- Monitor for complications associated with nutritional support
- Evaluate patient's response to nutritional interventions, monitoring weight and other relevant parameters
- Support and reassure patient and family.

The successful management of altered nutritional status requires the commitment of patients and their carers. In a situation where much choice and control is lost, the planning and preparation of food and drink provide an opportunity for patients and carers to be centrally involved. Carers often feel helpless when the meals they have prepared are rejected because patients cannot swallow them, or have developed taste changes that alter their usual likes and dislikes. Although it is not always possible to tempt a failing appetite (and this can be very distressing for carers), the provision of dietary information can enable carers to prepare foods that are more likely to be tolerated. Patients will adopt their own eating strategies (Wilson et al 1991) but many of these arise through trial and error. Several excellent booklets exist for patients and carers, containing general advice, self-care measures and recipes for patients with specific nutritional needs.

All patients undergoing radiotherapy should be given information and advice about the actual and potential side effects of their treatment, so that they are pre-pared for any nutritional problems they may experience. Although not all patients will encounter difficulties with eating and drinking as a result of radiotherapy, an initial nutritional assessment provides the opportunity to advise about healthy eat-ing during and after treatment, so as to promote tissue recovery.

Table 11.3 illustrates self-care strategies and dietary advice for patients suffering from particular symptoms induced by cancer or radiotherapy treatment. It is important that patients' symptoms and ability to self-care are regularly reviewed during treatment so that further nutritional support using dietary supplements or enteral/parenteral feeding can be initiated promptly. Cultural and religious beliefs must also be taken into account, as it may be more difficult for certain ethnic groups to modify their diets. For example, patients who are used to eating very spicy food may require particular support and guidance to accept and prepare a bland diet.

Some areas of controversy exist in relation to the most appropriate dietary advice for certain groups of patients undergoing radiotherapy. Many departments still recommend low-fibre diets for patients who are receiving pelvic treatment, despite there being no real evidence that radiation-induced diarrhoea improves as a result (Faithfull 2001). There is, however, increasing evidence that elemental and low-fat diets are effective at reducing diarrhoea. Bile acid malabsorption is impaired as a result of pelvic radiotherapy, thus a diet low in fat tends to be better tolerated by the damaged gut mucosa. An example of a low-fat diet is shown in Table 11.4.

NUTRITIONAL SUPPORT

When patients have lost weight unintentionally, or their ability to eat and drink is impaired, nutritional support may be required. Although a meta-analysis conducted in the 1990s failed to demonstrate specific benefits associated with enteral and parenteral nutrition in cancer patients (Klein & Koretz 1994), a number of studies show the benefits of oral nutritional support during radiotherapy. Nayel et al (1992) randomly allocated 23 patients with head and neck cancer to receive either radiotherapy alone or radiotherapy with oral nutritional supplementation using high-protein supplements. Although there were no differences in the fre-quency of dry mouth, taste changes or loss of appetite, those who did not receive nutritional supplements experienced greater difficulty swallowing. Radiotherapy had to be suspended in five of the 12 patients in this group because of severe mucosal reactions, and 58% also experienced weight loss. However, there were no interruptions to treatment in the group who took supplements, and all patients experienced an increase in weight and triceps skinfold thickness.

Table 11.3   Dietary advice and self-care measures to alleviate specific symptoms associated with altered nutritional intake

Symptom	Dietary advice and self-care measures
Anorexia	Provide small, frequent, high-calorie meals and snacks throughout the day Encourage favourite foods Use high-energy foods to enhance calorie intake, e.g. cream, butter, full-fat milk, cheese, eggs Use gentle exercise, relaxation or alcohol to stimulate the appetite Try to make the environment as normal as possible for eating, encouraging family meals where possible Encourage attractive presentation of foods, using colours and textures as appropriate Modify the consistency and temperature of food as necessary (cold foods have less odour so tend to be better tolerated if nausea or smell is a problem)
Mucositis, stomatitis or xerostomia (dry mouth)	Encourage regular mouthwashes before and after food, avoiding commercial mouthwash preparations Ensure adequate analgesia and premeal medication are given as necessary Use a liquidiser or mouli, or choose soft or liquid foods such as soups, mashed potatoes, cooked/puréed vegetables and fruit, milk puddings, custard Provide bland foods, avoiding anything acidic, salty or spicy Avoid dry or coarse food Add extra sauces, gravy or cream to solid foods Use straws to avoid excessive irritation of the oral mucosa Avoid smoking and drinking alcohol (both are drying to the mucous membranes)
Taste changes	Use plastic cutlery if the patient has a metallic taste Experiment with herbs, flavourings and spices, marinades and sauces Try tart foods, including fruit and fruit juices, unless mucositis is a problem Try white meat and dairy products rather than red meats
Dysphagia	Use techniques for mucositis as above Refer to speech therapist for swallowing advice
Oesophagitis/gastritis	Offer bland, soft foods Avoid smoking, drinking and spicy or acidic foods Consider the use of antacids or coating agents to ease discomfort
Early satiety	Provide small frequent meals and nutritious snacks Avoid fatty foods which can delay gastric emptying Make the most of times of the day when the appetite is greater (this is often breakfast) Avoid drinking large amounts with meals Consider the use of drugs that enhance gastric emptying, e.g. metoclopramide
Nausea and vomiting	Give prescribed antiemetics half an hour before meals Provide small, frequent meals Dry, bland foods may be easier to take Try fizzy drinks and ginger-flavoured foods and drinks Sip drinks slowly through a straw Try foods at different temperatures – cold or room temperature may be best
Diarrhoea	Ensure fluids are replaced Encourage a low-fat diet Consider antidiarrhoeal medication Consider reducing dietary fibre if low-fat diet is ineffective Caution is required, as low-fibre diets can result in constipation and abdominal cramps

Table 11.4 Suggestions for a low-fat diet

Foods to avoid	Recommended foods
Whole milk, full-cream condensed milk, evaporated milk, cream, lard, dripping, vegetable oil	Fresh skimmed milk, skimmed condensed milk
Hard cheese, cream cheese	Dried skimmed milk, e.g. Marvel, Boots, Country Maid
Fatty and all red meats, liver and kidney, sausages, oily fish such as sardines, herrings, fish tinned in oil, paté, duck, meat pies	Cottage cheese, low-fat yoghurt, quark, skimmed-milk cheese
Crisps, chips, roast potatoes, fried vegetables	Chicken and turkey (no skin), white fish, smoked white fish, e.g. smoked haddock
Avocado pears	Vegetables – fresh, frozen or tinned
Pastry, whole-milk puddings, suet puddings, dumplings	Salad vegetables, potatoes
Cakes made with fat, chocolate biscuits, cream biscuits, shortbread	Fruit – fresh, tinned, frozen, dried, stewed, baked. Fruit juice, fruit squash, fizzy drinks
Chocolate, toffee, fudge, icecream, nuts, peanut butter, lemon curd, marzipan, butterscotch	Rice, spaghetti, macaroni, sago, semolina, tapioca, flour, cornflour, custard powder
Salad cream, mayonnaise, salad dressings containing oil	Instant desserts made with skimmed milk, table jellies, gelatine, sorbet
Cream soups	Egg white, meringues, fat-free cakes, e.g. Swiss roll, fatless sponge
	Bread, plain biscuits, crispbreads, water biscuits
	Breakfast cereals, porridge
	Sugar, jam, marmalade, honey, syrup
	Boiled sweets, mints, fruit gums, pastilles, water ice lollies
	Chutney, bottled sauces, pickles, vinegar, mustard, salt, pepper, herbs, spices
	Bovril, Oxo, Marmite, stock cubes
	Tea, coffee, essences, flavourings, Horlicks, Ovaltine, drinking chocolate, Carnation Build-up (made with skimmed or semiskimmed milk)

A larger study of patients undergoing radiotherapy to the head and neck, breast or abdomen/pelvis compared 62 patients who were given no dietetic instruction with 30 patients who received specific dietary advice tailored to their nutritional needs and preferences (Macia et al 1991). Although the design of this study is somewhat flawed, there are some interesting aspects to the dietary advice given and the results achieved. The experimental groups were given natural-food supplements using stewed fruit, nuts, jam, honey and mixed preparations, as well as advice on foods they could obtain easily in their area. Those receiving radiotherapy to the head and neck were given advice on soft or liquidised diets, and those having abdominal radiotherapy followed a gluten- and lactose-free diet. There were no real differences between the two breast groups as neither had specific nutritional problems, but the control groups for both head and neck and abdominopelvic patients experienced a deterioration in their symptoms compared with the experimental groups. Radiotherapy had to be suspended for a total of 96 days in the head and neck control group because of severe mucosal and skin reactions, whereas there were no treatment breaks in the experimental group.

The efficacy of enteral and parenteral feeding in cancer patients remains controversial (Shaw 2002). Some studies have shown benefits in surgical patients, but fewer studies have been conducted in those undergoing radiotherapy or chemotherapy. However, one study of 50 dysphagic patients with oesophageal cancer who were undergoing combined chemoradiotherapy found that enteral nutrition during treatment resulted in stable weight, visceral proteins and serum albumin, whereas a standard oral diet was associated with a decrease in all these outcomes (Bozzetti et al 1998).

The overall goal of treatment and care must be kept at the forefront of any decisions made to instigate nutritional support (Pennell 2001). Enteral and parenteral feeding are associated with complications (Klein & Koretz 1994), and may be inappropriate in patients with advanced disease, for whom the goal of treatment is palliative. The aims of nutritional support should be to increase tolerance so as to enable treatment to be completed, and to improve quality of life (Shaw 2002). If aggressive nutritional support is likely to necessitate hospitalisation, induce complications or create difficulties for patients and families in coming to terms with their situation, it is probably inappropriate. In this case, the aim of nutritional support should be adaptive rather than restorative, based upon the needs of the patient and family.

Oral supplementation

A wide variety of oral nutritional supplements are available commercially, although they are expensive for patients to buy over the counter, and many require a prescription from the dietician and general practitioner (GP). Most are high in protein and energy, and they offer a useful means of increasing nutritional intake for patients who are reluctant to eat. Many liquid supplements (e.g. Ensure Plus, Fresubin, Enlive) are available in cartons, making them very convenient to use, although not always to patients' taste. Others such as Build-Up, Complan or Scandishake are in powdered form and have to be mixed with milk. Fortified soups and puddings are also available, and tasteless powders such as Maxijul can be added to any food or drink to boost calorie intake. If patients have difficulty with thin liquids because they are more likely to aspirate, products such as Thick 'n' easy can be added to thicken the consistency of drinks and make them easier to swallow.

Although nutritional supplements can be extremely helpful, not all patients like the taste, and over time, many experience taste fatigue, where they become tired of the same flavours, and become uninterested in supplementing their diet. McCarthy & Weihofen (1999) also questioned whether taking supplements between meals might ruin the appetite, thus reducing patients' intake of solid food. Their study investigated dietary intake in 40 patients undergoing radiotherapy, half of whom were randomly assigned to take a liquid nutritional supplement between each meal and at bedtime. Those who took supplements had a higher calorie and protein intake each day than those who did not, but their normal food intake did not diminish as a result.

This small study included patients having radiotherapy to a variety of sites, and excluded those who might have been more vulnerable to nutritional problems, such as patients with head and neck cancer. It cannot be assumed, therefore, that the effect of nutritional supplements would be the same with patients who were initially malnourished or specifically at risk. However, one interesting finding was that the group who did not take supplements maintained their baseline level of food intake throughout the first 4 weeks of radiotherapy, a period during which they might have been expected to have less of an appetite. The authors propose that this effect may have been associated with the weekly dietary 'counselling' received by all patients in the study, suggesting that regular input from the dietician is worthwhile. Another study by Ireton-Jones et al (1995) also suggests that nutritional outcomes in cancer patients are improved as a result of referral to the dietician, but there are no large well-designed studies to confirm these findings. Until malnutrition is sufficiently appreciated and recognised, such evidence is unlikely to be available. McWhirter & Pennington (1994) found that, although 40% of the 500 patients admitted to general wards during their prospective study were malnourished, less than half of these had any nutritional information recorded in their case notes, and only 2% were referred for nutritional support. A significantly greater proportion of those who received nutritional support gained weight, demonstrating that malnutrition can be effectively managed, provided it is recognised in the first place.

Enteral tube feeding

Patients who are unable to meet their protein, carbohydrate, fats, vitamin and calorific needs orally may benefit from enteral tube feeding, provided their gut is functioning normally. As Shaw (2002) states, the choice of tube depends on the patients' wishes, their physical condition and the likely duration of feeding. Nasogastric tubes are a useful short-term measure, but they frequently become dislodged and can be difficult to pass in some patients with oropharyngeal or oesophageal tumours. Many patients also find the appearance of a nasogastric tube unacceptable. Other forms of enteral feeding are more invasive, requiring surgical or endoscopic insertion. Probably the most popular form of enteral feeding for head and neck cancer patients is via a percutaneous endoscopic gastrostomy (PEG) tube, whereby a feeding tube is placed endoscopically through a fistula created between the stomach and the anterior abdominal wall (Liddle & Yuill 1995). Jejunostomy tubes can be useful after upper gastrointestinal surgery. Feeds can be delivered at home or in hospital, and can be given intermittently, continuously or by bolus, depending on the patient's nutritional needs and wishes. Although the majority of cancer patients require whole-protein feeds (Shaw 2002), patients with malabsorption problems such as those receiving radiotherapy to the pelvis can safely receive elemental, low-fat or defined formula feeds (Holmes 1999).

Unfortunately, enteral feeding does have side effects and complications. Some patients develop diarrhoea, although the composition of feeds can sometimes be changed to overcome this problem. Nausea and vomiting, dumping syndrome, aspiration, infection, fluid and electrolyte imbalances, abdominal pain, constipation, migration or blockage of the tube can also occur (Brown 1999, Klein & Koretz 1994). PEG tubes that leak or are badly positioned can cause daily discomfort and misery, so it is vital that they are regularly reassessed. Successful enteral feeding requires education of the patient and family, close monitoring and regular communication between all members of the multidisciplinary team, both in hospital and the community.

Parenteral feeding

Parenteral feeding is rarely indicated in radiotherapy patients, and its use must be considered carefully as it is associated with life-threatening complications such as sepsis, air embolism, venous thrombosis and serious metabolic disorders. If a patient's gastrointestinal tract is not functioning, parenteral feeding may be the only option. The toxic effects of combined chemoradiotherapy, bone marrow transplantation and total body irradiation may necessitate parenteral feeding if gastrointestinal symptoms are very severe. Total parenteral nutrition (TPN) is usually administered via an indwelling venous access device, such as a Hickman line. Although it can be given at home, this can present a major burden to patients and families and requires significant dietetic and medical support (Brown 1999). It is also very expensive, and its efficacy during radiotherapy and chemotherapy has not been proven (Klein & Koretz 1994).

Pharmacological interventions

The use of drugs to stimulate appetite in cancer patients remains controversial. There is insufficient evidence to support the routine use of appetite stimulants (Fainsinger 1996, Tait 1999) but several drugs appear to have beneficial effects on nutritional status and the symptoms of cachexia (Bruera 1997). Corticosteroids, progestational and prokinetic drugs are the drugs of choice, but each has limitations and side effects. Corticosteroids are only advisable for short periods due to their long-term complications (Herrington et al 1997). Although they can improve anorexia and weakness in cancer patients, they do not appear to be associated with a corresponding improvement in weight or nutritional status. They do, however, have antiemetic and analgesic effects, and may inhibit the release of metabolic products by the tumour or immune system, so they can be useful in patients with advanced disease (Bruera 1997).

Progestational drugs such as medroxyprogesterone acetate (MPA) have been specifically tested in radiotherapy patients and do seem to result in improvements in appetite, weight loss and quality of life (Chen et al 1997, Fietkau et al 1997), although they are expensive. They are also associated with side effects, namely oedema and thrombosis (Bruera 1997). Prokinetic agents such as Metoclopramide, cisapride and domperidone increase gastric emptying and thus can be effective if the patient is suffering from nausea and/or early satiety. There is currently insufficient evidence for most other drugs, although clinical trials are ongoing (Bruera 1997). A recent study by Ripamonti et al (1998) has, for instance, demonstrated that zinc sulphate supplements can improve taste changes, and therefore has a positive effect on nutritional intake.

Alternative diets

Many patients now choose to follow alternative diets, which they believe may improve their well-being or have a positive impact on their cancer. The beneficial effect of these diets is generally unproven (Shaw 2002) and controversies exist over the safety of some dietary regimens (Brown et al 2001). Healthcare professionals can help patients to make an informed choice by providing information about the nutritional value, ease and practicality, cost and appropriateness of alternative diets, considering the potential benefits for the individual along with any areas of concern in relation to their cancer treatment.

CONCLUSION

Nutrition is fundamental to our well-being, but the maintenance of an adequate nutritional intake can pose an enormous challenge to patients with cancer and those who care for them. Metabolic changes, physical and psychological symptoms and the side effects and consequences of cancer therapy can all compromise nutritional status. The multifactorial nature of most nutritional problems explains why most patients experience alterations in their nutritional status at some stage of the cancer trajectory. Studies show that a significant number are malnourished, and that the impact on quality of life can be profound. Many of the toxicities associated with radiotherapy cause particular nutritional problems. The anticipation and management of such problems rely on an initial assessment of nutritional needs and the provision of appropriate dietary information and education about self-care strategies. Patients who are particularly at risk, such as those with cancers of the head and neck, lung and gastrointestinal tract, should be considered for dietetic referral at the beginning of treatment. Others should be assessed regularly so that early intervention and nutritional support can be instigated at the appropriate time. A multidisciplinary approach to altered nutritional status is likely to be most effective, with the dietician playing a central role. Further research is required to explore the full nature and impact of specific nutritional problems. Nutritional assessment should, however, be considered pivotal to the supportive care of patients undergoing radiotherapy.

SUMMARY OF KEY CLINICAL POINTS

- Nutrition is not only important for health, but also has psychosocial and cultural significance.
- Malnutrition is extremely common in patients with cancer. Altered nutritional status arises as a result of metabolic changes, physical and psychological effects of cancer and its treatment.
- Weight loss, anorexia and cachexia affect many patients with cancer, particularly those with metastatic disease and those with cancers of the lung, head and neck and gastrointestinal tract.
- Radiotherapy causes particular nutritional problems, especially when the head and neck or gastrointestinal tract are included in the treatment field.
- Assessment is the key to adequate nutritional support, but relatively little attention is paid to assessing the nutritional status of patients undergoing radiotherapy.
- Screening and assessment tools should be more widely used in radiotherapy. Any assessment should take account of physical, functional and psychosocial symptoms, as well as weight loss and BMI.

- A multidisciplinary approach to the management of nutritional problems is essential. The dietician plays a particularly important role, and should be involved at an early stage when nutritional support is required.
- Patient information and education are important components of nutritional management. Wherever possible, carers should also be involved.
- The management of nutritional problems should include symptom management, promotion of self-care strategies and dietary advice relevant to individuals and family as well as pertinent to their particular treatment.
- Oral, enteral and parenteral feeding or supplementation may be required for certain patients. Early intervention is crucial, if nutritional support is to be effective.
- Pharmacological interventions may have a place in the management of nutritional problems. It must also be recognised that certain drugs can interfere with appetite and nutritional intake.

AREAS FOR FURTHER RESEARCH

- The incidence, nature and severity of nutritional problems in radiotherapy patients
- Educational/action research to improve the recognition and management of nutritional problems amongst ward and outpatient staff
- The development and evaluation of assessment tools specific to oncology and radiotherapy patients
- The experience of weight loss and anorexia
- The development and evaluation of nutritional interventions aimed at educating and facilitating patients and carers to improve nutritional status
- The efficacy of low-fat versus low-fibre diets in patients undergoing pelvic radiotherapy
- The evaluation of nurse/dietician-led clinics aimed at minimising alterations to nutritional status during radiotherapy
- The use of pharmacological and non-pharmacological methods to improve appetite and enhance nutritional intake.

FURTHER INFORMATION

Sources of information and dietary advice

Diet and the cancer patient (1997)
Cancer BACUP
3 Bath Place
Rivington Street
London
EC2A 3DR
Tel: 0800 18 11 99
Tel: 0207 696 9003 (publications)
http://www.cancerbacup.org.uk

Eating hints for cancer patients before, during and after treatment (1997)
National Cancer Institute
http://www.cancernet.nci.nih.gov/peb/eating_hints/index.html

Eating: helping yourself (1997)
Department of Clinical Audit and Quality Assurance
Centre for Cancer Epidemiology
Christie Hospital NHS Trust
Kinnaird Road
Withington
Manchester
M20 4QL
Tel: 0161 446 3576
http://christie.man.ac.uk

Overcoming eating difficulties. A guide for cancer patients (1997)
Royal Marsden NHS Trust
Available from:
Hochland and Hochland
174a Ashley Road
Hale
Cheshire
WA15 9SF
Tel: 0161 929 0190

Helpful Hints Series 3 Appetite
Helpful Hint Series 5 Taste changes
Helpful Hints Series 4 Preventing weight loss
A guide to people having chewing and swallowing problems
Lynda Jackson Macmillan Centre
Mount Vernon Centre for Cancer Treatment
Mount Vernon Hospital
Northwood
Middlesex
HA6 2RN
Tel: 01923 844014
http://mountvernonhospital.co.uk

REFERENCES

Bozzetti F, Cozzaglio L, Gavazzi C et al 1998 Nutritional support in patients with cancer of the oesophagus: impact on nutritional status, patient compliance to therapy and survival. Tumori 84:681–686

Brookes G 1985 Nutritional status – a prognostic indicator in head and neck cancer. Otolaryngology Head and Neck Surgery 93:69–74

Brown P 1999 Nutrition and cancer. Medical Surgical Nursing 8:333–345

Brown J, Byers T, Thompson K et al 2001 Nutrition during and after cancer treatment: a guide for informed choices by cancer survivors. CA: A Cancer Journal for Clinicians 51:153–181

Bruera E 1997 ABC of palliative care: anorexia, cachexia, and nutrition. British Medical Journal 315:1219–1222

Chen H C, Leung S W, Wang C J et al 1997 Effect of megestrol acetate and prepulsid on nutritional improvement in patients with head and neck cancers undergoing radiotherapy. Radiotherapy and Oncology 43(1):75–79

Curtis E B 1991 Common symptoms in patients with advanced cancer. Journal of Palliative Care 7(2):25–29

Delmore G 1996 Nutrition in cancer patients: frustrating neglect and permanent challenge. Support Care Cancer 4:1–3

Delmore G 1997 Assessment of nutritional status in cancer patients: widely neglected? Support Care Cancer 5:376–380

Detoog S 1985 Identifying patients at nutritional risk and determining clinical productivity: essentials for an effective nutrition care program. Journal of the American Dietetic Association 85:1620–1622

Detsky A, McLaughlin J, Baker J 1987 What is subjective global assessment of nutritional status? Journal of Parenteral and Enteral Nutrition 11:8–13

De Wys W 1980 Nutritional care of the cancer patient. Journal of the American Medical Association 244:374–376

Donnelly S, Walsh D 1995 The symptoms of advanced cancer; identification of clinical research priorities by assessment of prevalence and severity. Journal of Palliative Care 11(1):27–32

Fainsinger R 1996 Pharmacological approaches to cancer and cachexia. In: Bruera E, Higginson I (eds) Cachexia – anorexia in cancer patients. Oxford University Press, Oxford, p 128–140

Faithfull S 2001 Radiotherapy. In: Corner J, Bailey C (eds) Cancer nursing: care in context. Blackwell Science, Oxford, p 222–261

Ferguson M, Bauer J, Gallagher B et al (1999a) Validation of a malnutrition screening tool for patients receiving radiotherapy. Australasian Radiology 43:325–327

Ferguson et al 1999 Development of a valid & reliable Malnutrition Screening Tool for adult acute hospital patients. Nutrition 15: 458–464.

Fietkau R, Riepl M, Kettner H et al 1997 Supportive use of megestrol acetate in patients with head and neck cancer during radio (chemo) therapy. European Journal of Cancer 33(1):75–79

French M 1999 A season in hell. Virago, London

Garron, J S, Janes W P T (eds) 1993 Human nutrition and dietetics, 9th edn. Churchill Livingstone, Edinburgh

Heber D, Byerley L, Jocelyn C et al 1986 Pathophysiology of malnutrition in the adult cancer patient. Cancer 58:1867–1873

Herrington A, Herrington J, Church C 1997 Pharmacologic options for the treatment of cachexia. Nutrition in Clinical Practice 12:101–113

Hespanhol V, Queiroga H, Magalhaes A et al (1995) Survival predictors in advanced small cell lung cancer. Lung Cancer 13: 253–267

Holden C M 1991 Anorexia in the terminally ill cancer patient: the emotional impact on the patient and the family. Hospice Journal 7(3):73–84

Holmes S 1999 Nutrition and radiotherapy. Nursing Times Clinical Monographs no. 20. NT Books/Emap Healthcare, London

Hunter A 1996 Nutrition management of patients with neoplastic disease of the head and neck treated with radiation therapy. Nutrition in Clinical Practice 11:157–169

Ireton-Jones C, Garritson B, Kitchens L 1995 Nutrition intervention in cancer patients: does the registered dietician make a difference? Topics in Clinical Nutrition 10:42–48

Klein S, Koretz R 1994 Nutrition support in patients with cancer: what do the data really show? Nutrition in Clinical Practice 9:91–100

Lees J 1999 Incidence of weight loss in head and neck cancer patients on commencing radiotherapy treatment at a regional oncology centre. European Journal of Cancer Care 8:133–136

Liddle K, Yuill R 1995 Making sense of percutaneous endoscopic gastrostomy. Nursing Times 9(18):32–33

McCarthy D, Weihofen D 1999 The effect of nutritional supplements on food intake in patients undergoing radiotherapy. Oncology Nursing Forum 26:897–900

McClement S E, Woodgate R L 1997 Care of the terminally ill cachectic cancer patient: interface between nursing and psychological anthropology. European Journal of Cancer Care 6:295–303

McNamara M J, Alexander R, Norton J A 1992 Cytokines and their role in the pathophysiology of cancer cachexia. Journal of Parenteral and Enteral Nutrition 16 (suppl.):50–55

McWhirter J P, Pennington C 1994 Incidence and recognition of malnutrition in hospital. British Medical Journal 308:945–948

Macia E, Moran J, Santos J et al 1991 Nutrition. Nutritional evaluation and dietetic care in cancer patients treated with radiotherapy: prospective study. Nutrition 7:205–209

Macqueen C, Frost G 1998 Visual analog scales: a screening tool for assessing nutritional need in head and neck radiotherapy patients. Journal of Human Nutrition and Dietetics 11:115–124

Mattes R, Curran W, Powlis W et al 1991 A descriptive study of learned food aversions in radiotherapy patients. Physiology and Behaviour 50:1103–1109

Mercadante S 1996 Nutrition in cancer patients. Support Care Cancer 4:10–20

Nayel H, El-Ghoneimy E, El-Haddad S 1992 Impact of nutritional supplementation on treatment delay and morbidity in patients with head and neck tumours treated with irradiation. Nutrition 8(1):13–18

Naylor W, Laverty D, Mallett J (eds) 2001 The Royal Marsden book of wound management in cancer care. Blackwell Science, Oxford

Ottery F 1994 Cancer cachexia: prevention, early diagnosis, and management. Cancer Practice 2:123–131

Pennell M 2001 Compromised nutrition. In: Corner J, Bailey C (eds) Cancer nursing: care in context. Blackwell Science: Oxford, p 409–413

Ripamonti C, Zecca E, Brunelli C et al 1998 A randomised controlled clinical trial to evaluate the effects of zinc sulphate on cancer patients with taste alterations caused by head and neck irradiation. Cancer 82:1938–1945

Shaw C 2002 Therapeutic aspects of nutrition in cancer patients. In: Souhami R, Tannock I, Hohenberger P et al (eds) Oxford textbook of oncology, vol. 1. Oxford University Press, Oxford, p 1007–1015

Tait S N 1999 Anorexia – cochexia symdrome. In: Yarbro C H, Frogge M H, Goodman M (eds) Cancer symptom management, 2nd edn. Jones and Bartlett, Boston, p 183–197

Vianio A, Auvinen A 1996 Prevalence of symptoms among patients with advanced cancer; an international collaborative study. Journal of Pain and Symptom Management 12(1):3–10

Wells M 1995 The impact of radiotherapy to the head and neck: a qualitative study of patients after completion of treatment. Centre for cancer and palliative care studies. Institute of Cancer Research, London

Wilson P, Herman J, Chubon S 1991 Eating strategies used by persons with head and neck cancer during and after radiotherapy. Cancer Nursing 14:98–104

Wilson R 2000 Optimising nutrition for patients with cancer. Clinical Journal of Oncology Nursing 4:23–28

12

Urinary symptoms and radiotherapy

Sara Faithfull

INTRODUCTION

Radiation to any site within the pelvis can cause acute damage to the many adjacent pelvic structures. Although such damage may be intentional, for example in the case of irradiating the bladder for transitional cell carcinoma, it also occurs unintentionally when treating prostate, rectal and gynaecological cancers. Because pelvic tumours commonly sit close to or invade surrounding organs, incidental irradiation of bladder tissues is often unavoidable. The close proximity of bladder, ureter and urethral tissues in the pelvis means that urinary problems are a common consequence of radiotherapy treatment (Marks et al 1995). Incidence figures for bladder symptoms vary widely in the reported literature from 23 to 80% (Klee et al 2000, Pilpepch et al 1987, Raghavan 1992). This wide variance partly reflects the different time–dose–volume factors inherent in different treatment regimes but also the hidden and embarrassing nature of such symptoms and possible underreporting. Acute symptoms include pain or burning on micturition (dysuria), increased frequency and urgency of passing urine (passing urine more than every 2 h), incontinence or leakage and nocturia (getting up at night to pass urine) (Berry 1999). These symptoms can continue for many weeks to months during and following radiotherapy. The resulting pattern of symptoms is uncomfortable, causes disruption to sleep, results in isolation and influences quality of life. Relatively few studies have been published concerning the management of urinary problems following radiotherapy. This chapter explores the current evidence and uses wider urological literature to explore possible management strategies that may be of benefit to patients undergoing radiotherapy.

THE AETIOLOGY OF ACUTE BLADDER SIDE EFFECTS

Urinary symptoms resulting from radiotherapy to the pelvis occur for a number of reasons. Symptoms can arise as a result of mechanical obstruction secondary to

227

swelling of the prostate, contraction of smooth-muscle tissue at the bladder neck or through inflammation of the bladder lining. Understanding the aetiology of urinary symptoms is important for assessment and management. In order to explain symptoms, an understanding of normal bladder function is necessary. The epithelial lining of the bladder is composed of three to seven layers of transitional cells (urothelium), resting on a basement membrane (Fig. 12.1). The surface urothelium is coated with sulphated polysaccharides (glycosaminoglycans) that act as a permeability barrier and prevent attachment of substances such as bacteria and proteins but allow certain ions to pass through (this acts rather like a Goretex layer on a coat stopping rain coming through but allowing air to pass out) (Dorr et al 1998). Beyond the superficial layers lies smooth connective tissue with smooth-muscle fibres. The muscle wall (detrusor muscle) has many bundles of fibres layered in different directions so that they converge to form three distinct layers that extend down the urethra, finishing at differing levels. An external sphincter controls the voluntary mechanisms of the bladder and acts rather like a tap holding the urine in or letting it out as required. In infants where cerebral control is lacking, a sustained detrusor contraction can initiate the passing of urine. In adults the control of the bladder is via suppression of this reflex (Fig. 12.2). Normal bladder capacity is 400–500 ml of urine. Damage to the bladder or urethra may reduce storage capacity and influence when and how urine is expelled.

The effects of radiotherapy treatment may vary depending on the dose delivered to the bladder (Marks et al 1995). The early reactions of tissues to radiation in the bladder are related to inflammation and injury to the epithelial cell layer.

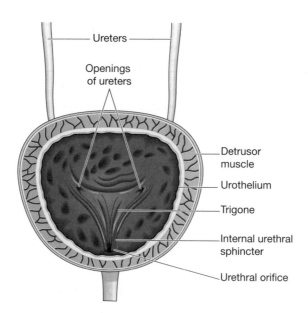

Figure 12.1 Section of the bladder and bladder wall (Adapted with permission from Waugh & Grant 2001.)

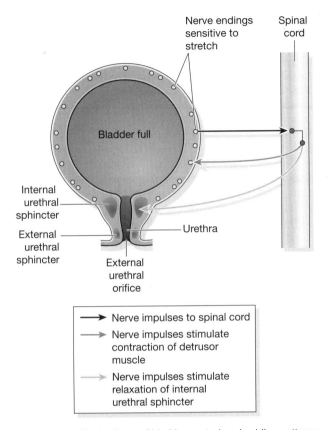

Figure 12.2   Mechanisms of bladder control and voiding patterns. (Adapted with permission from Waugh & Grant 2001.)

Computerised tomography (CT) of the bladder shortly after irradiation shows increased bladder wall thickness and reduction of bladder volume, possibly as a result of inflammation (Lundbeck 1993, Sager et al 1990). However, a similar study using CT planning scans found that bladder volume increased in some men with prostate cancer during pelvic treatment and this was considered to be as a result of partial bladder outflow obstruction (Scrase et al 1999). Radiation damage occurs at a dose of around 15–30 Gy, usually 2–3 weeks into treatment (Woodhouse 1990). Microscopic changes seen in experimental studies include inflammation, oedema, lymphocytic infiltration and degeneration of the epithelium, partially due to the high mitotic activity of superficial cells (Dorr et al 1998). Further damage causes ulceration, submucosal petechiae and loss of protein into the urine, sometimes resulting in haematuria detected within a urine specimen. The impairment of the permeability barrier by the superficial layer of glycosaminoglycans and urothelial cells may also contribute to some of the functional changes. Leakiness of the bladder lining may bring cells in contact with urine causing subsequent sublethal damage. As radiation dose increases, the inflammatory changes become worse. This causes increased sensitivity of the bladder lining, pain and instability of the bladder muscles, resulting in reduced bladder capacity and further symptoms of frequency and dysuria. The presence of tumour or surgical damage in the bladder may also make the symptoms following radiotherapy more pronounced (Marks et al 1995). Bladder tone is regulated by prostaglandins produced in the urothelium. Changes in prostaglandin synthesis as a result of these inflammatory changes could result in increased baseline tone and reduced storage capacity, however the exact mechanisms are unclear (Dorr et al 1998).

The radiation changes referred to form a cluster of urinary symptoms which in reality overlap, although they are often grouped as 'obstructive' or 'irritative'. The incidence of these symptoms for different treatment groups is shown in Table 12.1. Acute symptoms usually subside several weeks following radiotherapy, but the exact mechanisms and sequence of events are not clearly understood. Detailed clinical data of the factors influencing radiation changes in the bladder are scarce, as few techniques are available for objective measurement of bladder function (Hanfman et al 1998).

RISK FACTORS FOR URINARY PROBLEMS

The likelihood of acute radiation changes depends on the actual dose received by each structure of the bladder and prior damage that has occurred (Table 12.2). Curative treatment to the bladder is more likely to cause symptoms, since acute side effects may begin as early as 15 Gy and are likely at doses of 30–40 Gy. Urinary complications are directly related to the size of the radiation field and radiation dose (Ames & Gray 2000). The likelihood of urinary problems is increased if radiotherapy is delivered following adjuvant cancer treatment such as

Table 12.1 Incidence of urinary symptoms following pelvic radiotherapy

Site of therapy	Incidence and pattern of urinary symptoms
Prostate cancer	External beam: pretreatment urinary frequency 20%, 16% at 3 months and 9% at 12 months. Nocturia pretreatment 41%, 60% at 3 months and 43% at 12 months (Beard et al 1997) Brachytherapy: 79% experienced urinary problems initially after treatment. At 12 months 22% of men had persistent urinary morbidity (Brown et al 2000)
Bladder cancer	External beam radiotherapy: 30–80% of patients experience urinary symptoms (Lynch et al 1992, Quilty et al 1985)
Gynaecological cancer	During radiotherapy the most common urinary symptom is frequent voiding and pain or soreness at voiding (Klee et al 2000). The overall rate of urinary sequelae posttreatment is 8–12%. Incontinence is a common problem posttreatment: 45% of women in a survey complained of this symptom (Parkin et al 1987)
Rectal cancer	A decrease in micturition volume of 20% between week 2 and 5 of radiotherapy, resulting in frequency (Hanfman et al 1998)

Table 12.2 Risk factors for radiation-induced urinary symptoms

Treatment-related risk factors
Dose of radiotherapy
Volume
Brachytherapy
Adjuvant chemotherapy
Intravesical BCG (Bacillus Calmette-Guérin)
Previous neurological deficits
Comorbid disease
Surgery to bladder
Transurethral resection of the prostate (TURP)
Hysterectomy
Predisposition to urinary tract infections

surgery or chemotherapy (Marks et al 1995). Interstitial brachytherapy for prostate cancer leads to a higher incidence of acute urinary symptoms than external beam therapy; side effects last for up to 12 months following treatment (Kang et al 2001). With brachytherapy, urinary morbidity is associated with the total number of sources implanted and the total dose (Brown et al 2000).

The risk of incontinence is a major consideration for those men who have prostate cancer, with incidence rates ranging from 2 to 42% following radical prostatectomy. One of the reported benefits of radiotherapy over surgery is that urinary incontinence is not such a problem. Indeed, the literature suggests that urinary incontinence is uncommon, occurring in only 6% of men 3 months following pelvic irradiation (Talcott et al 1998). Lee et al (1996) found that 0.3% of men had subacute incontinence up to 3 months post-treatment, defining this as leakage once during a week. They concluded that the development of incontinence during radiation therapy was a direct result of surgical injury to the bladder neck; men who had previous transurethral resection of the prostate (TURP) were significantly ($P = 0.02$) more likely to have incontinence compared with those who did not have surgery. In gynaecological malignancies the link between bladder injury and symptoms is clearer, with 11–45% of women reporting urinary incontinence 3 months after radiotherapy (Parkin et al 1987, Pourquier et al 1987). This may be an underestimate, as many toxicity-grading schemes do not explicitly include this symptom. In gynaecological treatments the dose to the anterior wall of the bladder is high, usually as a result of intracavitary treatment in combination with external beam radiotherapy (Marks et al 1995). Prior surgery such as hysterectomy is suggested as a major factor in the development of urinary problems postgynaecological radiotherapy (Klee et al 2000, Parkin et al 1987).

Bacterial infection of the urinary tract is also considered to be a major factor in the development of urinary symptoms following radiotherapy. Infection can delay healing and make urinary symptoms worse. In a study of the incidence of urinary tract infection with pelvic radiotherapy, Bialas et al (1989) found that 17% of those reviewed ($n = 172$) had bladder infections prior to starting and a further 17% developed infections during treatment. Bessell & Granville-White (1994) in a further study found that 24% of those planning to have pelvic radiotherapy already had an existing urinary tract infection. Roberts et al (1990), who looked more specifically at men with prostate cancer, found that 7% of those being planned for pelvic radiotherapy had urinary tract infections, and that this increased to 11% prior to radiation. Furthermore, 1–2% of men per week developed an infection during treatment. This difference in infection rates at different times may be a result of invasive planning techniques. In total, 14% of men in this study had a significant urine culture detected during the course of treatment. Women with cervical cancer having pelvic treatments are more likely to develop urinary tract infections due to the insertion of urinary catheters during intra-cavitary treatment.

The true extent of urinary tract infection is unclear, and the degree to which infections are reflected in symptoms is even less clear. Symptoms prior to treatment may also add to the risk of developing urinary problems during radiotherapy. Previous studies suggest that up to 50% of men undergoing pelvic radiotherapy have urinary frequency and/or dysuria prior to radiotherapy (Beard et al 1997, Faithfull et al 2001, Talcott et al 1998). If symptoms are already severe then these can be further exacerbated by radiation damage.

PATTERN OF SYMPTOMS

The incidence and pattern of urinary symptoms vary over the course of radiotherapy. Very few studies distinguish between distinct urinary symptoms; instead, they are usually described together as bladder toxicity over the course of treatment. Clinical studies that describe the pattern of symptoms in detail are rare. Tait et al (1997) in a study of conformal radiotherapy for pelvic cancer found a clear pattern of increasing symptoms from baseline during treatment with maximum symptom scores occurring around the sixth week from start of radiotherapy. This was followed by a gradual decrease up until 3 months after therapy. Bladder symptoms affected 75% of patients 'a little', 28% 'quite a bit' and 7% were 'very severe'. Fieler (1997) in a descriptive study of the side effects of high-dose brachytherapy documented the symptoms of 96 women undergoing radiotherapy for gynaecological cancer. The incidence of urinary symptoms varied over the course of treatment, with 50% of women experiencing urinary frequency and 40% pain at 1 week after treatment; both diminished by 3 months. Eardley (1990) found that men and women having completed radiotherapy for bladder cancer still complained of urinary symptoms 2 months after treatment. The duration of bladder symptom occurrence postpelvic radiotherapy has been described in other studies of men with pelvic cancer (Crook et al 1996). Widmark et al (1994) found that in an age-matched population men without cancer had similar urinary problems to those described in men following radiotherapy. Hence the incidence of side effects needs to be considered as a change from baseline rather than a simple number of people experiencing symptoms.

The pattern of urinary symptoms from brachytherapy is distinct from those experienced as a result of external beam treatment. Kleinberg et al (1994) found that nocturia was the most common problem, occurring in 80% of their patients within 2 months of implantation. Obstructive urinary symptoms such as frequency, urgency and leakage of urine appear to be the most common and can be prolonged following prostate brachytherapy. Data from Kang et al (2001) identify that urinary symptoms are still a common problem for patients up to 12 months after brachytherapy.

THE IMPACT OF URINARY SYMPTOMS

There has been little systematic study of how individuals react to urinary symptoms. King et al (1985) in their survey of radiation symptoms failed to include urinary symptoms in the assessment criteria for pelvic treatment until later in the study, but did recognise that they caused patients distress. The discomfort, stinging or pain that is associated with dysuria can be profound. Faithfull (1995) interviewed men following pelvic radiotherapy for prostate and bladder cancer and found that urinary symptoms caused considerable difficulty. In order of symptom concern, symptoms were ranked and urinary problems were placed first pre- and post-treatment and ranked second to diarrhoea during radiotherapy. Pain linked to radiation-induced dysuria was considered difficult to manage because of its transient nature; patients felt that there was little that could be done. One man described his pain as a result of bladder cancer irradiation:

> I started [radiotherapy] and then it was really painful going to the toilet. I used to, you know, do the wrong thing, which is refrain from drinking because it meant that I had to go to the toilet. It was so painful, I mean I had to, you know go and sit down, effort and literally just grind my teeth as I went as it was so bad
>
> (Faithfull unpublished data).

Analgesia was the main strategy for managing such pain; however, this often proved ineffective, as patients would either find medication did not work or they kept tablets back for extreme pain. The men in this study would only use medication if they were in 'dead trouble'. One reason that they felt that the analgesics were not that useful was that once the pain had gone they were left feeling dizzy or disoriented. Side effects of analgesics such as constipation were also cited as a reason for not taking medication.

Urinary frequency had a significant impact on travel, as patients needed to plan trips around the availability of public toilets. This led to a lack of confidence in the ability to go out of the home, even when treatment had ended several months before. One man described these problems as a 'social evil' affecting his ability to go down the pub, work or shop, because of the frequency and uncertainty of urinary function. He described how this influenced his social life during radiotherapy:

> I wanted to go and play golf of course, because I feel perfectly fit but I just didn't fancy being rather like a dog at every other tree
>
> (Faithfull 1995).

Poor urinary flow could also be embarrassing and was not something that could be shared or discussed with friends.

> I don't like to go in the big men's toilet because I stand there and not be able to do anything, so I have to creep in one of the cubicles
>
> (Faithfull 1995).

Changes in bladder tone sometimes resulted in leakage of urine, either after passing urine or with the feeling of urgency prior to urinating. One patient described his bladder as:

Weakened somehow because one thing that you tend to do is you dribble a lot, there's slight incontinency ... it really is horrible and of course it's the smell and everything like that it's pretty bad but you know

(Faithfull unpublished data).

Urinary problems are a taboo subject in society; the inability to control passing urine creates feelings of uncertainty and embarrassment and is linked with senility or childhood. Incontinence is also seen as a problem of personal control and a sign of ageing. Patients may feel horribly unique and also worry that incontinence is their fault (Ashworth & Hagan 1993, Lawler 1991). Healthcare professionals may underestimate the extent of the problem. In a national survey of men undergoing prostate cancer treatment in Canada, 35% of men indicated that they had not received adequate support for symptoms and 30% indicated that they had experienced lifestyle changes as a result of treatment. These aspects included relationships, employment opportunities, leisure time, mental health and household responsibilities (Fitch et al 1999). Quality-of-life studies also identify social and lifestyle changes (Janda et al 2000, Joly et al 1998). Fossa et al (1997) in a study of urological morbidity following prostate cancer treatment found that lower urinary tract symptoms and fatigue were correlated with changes in global quality of life. The impact of gynaecological treatment on women is also profound with similar impairment of social life, daily activities and quality of life (Klee et al 1999, 2000).

MANAGEMENT OF URINARY SYMPTOMS

Providing effective care for individuals undergoing pelvic radiotherapy is an important issue for healthcare professionals. However the implementation of strategies to manage radiation-induced urinary symptoms is limited by the paucity of evidence. Furthermore urological studies focus on surgical rather than pharmacological and behavioural strategies. Therefore the evidence base is limited and the suggestions given in this chapter are based mainly on clinical experience.

Assessment of urinary symptoms

One of the most important aspects of management is a full assessment of urinary symptoms. This should include not only physical problems but also the extent and impact of symptoms. Bladder complications arising from radiation therapy can be graded using the Radiation Therapy Oncology Group (RTOG) classification scheme (Ch. 6). However most symptoms fall into category 1 and 2 and therefore this scoring system does not provide the detail necessary to distinguish between different urinary symptoms. The subjective nature of symptoms may also make observer rating difficult; patients may feel that pre-existing urinary symptoms are not necessary to report (Ashworth & Hagan 1993). Patient self-assessment tools therefore provide greater symptom definition and give a personal perspective of the physical impact of symptoms. Examples of urinary assessments are those of the American Urological Association (AUA) symptom index (Abel et al 2000) and the International Prostate Symptom Score (IPSS) (Cockett et al 1991) (Fig. 12.3). The AUA index was designed to discriminate between patients with benign prostate hyperplasia and those with more general urinary problems (Hines 1996), although it has also been used successfully in women (Chancellor & Rivas 1993). The IPSS is very similar but includes a quality-of-life question. The IPSS contains both obstructive symptom items such as hesitancy, incomplete emptying, intermittent flow and weak stream as well as irriative symptom items such as urinary frequency, urgency and nocturia. Although useful for monitoring symptoms over time, this scale does not include dysuria, which limits its application to patients with bladder cancer and those with pain as a result of inflammatory bladder changes.

A simpler but effective assessment tool is to ask patients to complete a voiding diary, an example of which is shown in Figure 12.4. This is a written record kept over a few days. A more detailed diary could include information on leakage, fluid intake, urgency and pain, thus providing useful information as to the pattern, severity and impact of symptoms. The information from such a diary can be used to assess the possible cause of symptoms and therefore direct their management. If individuals who have completed the diary have passed several small amounts of urine with small volumes, then their symptoms may be indicative of obstruction. If over the course of the day they have passed urine frequently but with occasional large volumes, the pattern is likely to be indicative of irritative symptoms. The bladder is sensitised by the inflammation and, despite not being full, is constantly sending signals to the brain that the bladder needs emptying. If the person is distracted, those signals fade into the background as the bladder is not really full, and hence a larger volume is passed later in the day.

Physical examination is also necessary so as to identify any signs of urinary obstruction. This requires clinical skill and experience in palpating the abdomen and looking for signs of distension following voiding. General observations should also be conducted as part of the assessment; weight changes following voiding can also map symptom changes (Hanfman et al 1998). Injury to the spinal cord due to bony metastasis can lead to detrusor paralysis. Urinary incontinence with pain and leg weakness is a symptom of spinal cord compression (Peterson 1993). Assessment of medications should also be made as narcotics taken for pain relief can reduce bladder muscle contractility and cause urinary retention. Many patients with bladder cancer lose small amounts of blood from their bladder during radiotherapy, as haematuria (pink-tinged urine). Microscopic amounts of blood can also be detected in urinalysis. Women undergoing pelvic treatments often experience rashes or sores around the perineum or vulval areas, which can contribute to urinary problems (Berry 1999). Routine assessment for urinary tract infection and anaemia should be carried out prior to radiotherapy and if symptoms indicate.

Prevention

The use of antibiotics for established urinary tract infections during the course of treatment is customary clinical practice but has little basis in research evidence.

Question	Not at all	Less than one time in five	Less than half the time	About half the time	More than half the time	Almost always
1. Incomplete emptying Over the past month, how often have you had a sensation of not emptying your bladder completely after you finished urinating?	0	1	2	3	4	5
2. Frequency Over the past month, how often have you had to urinate again less than 2 h after you finished urinating?	0	1	2	3	4	5
3. Intermittency Over the past month, how often have you found you stopped and started again several times when you urinated?	0	1	2	3	4	5
4. Urgency Over the past month, how often have you found it difficult to postpone urination?	0	1	2	3	4	5
5. Weak stream Over the past month, how often have you had a weak urinary stream?	0	1	2	3	4	5
6. Straining Over the past month, how often have you had to push or strain to begin urination?	0	1	2	3	4	5
7. Nocturia Over the past month, how many times did you most typically get up to urinate from the time you went to bed at night until the time you got up in the morning?	0	1	2	3	4	5
Total IPSS						

Figure 12.3 International Prostate Symptom Score (IPSS).

	Delighted	Pleased	Mostly satisfied	Mixed	Mostly dissatisfied	Unhappy	Terrible
Quality of life due to urinary symptoms If you were to spend the rest of your life with your urinary condition the way it is now, how would you feel about that?	0	1	2	3	4	5	6

The severity of urinary symptom can be assessed by means of the IPSS: < 8 mild; 8–20 moderate, > 20 severe.

Figure 12.3   Continued.

Bessell & Granville-White (1994) used the antibiotic trimethoprim to prevent urinary tract infection during radiotherapy. The antibiotic was prescribed routinely at a lower than standard dose of 200 mg as prophylaxis for patients undergoing pelvic radiotherapy ($n = 210$). These authors found that, despite antibiotics, 25 patients went on to develop infection and, in seven cases, the infections were due to organisms resistant to trimethoprim. They conclude that prophylactic antibiotics were of no value in reducing the incidence of urinary tract infection.

Changing the pH of urine and making it more acidic has been one strategy to prevent urinary infections. Although studies have found that pH changes can be induced by using agents such as ascorbic acid (Kinney & Blount 1979, Schultz 1984), few look at how effective this change is in preventing infection.

Another strategy, popular with women, is the use of cranberry juice to prevent urinary tract infection. Previous studies of the effect of cranberry juice have been small and uncontrolled, thus yielding conflicting results. The ability of cranberries and blueberries to reduce bacterial adherence to mucosal surfaces has been established in experimental studies (Sobota 1984). Rather than changing the acidity, the compounds excreted in the urine provide an environment that prevents bacterial growth. Avorn et al (1994), in a randomised, double-blind, controlled trial of prophylactic cranberry juice in an elderly population of women ($n = 153$), found that cranberry juice significantly ($P = 0.004$) reduced frequency of infection, but was effective only after 4–8 weeks of taking the juice. This effect was more pronounced in preventing reinfection. Using higher and lower quantities of juice assessed the optimal amount. Larger amounts had little effect and so the optimal amount of cranberry juice was defined as 300 ml/day. This may be a preventive strategy for those at risk from urinary tract infection such as those who have had invasive bladder procedures.

Day		Day time							Night time						Total daily volume
1	Time														
	Volume														
2	Time														
	Volume														
3	Time														
	Volume														
4	Time														
	Volume														
5	Time														
	Volume														

Suggested plan for assessment:

- Obtain a suitable measuring jug marked in fluid ounces or millilitres.
- Record the time and the amount of urine that is passed at each visit to the toilet over a period of 5 days.
- If you pass urine more times than that available on the chart, go on to the next day or night and add the correct day in the left-hand column.
- Make a particular note of the largest volume passed at any one time, to get an indication of the capacity of your bladder.
- Check the total amount of urine over a 24-h period.
- From this you can see how much is passed during the day and night.

Figure 12.4 Voiding diary.

Orgotein (superoxide dismutase), an antioxidant, has also been used to prevent the occurrence of acute side effects by counteracting the free radicals produced by radiation damage (Sanchiz et al 1996). In a randomised study, patients who received Orgotein after radiotherapy to the pelvis were compared with those who did not. Acute toxicity was monitored using the World Health Organization observer rating toxicity scale (similar to the RTOG). There were significant differences in urinary symptoms between groups, with those receiving Orgotein having fewer urinary problems. Such pharmacological management requires further experimental testing.

Pharmacological management of urinary symptoms

There is little consensus in how to provide relief for urinary symptoms as a result of radiation, as pharmacological and practical strategies have not been rigorously evaluated. Anticholinergic drugs such as α_1-blockers are frequently used in clinical practice, to block α_1-adrenergic receptors in smooth-muscle cells within the bladder and prostate stroma, thus decreasing muscle tone. The theory is that this reduces sensitivity and resistance, so decreasing obstruction to urinary flow. However, drugs such as oxybutynin currently in clincial use are unselective α_1-blockers and result in side effects such as mouth dryness, drowsiness and headaches. Caution also needs to be taken when prescribing such medication for those with impaired renal and hepatic function, cardiac disease or hypertension, which are all common comorbid diseases in the older population. This effectively limits the use of such medication. In recent years selective α_1-blocker drugs have become available and a number of research studies have investigated their potential to reduce urinary symptoms. Prosnitz and colleagues (1999) in a pilot study evaluated the effectiveness of tamsulosin hydrochloride (Flomax) in the management of acute radiation urinary symptoms. The sample consisted of 26 men undergoing radiotherapy for prostate cancer. Flomax was found to be effective in relieving urinary symptoms, reducing them from predicted levels of 78% to that of 25%. A further descriptive study of 743 patients comparing terazosin hydrochloride (THC) with non-steroidal anti-inflammatory drugs (NSAIDs) found that THC resulted in an overall significant reduction in symptoms compared to those prescribed NSAIDs (Zelefsky et al 1999). Of the patients taking THC, 66% had significant improvement, 22% had moderate improvement and 14% had minimal response. In comparison with the patients taking NSAIDs, 16% experienced significant relief, 28% had moderate improvement and 56% had minimal response.

Unfortunately, neither of these studies randomised patients to treatment groups or assessed patients' perceptions of symptoms or distress. Neither did they target therapy specifically for irritative or obstructive symptoms, perhaps explaining the diverse results in relation to response to NSAIDs. At present there is no consensus as to the best pharmacological management for urinary symptoms; however, therapy can be more effectively targeted and individualised if assessment is carried out (Fig. 12.5). Further studies are needed to confirm pharmacological management. Although research has focused on men's urinary symptoms as a result of prostate cancer, there is also a need to explore women's urinary symptoms and how they are affected by pharmacological strategies.

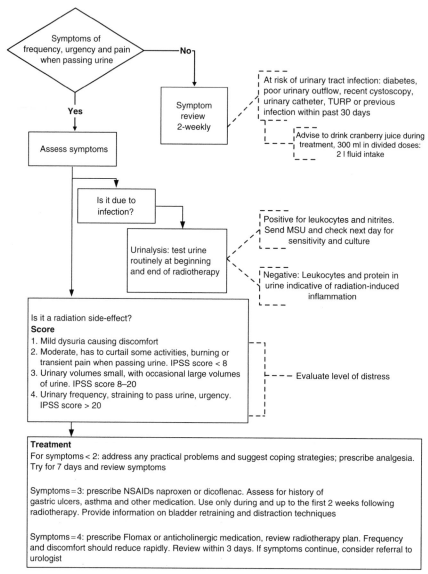

Figure 12.5 Algorithm of managing urinary frequency, dysuria and urgency. IPSS, international prostate symptom score; TURP, transurethral resection of the prostate; MSU, midstream specimen of urine; NSAIDs, non-steroidal anti-inflammatory drugs.

Non-pharmacological approaches to urinary symptoms

One aspect of care which has not been evaluated is that of behavioural and coping strategies to help patients manage urinary symptoms. Alternative strategies such as acupuncture or bladder retraining techniques are infrequently utilised in oncology, but have been found to benefit patients with longer-term bladder symptoms. Bladder-retraining techniques are widely used to treat urinary incontinence, particularly for people with stress incontinence or detrusor instability, although they are also thought to be of use in men with prostate problems following radiotherapy and surgery. A Cochrane systematic review (Roe et al 2001) found that, although there may be some benefit for patients, this conclusion can only be tentative because of the poor quality of the evidence available. Bladder-retraining techniques, pelvic floor exercises and behavioural coping strategies may have some benefits for patients following treatment but the efficacy of these approaches is uncertain (Table 12.3). It is important that patients' needs for urinary symptom management are assessed and appropriate analgesics or practical advice given (Fig. 12.6).

In a randomised controlled trial of 115 men with prostate and bladder cancer (Faithfull et al 2001), in the first week of treatment urinary symptoms were significantly less for those who received nursing intervention. This comprised patient self-assessment, specific urinary advice and practical information about

Table 12.3 Non-pharmacological management strategies for urinary symptoms

Intervention	Evidence
Bladder-retraining techniques Patients are asked to delay bladder emptying for as long as possible whenever they experience the need to pass urine. Advise to pass urine by the clock: feel confident and pick an interval they know they can meet, i.e. 1–2 h. Advise distraction, take a walk, phone a friend, do something in the house. As each interval becomes more manageable, increase it once more. Relaxation can also take the mind off the feeling of urgency and can be especially helpful if patients feel anxious or depressed. Most patients with urinary incontinence are highly motivated to participate in bladder retraining, but need support and encouragement (McCreanor et al 1998)	Bladder retraining is successful, with high reported success rates (Cardozo 1991) in women with incontinence. Wiseman et al (1991) in an RCT found that bladder retraining provided similar results to that of medication – overall, a 12% improvement in function. Szonyi et al (1995) in another RCT found that bladder retraining with oxybutynin was superior to that of bladder retraining alone. A 23% treatment effect was found with the intervention. McCreanor et al (1998) found that bladder retraining was superior to oxybutynin in a small non-randomised study. There is no research evidence available to confirm its effect in patients who are symptomatic following pelvic radiotherapy
Pelvic floor exercises The physiotherapist can advise on pelvic floor exercises. These exercises involve tightening and contracting pelvic floor muscles. If used with biofeedback techniques, this can be more successful	O'Brien et al (1991) conducted a randomised trial of men and women at a general practice experiencing urinary incontinence. Intervention was by the nurse with bladder-retraining techniques and physiotherapy: 68% of the sample reported improvement or cure of symptoms. Burgio et al (1998) found that biofeedback reduced symptoms by 35%
Acupuncture The use of acupuncture has been utilised for the management of irritative bladder symptoms	Acupuncture has been shown to be as effective in the management of irritative bladder symptoms as conventional anticholinergic drugs, with few side effects

RCT, randomised controlled trial.

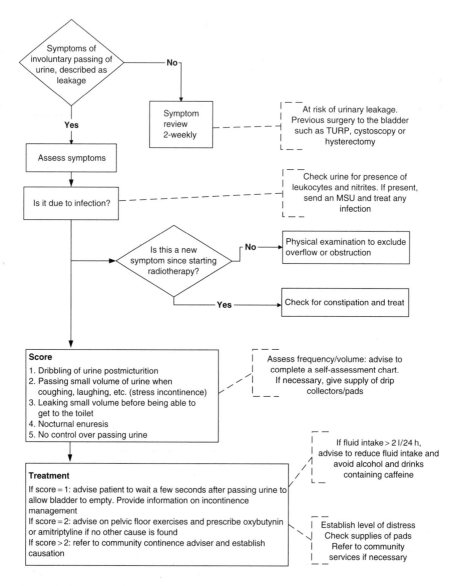

Figure 12.6 Algorithm of managing urinary incontinence. TURP, transurethral resection of the prostate; MSU, midstream specimen of urine.

symptoms. Once side effects from radiotherapy occurred, both intervention and control groups had similar levels of acute urinary symptoms; however, differences were again seen after completion of treatment. Further work is needed to clarify the longer-term benefits of such an individualised approach. Practical strategies such as incontinence pads or coping strategies for travel or social events are often neglected in the high-tech environment of radiotherapy care but these can prove very effective in reducing distress. Supportive care can help to reduce the impact of these symptoms even if the physical problem cannot be reversed.

CONCLUSION

Although there is a growing recognition of the quality-of-life issues affecting patients receiving pelvic radiotherapy, the management of physical symptoms such as urinary problems remains poor. Urinary symptoms produce a range of difficulties for patients, from urinary frequency to pain and incontinence. The varied needs of these patients are rarely assessed and are more often considered a nuisance than a legitimate symptom concern, as they rarely necessitate treatment to be stopped. Current interventions do not relieve the distress that patients experience. So far, healthcare strategies have focused on pharmacological management, neglecting the fact that much of the impact of these urinary symptoms is felt in relation to daily activities and roles. Rarely do urinary symptoms occur as a result of urinary tract infection; more commonly they are caused by radiation-induced inflammatory changes that result in irritation or obstruction. The most difficult problems to resolve are those that are chronic and inconsistent in occurrence, such as urinary symptoms. Sensitivity is required in order to recognise the problems they may cause for individuals and it is important that we listen and respond in a practical and sympathetic way. It is vital that new and existing approaches to the management of urinary symptoms are rigorously evaluated and that a combination of interventions is utilised so as to suit an individual's healthcare needs.

SUMMARY OF KEY CLINICAL POINTS

- Radiation-induced urinary symptoms are a common side effect of pelvic radiotherapy for both men and women.
- Risk factors for the development of urinary symptoms are existing urinary problems and adjuvant therapy such as surgery.
- The degree of urinary symptoms experienced is related to dose and volume of bladder treated.
- Damage is caused by inflammation to the urothelium layers, resulting in both 'irritative' and 'obstructive' urinary symptoms.
- Urinary symptoms such as frequency, nocturia, dysuria and incontinence increase over the course of radiotherapy and gradually diminish after treatment but may continue to cause problems for a minority of patients up to 12 months after completion of radiotherapy.
- Assessment of urinary symptoms is essential, either using a voiding diary or a specific urinary assessment tool such as the AUA or IPSS.
- Physical assessment to exclude urinary tract infection or physical obstruction is also important.
- There are limited data available as to the most suitable intervention approaches. For short-term inflammatory or obstructive symptoms, anticholinergic drugs and NSAIDs do seem to reduce acute symptoms.
- For longer-term symptoms occurring after treatment is complete, behavioural interventions may be more appropriate.

Most intervention studies for both pharmacological and non-pharmacological approaches to the management of radiation-induced urinary symptoms have utilised small samples and non-randomised designs. The lack of clear evidence makes it difficult to be prescriptive, but it appears that an individualised approach may be beneficial.

FURTHER INFORMATION

Continence Foundation Helpline
2 Doughty Street
London
WC1N 2PH
Tel: 0191 213 0050

http: www.prostate-ca.com/patientinfo.html
http: www.cancersourcer.com

www.vh.org/Patients/IHB/uro/Incontinence/Urinaryincontinence.html
www.vh.org/Patients/IHB/HealthProse/Urology/Urinaryproblems.html

REFERENCES

Abel L, Blatt H, Spetich R et al 2000 The role of urinary assessment scores in the nursing management of patients receiving prostate brachytherapy. Clinical Journal of Oncology Nursing 4:126–129

Ames C, Gray M 2000 Voiding dysfunction after radiation to the prostate for prostate cancer. Wound Ostomy and Continence Nurses Society 27:155–167

Ashworth P, Hagan M 1993 The meaning of incontinence: a qualitative study of non-geriatric urinary incontinence sufferers. Journal of Advanced Nursing 18:1415–1423

Avorn J, Monane M, Gurwitz J et al 1994 Reduction of bacteriuria and pyuria after ingestion of cranberry juice. Journal of the American Medical Association 271:751–754

Beard C, Propert K, Rieker P et al 1997 Complications after treatment with external beam irradiation in early stage prostate cancer patients: a prospective multi-institutional outcomes study. Journal of Clinical Oncology 15:223–229

Berry D 1999 Bladder disturbances. In: Henke Yarbro C, Frogge M, Goodman M (eds) Cancer symptom management. Sudbury, Jones and Bartlett, Sudbury, MA, p 489–507

Bessell E, Granville-White M 1994 The effect of prophylactic trimethorprim on aerobic urinary tract infection during pelvic radiotherapy and the incidence of infections due to fastidious or anaerobic organisms. Clinical Oncology (Royal College of Radiologists) 6:116–120

Bialas I, Bessell E, Sokal M et al 1989 A prospective study of urinary tract infection during pelvic radiotherapy. Radiotherapy and Oncology 16:305–309

Brown D, Colonias A, Miller R et al 2000 Urinary morbidity with a modified peripheral loading technique of transperineal ^{125}I prostate implantation. International Journal of Radiation Oncology, Biology, Physics 47:353–360

Burgio K, Locher J, Goode P et al 1998 Behavioural vs drug treatment for urge urinary incontinence in older women. Journal of the American Medical Association 280:1995–2000

Cardozo L 1991 Urinary incontince in women: have we anything new to offer? British Medical Journal 303:1453–1456

Chancellor M, Rivas D 1993 The American Urological Association symptom index for women with voiding symptoms. Lack of specificity for benign prostate hyperplasia. Journal of Urology 150:1706–1709

Cockett A, Aso Y, Dennis L et al 1991 Recommendations of the international consensus committee. Progress in Urology 1:957–972

Crook J, Esche B, Futter N 1996 Effect of pelvic radiotherapy for prostate cancer on bowel, bladder, and sexual function: the patients' perspective. Urology 47:387–394

Dorr W, Eckhardt A, Koi S 1998 Pathogenesis of acute radiation effects in the urinary bladder. Strahlentherapie und Onkologie 174:93–95

Eardley A 1990 Patients' needs after radiotherapy: the role of the general practitioner. Family Practice 7:39–42

Faithfull S 1995 'Just grin and bear it and hope that it will go away': coping with urinary symptoms from pelvic radiotherapy. European Journal of Cancer Care 4:158–165

Faithfull S Corner J, Myer L et al 2001 Evaluation of nurse-led care for men undergoing pelvic radiotherapy. British Journal of Cancer 18:1853–1864

Fieler V 1997 Side effects and quality of life in patients receiving high-dose rate brachytherapy. Oncology Nursing Forum 24:545–553

Fitch M, Johnson B, Gray R et al 1999 Survivors' perspectives on the impact of prostate cancer: implications for oncology nurses. Canadian Oncology Nursing Journal 9:23–28

Fossa S, Woehre H, Kurth K et al 1997 Influence of urological morbidity on quality of life in patients with prostate cancer. European Urology 31:3–8

Hanfman B, Engels M, Dorr W 1998 Radiation-induced impairment of urinary bladder function. Strahlentherapie und Onkologie 174:96–98

Hines J 1996 Symptom indicies in bladder outlet obstruction. British Journal of Urology 77:494–501

Janda M, Gerstner N, Obermair A et al 2000 Quality of life changes during conformal radiation therapy for prostate cancer. American Cancer Society 89:1322–1328

Joly F, Rune D, Couette J et al 1998 Health related quality of life and sequelae treated with brachytherapy and external beam irradiation for localized prostate cancer. Annals of Oncology 9:751–757

Kang S, Chou R, Dodge R et al 2001 Acute urinary toxicity following transperineal prostate brachytherapy using a modified quimby loading method. International Journal of Radiation Oncology, Biology, Physics 50:937–945

Kelleher C, Filshie J, Khullar V et al 1994 Acupuncture and the treatment of irritative bladder symptoms. Acupuncture in Medicine 12:9–12

King K, Nail L, Kreamer K et al 1985 Patients' descriptions of the experience of receiving radiation therapy. Oncology Nursing Forum 12:55–61

Kinney A, Blount M 1979 Effect of cranberry juice on urinary pH. Nursing Research 28:287–290

Klee M, Thranov I, Machin D 1999 Life after radiotherapy: the psychological and social effects experienced by women treated for advanced stages of cervical cancer. Gynaecologic Oncology 76:5–13

Klee M, Thranov I, Machin D 2000 The patients' perspective on physical symptoms after radiotherapy for cervical cancer. Gynaecologic Oncology 76:14–23

Lawler J 1991 Behind the screens nursing. Churchill Livingstone, Edinburgh

Lee R, Schultheiss T, Hanlon A et al 1996 Urinary incontinence following external beam radiotherapy for clinically localized prostate cancer. Urology 48:95–99

Lundbeck F 1993 An experimental in vivo model in mice to evaluate the change in reservoir function of the urinary bladder due to irradiation alone or combined with chemotherapy. In: Hinkelbein W, Bruggmoser G, Frommhold H (eds) Acute and long term side effects of radiotherapy. Recent results in cancer research, vol. 130. Springer Verlag, Berlin p 90–101

Lynch W, Jenkins B, Fowler C et al 1992 The quality of life after radical radiotherapy for bladder cancer. British Journal of Urology 70:519–521

Marks L, Carroll P, Dugan T et al 1995 The response of the urinary bladder, urethra, and ureter to radiation and chemotherapy. International Journal of Radiation Oncology, Biology, Physics 31:1257–1280

McCreanor J, Aitchison M, Woods M 1998 Comparing therapies for incontinence. Professional Nurse 13:215–219

O'Brien J, Austin M, Sethi P et al 1991 Urinary incontinence: prevalence, need for treatment and effectiveness of intervention by nurse. British Medical Journal 303:1308–1313

Parkin D, Davis J, Symonds R 1987 Long term bladder symptomatology following radiotherapy for cervical carcinoma. Radiotherapy and Oncology 9:195–199

Peterson R 1993 Nursing intervention for early detection of spinal cord compressions in patients with cancer. Cancer Nursing 16:113–116

Pilpepch M, Krall J, Sause W et al 1987 Correlation of radiotherapeutic parameters and treatment related morbidity in carcinoma of the prostate – analysis of RTOG study 75-06. International Journal of Radiation Oncology, Biology, Physics 13:351–357

Pourquier H, Delard R, Archille E et al 1987 A quantified approach to the analysis and prevention of urinary complications in radiotherapeutic treatment of cancer of the cervix. International Journal of Radiation Oncology, Biology, Physics 13:1025–1033

Prosnitz R, Schneider L, Manola J et al 1999 Tamsulosin palliates radiation-induced urethritis in patients with prostate cancer: results of a pilot study. International Journal of Oncology, Biology, Physics 45:563–566

Quilty P, Duncan W, Kerr G 1985 Results of randomized study to evaluate the influence of dose on morbidity in radiotherapy for bladder cancer. Clinical Radiology 36:615–618

Raghavan D 1992 Bladder cancer. In: Horwich A (ed.) Combined radiotherapy and chemotherapy in clinical oncology. Edward Arnold, London, p 113–126

Roberts F, Murphy J, Ludgate C 1990 The value and significance of routine urine cultures in patients referred for radiation therapy of prostatic malignancy. Clinical Oncology (Royal College of Radiologists) 2:18–21

Roe B, Williams K, Palmer M 2001 Bladder training for urinary incontinence in adults (Cochrane review). Cochrane Database Systematic Review 2:CD001308

Sager E, Fossa S, Kaalhus O et al 1990 Computed tomography of the urinary bladder shortly after irradiation for rectal carcinoma. Acta Radiologica 31:585–588

Sanchiz F, Milla A, Artola N et al 1996 Prevention of radioinduced cystitis by Orgotein: a randomized study. Anticancer Research 16:2025–2028

Schultz A 1984 Efficacy of cranberry juice and ascorbic acid in acidifying the urine in multiple sclerosis subjects. Journal of Community Health Nursing 1:159–169

Scrase C, Perks J, Bidmead A et al 1999 Changes in bladder volume during radical beam radiotherapy for prostate cancer. Royal College of Radiologists Annual Scientific Meeting 16–17 September abstract

Sobota A 1984 Inhibition of bacterial adherence by cranberry juice: the potential use for the treatment of urinary tract infections. Journal of Urology 131:1013–1016

Szonyi G, Collas D, Ding Y et al 1995 Oxybutynin with bladder retraining for detrusor instability in elderly people: a randomized controlled trial. Age and Ageing 24:287–291

Tait D, Nahum A, Meyer L et al 1997 Acute toxicity in pelvic radiotherapy; a randomised trial of conformal versus conventional treatment. Radiotherapy and Oncology 42:121–136

Talcott J, Rieker P, Clark J et al 1998 Patient reported symptoms after primary therapy for early prostate cancer: results of a prospective cohort study. Journal of Clinical Oncology 16:275–283

Waugh A, Grant A 2001 Ross and Wilson anatomy and physiology in health and illness, 9th edn. Churchill Livingstone, Edinburgh

Widmark A, Fransson P, Tavelin B 1994 Self-assessment questionnaire for evaluating urinary and intestinal late side effects after pelvic radiotherapy in patients with prostate cancer compared with an age-matched control population. Cancer 74:2520–2532

Wiseman P, Malone-Lee J, Rai G 1991 Terodiline with bladder retraining for detrusor instability in elderly people. British Medical Journal 302:994–996

Woodhouse C 1990 Injuries to the bladder. In: Galland R, Spencer J (eds) Radiation enteritis. Edward Arnold, London, p 162–167

Zelefsky M, Ginor R, Fuks Z et al 1999 Efficacy of selective alpha-1 blocker therapy in the treatment of acute urinary symptoms during radiotherapy for localised prostate cancer. International Journal of Radiation Oncology, Biology, Physics 45:567–570

13

Gastrointestinal effects of radiotherapy

Sara Faithfull

INTRODUCTION

This chapter focuses on the pathophysiology and management of gastrointestinal symptoms. Like many acute side effects as a result of radiotherapy, gastrointestinal symptoms are often hidden. Problems such as diarrhoea or faecal leakage have a cultural stigma, they are very personal and private; therefore they are often concealed or neglected. Radiation-induced intestinal injury causes a wide range of physical problems from symptoms of nausea and vomiting to diarrhoea, abdominal cramps, frequency and proctitis, which incorporates tenesmus (straining when trying to go to the toilet), urgency and occasionally bleeding.

The gastrointestinal tract is particularly vulnerable to radiation damage as the fast turnover of cells results in both acute and late side effects (Busch 1990). Gastrointestinal toxicity occurs when radiotherapy is directed to sites covering the oesophagus, abdomen and pelvis (Fig. 13.1). The incidence of acute symptoms is high in patients receiving total body irradiation (80–100%) (Buchali et al 2000) or upper abdominal irradiation (50–80%) (Aass et al 1992, Prentice 1988, Roberts & Priestman 1993), with studies of general treatment groups suggesting that as many as 40% of patients experience some nausea and vomiting with radiotherapy treatment (Feyer & Titlbach 1998, The Italian Group 1999). The incidence of acute bowel symptoms as a result of pelvic treatment ranges from 56% of men following prostate cancer radiation (Yeoh et al 2000) to 86% of women receiving pelvic radiotherapy treatment (King et al 1985). Such symptoms can cause significant distress for patients, can be socially and emotionally isolating, and can influence nutrition, sexuality and cause fatigue (Klee et al 2000, Padilla 1990). Symptoms can also linger for months to years after radiotherapy is completed, resulting in chronic problems (Klee et al 1999). Data from clinical studies of pelvic cancers suggest that the majority of patients experience increased frequency of bowel motions in the long term following radiotherapy (Danielsson et al 1991, Yeoh et al 1984) and there

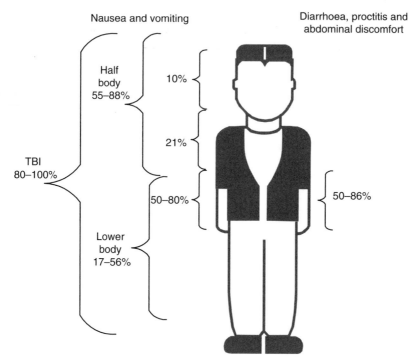

Figure13.1 Incidence by site of gastrointestinal symptoms. TBI, total body irradiation.

is a growing belief that a relationship exists between acute bowel toxicity and the incidence of late effects (Wang et al 1989).

Poor assessment of such symptoms has, in the past, led to an underestimation of the extent of bowel toxicity; however, the increasing use of subjective data has helped researchers map the extent of gastrointestinal problems experienced by patients. Patient self-report data suggest that 13% of men continue to have diarrhoea several times a week up to 3 months after completing radiotherapy for prostate cancer (Beard et al 1997). Follow-up studies for women treated with pelvic cancer also suggest that diarrhoea continues to be a problem up to 1 year after therapy is completed (Yeoh et al 2000). Chronic radiation enteritis is a late effect and can result in complications of stricture and fistula formation, which can be a major cause of morbidity and mortality for patients who have undergone pelvic radiotherapy (Beer et al 1985). These late symptoms are relatively rare but are explored in more detail in Chapter 19.

Modern techniques of delivery such as conformal radiotherapy have reduced some of the longer-term effects of radiation enteritis but have had little impact on acute symptoms (Tait et al 1997). Risk factors have been identified and preventive strategies for the occurrence of side effects have been developed; however, there is minimal evidence to support current management strategies for some symptoms such as diarrhoea.

If symptoms are severe they may lead to pathophysiological changes such as an imbalance of electrolytes, dehydration and malnutrition, which may necessitate treatment being interrupted. This can lead to the delivery of a biologically less effective dose, thus reducing the curative potential of the treatment (see Ch. 5). It is estimated that approximately 20% of patients undergoing pelvic irradiation who have experienced severe diarrhoea have required an interruption in their planned course of treatment (Amdur et al 1990, Yeoh et al 2000). These gastrointestinal symptoms rarely occur in isolation and may form a cluster of symptoms such as nausea, abdominal cramps and diarrhoea. In isolation these transient symptoms may not appear to be severe but in combination they can have a detrimental effect on the patients' quality of life.

AETIOLOGY

Acute symptoms may start within the first 2 weeks of radiotherapy treatment and reflect the radiosensitivity of the intestinal mucosa, whose tissues rapidly proliferate (Flickinger et al 1990, Yeoh & Horowitz 1988). Histopathological changes can be observed within hours of irradiation, such as abnormal mitotic activity in the epithelium, reduction in number of epithelial cells, presence of epithelial nuclear fragments, degeneration and necrosis of small epithelial cells, oedema, presence of lymphocytes and altered crypt size (Busch 1990). The stem cells are most affected by the irradiation and are located at the base of the crypts in the small bowel (Fig. 13.2). The number of cell divisions falls progressively during a course of radiotherapy and does not increase until the cessation of treatment. In the normal bowel, cell transit time from the crypt to the villus tip takes from 1 to 8 days, with the intestinal lining being replaced every 3–5 days (Claben et al 1998). Following irradiation the intestinal villi become shortened and flatter, reducing the surface area available for absorption (Churnratanakul et al 1990, Kinsella & Bloomer 1980) and the epithelial surface is reduced as cell loss exceeds repopulation (Flickinger et al 1990). The combination of these changes results in malabsorption of bile salts, vitamin B_{12} and lactose (Danielsson et al 1991, Yeoh et al 1993).

There are a number of possible reasons why patients experience diarrhoea; there is growing evidence that malabsorption and a subsequent increase in conjugated bile salts result in watery stools and diarrhoea. Under normal physiological conditions bile salts are almost totally reabsorbed in the small intestine. The colonic bacterial flora deconjugates the unabsorbed bile salts, resulting in water retention and diarrhoea (Stryker et al 1977, Sullivan 1962). Clinical studies show a significant decrease in bile salt absorption in 50–85% of patients receiving abdominal and pelvic irradiation (Bye et al 1995, Danielsson et al 1991). A decrease in mucosal surface area of the terminal ileum also results in malabsorption of vitamin B_{12}. Approximately 65% of patients clinically investigated for diarrhoea had a reduction in absorption of vitamin B_{12} (Fernandez-Barnes et al 1991). Few patients show obvious signs of malabsorption (Gray 1975).

The decline in the brush border of the epithelium may reduce enzymatic degradation of lactose, which accumulates in the intestine where it is subjected to bacterial fermentation causing flatulence, distension and diarrhoea. Bacterial overgrowth has been proposed as a factor in the occurrence of diarrhoea; however,

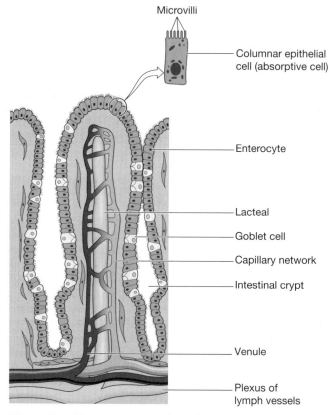

Microvilli

Columnar epithelial
cell (absorptive cell)

Enterocyte

Lacteal

Goblet cell

Capillary network

Intestinal crypt

Venule

Plexus of
lymph vessels

Figure 13.2 Highly magnified view of villi in the small intestine.
The epithelial cells (absorptive, columnar, goblet and endocrine cells)
arise from skin cells at the base of the crypts and gradually spread
up the villi, where they are shed from the villus tips. (Adapted with
permission from Waugh & Grant 2001.)

changes in the local flora of the ileum by colonic bacteria have not been correlated
with symptoms in experimental studies (Henriksson et al 1995).

Changes to gastrointestinal motility can also occur as radiation dose accumulates. However, during optimally fractionated radiotherapy, the loss of intestinal
mucosa can be compensated by repopulation, i.e. the regenerative response of the
surviving cells (see Ch. 5). Therefore only a few pathophysiological changes may
be seen in the superficial mucosal layers. More aggressive radiotherapy treatments
may result in greater damage, with subsequent cell loss and inflammatory
changes. In acute radiation proctitis, damage results in tissue hyperplasia and
subsequent ulceration to rectal tissues (Zimmermann & Feldmann 1998). Because
of the close proximity of rectal tissues, radiotherapy to the prostate often causes
feelings of tenesmus, urgency in defecation, pain, faecal incontinence, discomfort
and rectal bleeding (Colwell & Goldberg 2000).

Experimental studies on intestinal motility have revealed major disturbances in the physiological pattern of gut activity during radiotherapy. The contractions that cause peristalsis become irregular after irradiation, resulting in feelings of nausea, vomiting and overall a reduced intestinal transit time (Erickson et al 1994). Clinical studies have highlighted that patients have a more rapid small intestinal and colonic transit, thus reducing the time available for absorption. This may contribute to the diarrhoea and feelings of nausea associated with radiation enteritis; however, the explanation for these motility changes is far from clear.

The aetiology of nausea related to radiotherapy of the upper abdomen is poorly understood, but it is thought that degradation of products from normal or cancerous cells could stimulate efferent visceral fibres and initiate sensory signals to the medulla (Fig. 13.3). Nausea is often the earliest side-effect to develop; it usually appears 1–2 days after radiotherapy and persists for several hours afterwards.

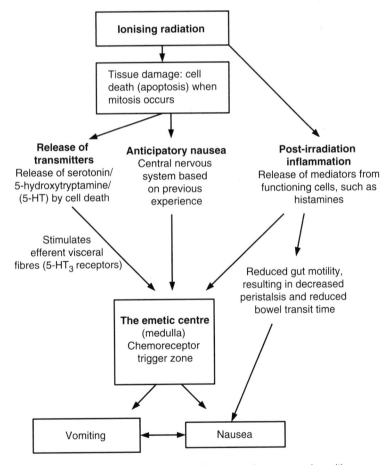

Figure 13.3   Aetiology of radiation-induced nausea and vomiting.

It can be most severe during the first few days of treatment and is more likely to be a problem where the treatment field includes the chest or oesophagus. During radiotherapy to the upper gastrointestinal tract, inflammation and denudation of the surface epithelium occur, potentially leading to oedema and ulceration. Feelings of epigastric pain, reflux, discomfort and pain when swallowing extremely hot, cold or coarse foods can discourage patients from eating, resulting in nutritional problems. These symptoms can occur within days of starting radiotherapy and may last 6–8 weeks. If untreated, they can be particularly distressing. The early onset of symptoms such as nausea or abdominal discomfort following initial treatment is not mirrored by observable biological changes, which may take several days to become apparent. This indicates that early changes in motility patterns are not dependent on the amount of damage to tissues but may occur in response to more individual factors (Claben et al 1998). Anticipatory nausea can occur prior to treatment as a result of anxiety or nervousness at the prospect of receiving radiotherapy or as a conditioned response to previous vomiting (Eckert 2001). However there is little research exploring why patients experience nausea with radiotherapy.

FACTORS INFLUENCING GASTROINTESTINAL SYMPTOM OCCURRENCE

Gastrointestinal changes, like many of the acute side effects from radiotherapy, are dose, field and quality-of-radiation-dependent (Busch 1990, Yeoh et al 2000). A few studies have examined the interaction between cancer chemotherapy and radiation damage; some drugs (Mitomycin C, Actinomycin D, 5-fluorouracil and Adriamycin) result in sensitisation and can produce greater bowel toxicity (Potish 1990, Potish et al 1979).

Factors that influence the occurrence of bowel symptoms have mainly been studied in relation to the incidence of late effects. Coexisting disease, surgery or patient characteristics may add to the chance of radiation damage (Table 13.1) (Potish 1990). Most small-bowel damage occurring in this context is thought to be

Table 13.1 Risk factors for the occurrence of radiation-induced gastrointestinal symptoms

Treatment factors	Patient factors
Fractionation regime	Thin physique
Irradiated volume	Diverticulosis
Radiation technique and beam energy	Hypertension
Organs included in the radiation field	Diabetes mellitus
Adjuvant chemotherapy	Gender: females have a higher incidence of
Prior abdominal surgery	lower-bowel symptoms, males have an
Single and total dose	increased risk of vomiting
	Vascular disease
	Old age
	The very young are more likely to have nausea and vomiting
	Pelvic inflammatory disease

secondary to vascular changes. Although pre-existing vascular changes may increase the risk of long-term damage following pelvic radiotherapy (Covens et al 1991), there is little evidence that they influence the incidence of acute bowel symptoms (Perez et al 1994). It is estimated that prior abdominal surgery increases nearly threefold the patient's risk of late side effects. The risk to a thin woman with hypertension is 16.8 times greater than someone without these conditions (Churnratanakul et al 1990). Unfortunately, as with most multimodality cancer therapies (irradiation, surgery or chemotherapy), it is difficult to predict all possible interactions and all factors which predispose patients to more severe side effects.

Radiation treatment using extended fields is more likely to include areas of small bowel, therefore acute bowel symptoms may be worse. Reducing the volume of small bowel within the treatment field may minimise the risk. Gallagher et al (1986) found that the severity of acute gastrointestinal effects positively correlated with the amount of small bowel within the treatment field, and that if this could be displaced, bowel symptoms were reduced. These findings have also been confirmed in radiotherapy for rectal carcinoma where field size and dose of radiotherapy to small bowel correlated with extent of late bowel injury (Miller et al 1999). In pelvic fields, the volume of the bladder may be important, as treating patients with full bladders helps push the small bowel out of the radiation field and hence may reduce the risk of bowel symptoms.

Risk factors for radiotherapy-induced nausea and vomiting are related to the treatment area, fraction size and total dose of radiation. Individual factors such as age, alcohol intake, anxiety or previous history of nausea and vomiting may also be important (Feyer et al 1998). However these data come from selected patient populations included in randomised trials of antiemetics. More convincing risk factors identified through a population survey found that previous experience of chemotherapy, field size and irradiated site (upper abdomen) were the only predictive risk factors for nausea and vomiting (The Italian Group 1999). Total body irradiation and radiotherapy to the upper part of the abdomen are those treatments most associated with nausea and vomiting.

PATTERN OF SYMPTOMS

The pattern of gastrointestinal symptoms varies over the course of treatment. Nausea and vomiting most often occurs 4–8 days from start of therapy and may continue throughout treatment. Vomiting can last between 1 and 37 days but its median duration was found to be 3 days in a recent Italian survey of cancer centres (The Italian Group 1999). This pattern may merely reflect prescribing habits if patients initially complaining of vomiting are prescribed antiemetics, which may take several days to be effective. In this survey, 57% of patients who experienced the symptom had mild nausea (which did not interfere with their daily activities) and 43% had moderate to severe nausea (which was defined as interfering with their lives). The median time for the onset of nausea was 5–8 days from start of radiotherapy (The Italian Group 1999). Nausea and vomiting as a result of total body irradiation have a higher incidence, with 26% of patients experiencing symptoms after the fourth fraction of treatment and over 42% experiencing nausea and 23% vomiting by the completion of radiotherapy (Buchali et al 2000). Nausea and vomiting are almost universal after total body irradiation and the high dose per fraction may be a contributing factor. Patients receiving palliative radiotherapy may also be given single exposures of 8–15 Gy, greatly increasing the risk of nausea and vomiting. Nausea also tends to last longer than vomiting and is a more persistent symptom.

Diarrhoea can occur within the first 2 weeks of radiotherapy but the incidence tends to increase over the course of treatment. Tait et al (1997) reported symptoms from a sample of 274 patients with pelvic cancer, one large subset of whom had prostate cancer. They provide a comprehensive analysis of the acute side effects of pelvic radiotherapy, illustrating that the incidence of acute symptoms was 30% within the first week of treatment and 70% by the end of radiotherapy. King et al (1985) followed 30 patients receiving pelvic radiotherapy on a weekly basis during treatment and found that over 50% had developed diarrhoea by the last week of therapy and that, for some patients, diarrhoea was still a problem 3 months after treatment had been completed. Klee et al (2000) in a population comparison study of 118 women treated with radiotherapy for cervical cancer describe how 46% of women recorded diarrhoea as having a severe impact on their lives. Such symptoms can be extremely personal and they impinge on many aspects of quality of life (Bye et al 1995).

IMPACT OF GASTROINTESTINAL SYMPTOMS

Nausea and vomiting are often reported as some of the most distressing of cancer treatment side effects (Rhodes et al 1995, Welch 1980). The feelings of nausea, which can accompany patients for many weeks during upper abdominal radiotherapy, can make treatment intolerable and quality of life poor. Often nausea and vomiting are treated as a single entity; however, they are two separate conditions and as such impact on people differently. Nausea is a subjective feeling that is described as an unpleasant sensation in the back of the throat and epigastrium, or by patients as feeling 'sick in the stomach' (Rhodes et al 1995). Nausea has been described as worse following treatment in the morning than in the afternoon (Welch 1980). Vomiting is the forceful expulsion of stomach, duodenum or jejunum contents through the oral cavity; patients often describe this as 'throwing up' (Krishnasamy 2001). The retching associated with vomiting can cause a sore, dry mouth and abdominal cramping. The persistent nausea associated with radiotherapy treatment can be more distressing than actual vomiting, as continuous nausea results in anorexia and feelings of weakness and can be isolating. Few studies have explored how enteritis symptoms are experienced. Most have focused on the extent of symptoms rather than the distress or impact they have on the individual.

Padilla (1990) in a study of 101 patients from four radiotherapy centres describes the impact of gastrointestinal side effects on psychological well-being, linking the two in 21.5% of patients. Although this study highlights some of the psychosocial issues related to enteritis, the quantitative design precludes exploration of what impact the symptoms had on the individual.

Diarrhoea from radiation treatment is often considered to be an inevitable consequence of radiation therapy – something that is to be suffered. Patients often describe the impact of diarrhoea as profoundly influencing activities:

> Basically I had diarrhoea … it was bad news because no sooner had you put a clean pair of underpants on, then I would need to go again and, you know, unfortunately you missed and they were messed again. This was very difficult to take

(Faithful unpublished data).

Diarrhoea disrupts sleep, journeys and social activities and patients can be fearful to leave the house in case they need a toilet.

> I needed to be near a toilet and to be perfectly honest some of the times I would go would be quite unusual

(Faithful unpublished data)

Medication for diarrhoea can also cause its own problems, with feelings of dizziness or constipation.

> The diarrhoea hasn't really gone it's a little naughty but the tablets cause a stalling they certainly help. The tablets leave me with a funny feeling I don't know what it is erm … a bit woozy it's a bit hard to explain

(Faithfull 2001).

Patients describe the uncertainty of gastrointestinal symptoms as the possibility of being let down by their bowels in a public place, making a mess of their pants or not being able to reach a toilet in time. The distress and loss of control felt by individuals who have always taken continence for granted can add to treatment anxieties.

MANAGEMENT OF GASTROINTESTINAL SYMPTOMS

A number of management approaches to radiation-induced gastrointestinal symptoms have been reported. There is a clear distinction between the management of nausea and vomiting and that of lower-bowel symptoms such as diarrhoea. Good assessment is fundamental to the management of both upper- and lower-bowel symptoms; strategies vary widely depending on the aetiology or contributing factors. Asking patients about their symptoms or requesting that they keep a diary or log over a week can give valuable information as to the extent and pattern of the problem, as well as contributing factors. For example, patients receiving pelvic radiotherapy for prostate cancer often complain that they are experiencing diarrhoea, but when men are asked to describe their stools and with what frequency they go to the toilet, they complain of small amounts of faeces, blood on the tissue paper, frequency and urgency. What they are describing is usually proctitis, as diarrhoea involves copious amounts of fluid, mucus-like stools, often accompanied by abdominal discomfort. Each symptom has different management strategies and requires careful assessment. Figure 13.4 gives key assessment points for exploring gastrointestinal symptoms.

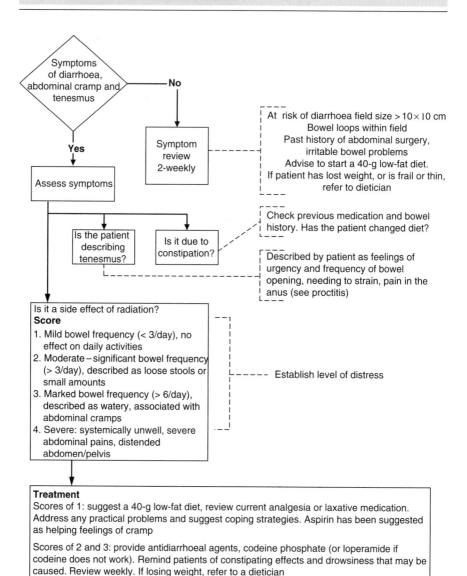

Figure 13.4 Assessment and management algorithm for bowel symptoms: part 1.

Managing nausea and vomiting

Prevention of radiation-induced nausea and vomiting is important, as the initial experience of treatment can induce anticipatory nausea and complicate recovery. In general, antiemetic drugs are rarely administered prophylactically to

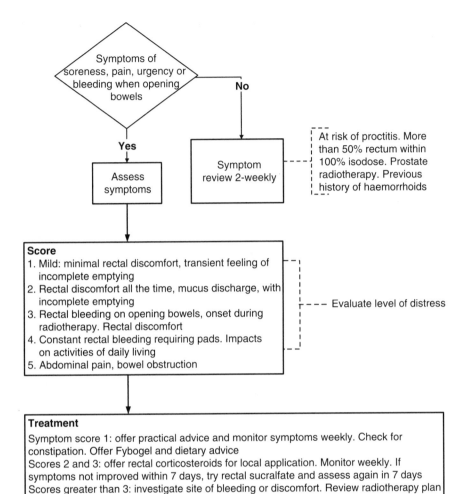

Figure 13.5   Assessment and mangement algorithm for bowel symptoms: part 2.

radiotherapy patients. The Italian study previously mentioned found that only 14% of patients received antiemetics during radiotherapy, 5% of these prophylactically and 9% following symptom episodes. This pattern of utilization of antiemetics may reflect an underestimate of the extent of nausea and vomiting experienced by patients undergoing radiotherapy, or perhaps a 'wait-and-see' attitude of clinicians who only prescribe antiemetics once symptoms occur. Although the severity of nausea and vomiting in patients undergoing radiotherapy is lower than that associated with chemotherapy regimes, its duration can be longer and therefore more challenging to control (Roila et al 1998). Many antiemetic agents may be useful in the control of radiotherapy-induced nausea and vomiting and some of these are listed in Table 13.2. However there is evidence that the newer 5-HT$_3$-antagonist drugs

Table 13.2 Antiemetic agents for the management of radiation-induced nausea and vomiting

Agents	Critique
Phenothiazines Prochlorperazine Chlorpromazine	These drugs exert their effect as dopamine antagonists, inhibiting transmission in the CTZ. The phenothiazines are often used for extrapyramidal reactions that result in nausea and vomiting. Phenothiazines are infrequently used with radiation-induced nausea and vomiting. Common side effects of these drugs are akatheisia, a sensation described by patients as feeling jittery with uncontrolled tremor and sleepiness
Substituted benzamide Metoclopramide	Metoclopramide is frequently used in radiation therapy. This drug acts both as a dopamine antagonist and also promotes gastric emptying, limiting reflux and retching. Side effects are dystonia, diarrhoea and sedation.
Corticosteroids Dexamethasone	Dexamethasone is frequently used in conjunction with other antiemetics such as metoclopramide and ondansetron for aggressive treatment regimes such as radiotherapy for total body irradiation. Its exact action is unknown but it is thought to influence and reduce prostaglandins
Benzodiazepines Lorazepam Diazepam	The exact antiemetic action of these drugs is not clear; however, they influence the central nervous system by producing anxiolytic and sedative effects. They should be used with caution
5-HT$_3$-antagonists Ondansetron, granisetron, tropisetron	This class of drug was developed to treat nausea and vomiting associated with chemotherapy. They work on the CTZ. They act by blocking the serotonin receptors. Although 5-HT$_3$-antagonists have become main-line therapy for the treatment and prevention of acute radiation-induced nausea and vomiting, their ability to influence longer-term nausea and delayed symptoms is far from clear. These antiemetics have only mild side effects, such as headaches and constipation, but are expensive

CTZ, chemoreceptor trigger zone; 5-HT$_3$, 5-hydroxytryptamine (serotonin).

are most successful at preventing nausea and vomiting as a result of radiotherapy and these are becoming the treatment of choice (Collis et al 1991, Roberts & Priestman 1993).

Support for the use of 5-hydroxytryptamine (5-HT$_3$)-antagonists mainly arises from trials of patients undergoing total body irradiation, and does not represent those patients having local external beam radiotherapy. Franzen and colleagues (1996) tested ondansetron in a randomised controlled trial of 111 radiotherapy patients, a substantial subgroup of whom received treatment to the abdomen.

Of the patients who received ondansetron, 67% had their nausea and vomiting completely controlled, compared to 45% in the placebo group. Patients taking the antiemetic had fewer days of nausea and vomiting and experienced significant benefits in quality of life; however these differences were not sustained over time (Hainsworth & Hesketh 1992). The Italian Group (1999) found that widespread use of 5-HT_3-antagonists in radiotherapy departments did not have a significant effect on nausea and vomiting. There was a wide range of doses and schedules used and, despite the use of prophylactic antiemetics, 46% of patients had vomiting and 58% experienced nausea. This relatively high failure rate raises several issues: firstly, that suboptimal dosages of antiemetics were administered compared to that given in clinical trials (for example, in the survey ondansetron 8 mg was given only once per day compared to two to three times per day in clinical trials). Secondly, patients most likely to receive prophylactic antiemetic treatment were those at high risk, such as patients receiving total body irradiation, rather than those with a more moderate risk. The data from studies of these high-risk groups show that antiemetics alone are not completely effective in reducing nausea and vomiting. Additionally, it is not only the dose of antiemetics but the route of administration (oral or intravenous) that is important in optimising antiemetic control (Feyer & Titlbach 1998).

Behavioural techniques for managing radiation-induced nausea may have benefit. Many studies have examined the effects of behavioural techniques such as relaxation, guided imagery, hypnosis and acupressure (Eckert 2001); however these techniques have not been tested in radiotherapy populations.

The low rate of antiemetic use and wide variety of schedules adopted within clinical centres suggest that an evidence-based approach to radiotherapy-induced nausea and vomiting is required. Further research is needed in order to identify more effective strategies of managing radiation-induced nausea and vomiting.

The management of diarrhoea

A number of approaches to reducing radiation-induced bowel symptoms have been reported (Table 13.3). There are two areas of diarrhoea management explored in the literature: diet and medication.

Diet

A reduced-fat diet has been shown to be beneficial in reducing diarrhoea. Experimental research has indicated that specific and elemental diets, which reduce food to its component parts, are useful in protecting bowel cell function during radiotherapy (Levi & Hodgson 1990). Craighead & Young (1998) in a feasibility study of elemental diets in women with gynaecological cancer found that diarrhoea and late symptoms were reduced in those women taking the elemental diet. Such diets have been mainly used in gastroenterology, for patients suffering from Crohn's disease or severe intestinal injury whose symptoms may be profound. Many patients undergoing pelvic radiotherapy have no initial symptoms, thus the rationale for such a drastic diet may seem questionable. Elemental supplements are fairly unpalatable and their use in routine clinical practice needs to be evaluated.

Table 13.3 Summary of research studies investigating the prevention or management of radiation-induced enteritis

Management approach	Authors	Method/strength of evidence (no. of patients/site of treatment)	Results	Endpoints/clinical outcomes
Sucralfate	Henriksson et al (1992a)	Double-blind and placebo-controlled trial. Included 70 patients being treated with pelvic radiotherapy for prostate or urinary bladder cancer. Sucralfate granules (1 g 6x a day) given 2 weeks after start of treatment and for 6 weeks	The frequency of bowel movements and stool consistency were significantly improved. One year later the patients in the sucralfate group had fewer late bowel side effects	Daily diary of frequency, stool consistency, pain, occurrence of blood and mucus. These data were subsequently converted to a diarrhoea score. This may be a useful agent for reducing enteritis side effects but has not been replicated
Colestipol hydrochloride (bile acid-sequestering resin)	Stryker et al (1983)	Randomised clinical trial to colestipol or routine medical management. Thirty three patients were recruited, receiving whole pelvis radiotherapy for gynaecological cancer. There was poor compliance with taking the drug	Patients experienced side effects from the drug. The weekly stool frequency for patients was not significantly different from controls. The patients in the colestipol group took 50% less antidiarrhoeal medication	Diary sheets were used to record stool frequency and volume. The high level of side effects from the drug and poor compliance suggest that little benefit is associated with colestipol
Cholestyramine and low-fat diet (bile acid-sequestering resin)	Chary & Thomson (1984)	A randomised clinical trial to determine the value of a 40-g low-fat diet with or without cholestyramine. Sample of 35 patients receiving pelvic radiation	Diarrhoea control was almost complete in those receiving the cholestyramine as well, but patients experienced side effects	Symptoms recorded on a diarrhoea scale. Low-fat diet was well tolerated with little weight loss (less than 5%) and reduced the incidence of diarrhoea. Do not recommend use of drug
Low-fat, low-lactose diet	Bye et al (1995)	A randomised controlled trial design testing low-fat, low-lactose diets in 143 women being treated with pelvic radiotherapy for gynaecological cancer	Significant difference seen in those taking low-fat and lactose diet: 23% of those taking the diet reported diarrhoea during treatment compared to 48% in the control group	Daily diary cards recording number and consistency of stools, use of antidiarrhoeal agents and quality of life (EORTC core questions). Those using the diet had less diarrhoea and required less antidiarrhoeal medication

Elemental supplements	Craighead & Young (1998)	Phase II study assessing feasibility of elemental diets in 17 women being treated for gynaecological cancer and assessment of 45 comparison patients not receiving intervention	15% of those receiving elemental diet reported diarrhoea compared to 55% in the non-intervention group. Bowel changes were less at 1 year in the intervention group	Daily diaries were used to assess compliance with taking the elemental diet (76% compliance). Bowel symptoms were recorded through RTOG scores Those using the elemental diet had fewer symptoms and less late toxicity than the comparison group
Ispaghula husk (fibre bulking)	Lodge et al (1985)	A randomised crossover trial comparing codeine phosphate to that of ispaghula husk (Isogel/Fybogel): 10 women receiving pelvic radiotherapy for gynaecological cancer	Trial was stopped early due to worse diarrhoea experienced by women from ispaghula husk	Daily diaries and treatment sheets. This study is inconclusive but suggests that bulk-forming agents are not helpful in managing diarrhoea
Aspirin	Mennie et al (1975)	Double-blind randomised trial of acetylsalicylate in 28 women receiving pelvic radiotherapy for uterine cancer	Acetylsalicylate reduced the number of bowel motions and relieved abdominal pain and flatulence	Daily bowel and bladder diary. Aspirin was effective in reducing symptoms. However, this study only occurred for 72 h and the longer-term effect is unclear

EORTC, European Organisation for Research and Treatment of Cancer; RTOG, Radiation Therapy Oncology Group.

A low-fat diet may provide a more practical option. As previously stated, bile acid malabsorption is a possible cause of diarrhoea. Bile acids are released in response to fat in the diet, therefore by reducing dietary fat diarrhoea may be minimised. Clinical studies suggest that a 40-g low-fat diet can significantly reduce diarrhoea (Bosaeus et al 1979, Danielsson et al 1991)(see Ch. 11 for low-fat diet). A small randomised clinical trial using an intervention of a low-fat and low-lactose diet in women with gynaecological cancer found that the diet significantly reduced the severity of women's diarrhoea (Bye et al 1995). However, in clinical practice, low-fat diets are rarely used and often patients are advised to lower the fibre in their diet instead, based on the assumption that reducing bowel bulk will reduce symptoms. There is no clinical evidence to suggest that this advice is of value and it may in fact result in constipation. Low-fat diets are also controversial as they can contribute to weight loss.

The use of bacterial cultures in fermented milk has also been tested as a way of reducing overgrowth of pathogenic microorganisms (Henriksson et al 1995). There is little clinical evidence that this is effective and it may make acute symptoms worse.

Medications

Drugs that act to bind with bile acids in the intestine (cholestyramine, colestipol hydrochloride) have been successfully used in reducing diarrhoea from pelvic radiotherapy. However, the side effects of the drugs outweigh any benefit that comes from a reduction in diarrhoea (Stryker et al 1983). Chary & Thomson (1984) used a combination of a 40-g low-fat diet with cholestyramine. Those in the diet and cholestyramine group had significantly ($P < 0.05$) less diarrhoea (one out of 17 patients) compared to those who had diet alone (six out of 16). The researchers concluded that the cholestyramine was effective in preventing acute diarrhoea but that it also caused nausea and was found by some to be unpalatable. Antidiarrhoeal agents such as codeine phosphate or loperamide are more often used for symptom management. These medications influence intestinal motility, but they may also cause problems of constipation or dizziness and may only produce short-term relief.

Sucralfate, an agent used in inflammatory bowel disease, has been shown to have a protective coating effect on the gastrointestinal mucosa (Tarnawski 1984). Henriksson et al (1992a) in a double-blind trial of 70 patients receiving radiotherapy for prostate or bladder cancer found that sucralfate granules significantly reduced diarrhoea and also reduced late bowel disturbances up to 1 year after treatment. An animal study exploring the efficacy of systemic antiinflammatory agents (aspirin, indometacin, piroxicam) found that these agents had no observed biological effect on bowel damage (Nofthway et al 1988). In contrast, Mennie et al (1975) found that acetylsalicylate significantly reduced bowel cramps and bowel movements; however, these results have not been replicated. In a study using 5-HT$_3$-anatagonists Henriksson et al (1992b) demonstrated that diarrhoea was reduced and other studies show constipation as a side effect of this class of drugs. However, the clinical applicability of these findings remains unclear.

The management of proctitis

The pathophysiological characteristics of radiation proctitis are poorly understood; therefore its management relies on good symptom control. Local pain relief can be provided through the application of enemas or anal creams. Sucralfate enemas given twice daily have been shown to result in significant clinical and endoscopic improvements (Kochhar et al 1990). Corticosteroids given orally or rectally have also been used for their antiinflammatory properties. A recent Cochrane review (Denton et al 2002) of non-surgical interventions for late radiation proctitis indicates that rectal hydrocortisone is more effective than rectal betamethasone, but that rectal sucralfate results in the greatest clinical improvements. These interventions relate mainly to late problems and therefore need further testing in the management of acute proctitis.

CONCLUSION

There is confusion about the most appropriate interventions for radiation-induced bowel symptoms (Claben et al 1998). Many of the treatments mentioned have not been effectively tested on radiation-induced gastrointestinal symptoms. There is also a need to improve the clinical assessment of nausea, vomiting and bowel symptoms. The possible link between acute and chronic symptoms is suggested in several clinical studies (Craighead & Young 1998, Henriksson et al 1992a), with indications that effective control of acute symptoms may reduce the incidence of chronic radiation enteritis. More accurate assessment of toxicity during radiotherapy will help to clarify such links. Although modern radiotherapeutic techniques have reduced bowel side effects to a certain extent, the increasing use of adjuvant and multimodality therapy is associated with greater toxicity, highlighting the need to understand the interrelationships of symptoms and their causes more effectively. Gastrointestinal side effects can have a major effect on patients' quality of life but there is little evidence of these being addressed adequately. Although the evidence base is small, certain interventions, such as the use of low-fat diets, do show benefits, and should be taken more seriously by clinicians.

SUMMARY OF KEY CLINICAL POINTS

- The gastrointestinal tract is particularly vulnerable to radiation damage due to the fast turnover of cells.
- The incidence of gastrointestinal effects varies considerably depending on the treatment site, dose, volume and fractionation schedule.
- Gastrointestinal symptoms can have a detrimental effect on patients' quality of life.
- Assess risk factors for nausea and vomiting or gastrointestinal problems prior to start of radiotherapy.
- Consider patients' past medical history and comorbid disease to identify factors that may increase risk.
- Those at moderate to high risk of nausea and vomiting (treatment to upper abdomen, large single fractions, total body irradiation, hemibody or palliative irradiation) should be prescribed appropriate antiemetics prior to starting treatment.

• Wider strategies for managing nausea should be employed, such as patient education, information, relaxation and acupressure.
• The efficacy of antiemetics should be assessed on a daily basis throughout radiotherapy. If not effective, patients should be aware of how to seek help.
• Patients receiving wide-field pelvic radiotherapy should be encouraged, from the start of treatment, to maintain a low-fat diet. Monitoring of weight prior to and during treatment is important. If patients have already lost weight prior to therapy or have a pre-existing gastrointestinal problem, they should be referred to a dietician.
• Patients suffering from proctitis should be prescribed rectal sucralfate or corticosteroids and drug effectiveness should be assessed weekly.

AREAS FOR FURTHER RESEARCH

• Study and evaluation of assessment tools for determining risk of radiation-induced gastrointestinal symptoms
• Research to determine aetiology of radiation-induced nausea and vomiting
• Evaluation of an algorithm to manage nausea and vomiting as a result of radiotherapy
• Assessment of behavioural and pharmacological management for radiation-induced anticipatory nausea and vomiting
• Systematic review of existing evidence for the management of radiation-induced bowel problems
• Evaluation of special diets to control bowel symptoms and their effect on late toxicity.

FURTHER INFORMATION

NCI/PDQ Nausea and vomiting (PDQ®) (Health Professional)
http://www.cancer.gov/cancer_information/doc_pdq.

CancerNet supportive care statement: radiation enteritis
http://www.cancer.gov/cancer_information

REFERENCES

Aass N, Fossa S, Host H 1992 Acute and subacute side effects due to infra-diaphragmatic radiotherapy for testicular cancer: a prospective study. International Journal of Radiation Oncology, Biology, Physics 5:358–363
Amdur R, Parsons J, Fitzgerald L et al 1990 Adenocarcinoma of the prostate treated with external beam radiation therapy: 5 year minimum follow-up. Radiotherapy and Oncology 18:235–246
Beard C, Propert K, Rieker P et al 1997 Complications after treatment with external beam irradiation in early stage prostate cancer patients: a prospective multiinstitutional outcomes study. Journal of Clinical Oncology 15:223–229
Beer W, Fan A, Halstead C 1985 Clinical and nutritional complications of radiation enteritis. American Journal of Clinical Nutrition 41:85–91

Bosaeus I, Andersson H, Nystrom C 1979 Effect of low-fat diet on bile salt excretion and diarrhoea in the gastrointestinal radiation syndrome. Acta Radiologica Oncology 18:460–464

Buchali A, Feyer P, Groll J et al 2000 Immediate toxicity during fractionated total body irradiation as conditioning for bone marrow transplantation. Radiotherapy and Oncology 54:157–162

Busch D 1990 Pathology of the radiation-damaged bowel. In: Gallard R, Spencer J (eds) Radiation enteritis. Edward Arnold, London, 67–87

Bye A, Ose T, Kassa S 1995 Quality of life during pelvic radiotherapy. Acta Obstetrica Gynecologica Scandinavica 74:147–152

Chary S, Thomson D 1984 A clinical trial evaluating cholestyramine to prevent diarrhoea in patients maintained on low fat diets during pelvic radiation therapy. International Journal of Radiation Oncology, Biology, Physics 10:1885–1890

Churnratanakul S, Wirzba B, Lam T et al 1990 Radiation and the small intestine: future perspectives for preventive therapy. Digestive Disease 8:45–60

Claben J, Belka C, Paulsen F et al 1998 Radiation induced gastrointestinal toxicity. Strahlentherapie und Onkologie 174:82–84

Collis C, Priestman T, Priestman S 1991 The final assesment of a randomized double-blind comparative study of ondansetron vs. metoclopramide in the prevention of nausea and vomiting following upper abdomen irradiation. Clinical Oncology (Royal College of Radiologists) 3:341–343

Colwell J, Goldberg M 2000 A review of radiation proctitis in the treatment of prostate cancer. Journal of Wound Ostomy and Continence Nurses Society 27:179–187

Covens A, Thomas G, DePetrillo A 1991 The prognostic importance of site and type of radiation-induced bowel injury in patients requiring surgical management. Gynaecological Oncology 43:270–274

Craighead P, Young S 1998 Phase II study assessing the feasability of using elemental supplements to reduce acute enteritis in patients receiving radical pelvic radiotherapy. American Journal of Clinical Oncology 21:573–578

Danielsson A, Nyhlin H, Stendahl R et al 1991 Chronic diarrhoea after radiotherapy for gynaecological cancer: occurrence and aetiology. Gut 32:1180–1187

Denton A, Forbes A, Andreyev J et al 2002 Non surgical interventions for late radiation proctitis in patients who have received radical radiotherapy to the pelvis. Cochrane Library, Oxford

Eckert R 2001 Understanding anticipatory nausea. Oncology Nursing Forum 28:1553–1558

Erickson B, Otterson M, Moulder J 1994 Altered motility causes the early gastrointestinal toxicity of irradiation. International Journal of Radiation Oncology, Biology, Physics 28:905–912

Faithfull S 2001 Radiotherapy. In: Corner J, Bailey C (eds) Cancer nursing: care in context. Blackwell Science, Oxford, p 222–261

Fernandez-Barnes F, Villa S, Esteve M 1991 Acute effects of abdominopelvic irradiation on orocecal transit time: its relation to clinical symptoms and bile salt and lactose malabsorption. American Journal of Gastroenterology 86:1771–1777

Feyer P, Titlbach O 1998 Treatment of radiotherapy-induced nausea and vomiting. In: Dicato M (ed) Cancer treatment induced emesis. Martin Dunitz, London, p 103–129

Feyer P, Stewart A, Titlbach O 1998 Aetiology and prevention of emesis induced by radiotherapy. Support Cancer Care 6:253–260

Flickinger J, Bloomer W, Kinsella J 1990 Intestinal intolerance of radiation injury. In: Galland R, Spencer J (eds) Radiation enteritis. Edward Arnold, London, p 51–65

Franzen L, Nyman I, Hagberg H et al 1996 A randomised placebo controlled study with ondansetron in patients undergoing fractionated radiotherapy. American Oncology 7:587–592

Gallagher M, Brereton H, Rostock R et al 1986 A prospective study of treatment techniques to minimize the volume of pelvic small bowel with reduction of acute and late effects associated with pelvic irradiation. International Journal of Radiation Oncology, Biology, Physics 12:1565–1573

Gray G 1975 Carbohydrate digestion and absorption: role of the small intestine. New England Journal of Medicine 292:1225–1230

Hainsworth J, Hesketh P 1992 Single-dose ondanestron for the prevention of cisplatin-induced emesis: efficacy results. Seminars in Oncology 19:14–19

Henriksson R, Franzen L, Littbrand B 1992a Effects of sucralfate on acute and late bowel discomfort following radiotherapy of pelvic cancer. Journal of Clinical Oncology 10:969–975

Henriksson R, Lomberg H, Israelsson G 1992b The effect on ondansetron on radiation-induced emesis and diarrhoea. Acta Oncologica 31:767–769

Henriksson R, Franzen L, Sandstrom K et al 1995 Effects of active addition of bacteria cultures in fermented milk to patients with chronic bowel discomfort following irradiation. Support Care Cancer 3:81–83

King K, Nail L, Kreamer K et al 1985 Patients' descriptions of the experience of receiving radiation therapy. Oncology Nursing Forum 12:55–61

Kinsella T, Bloomer W 1980 Bowel tolerance to radiation therapy. Surgery, Gynaecology and Obstetrics 151:273–284

Klee M, Thranov I, Machin D 1999 Life after radiotherapy: the psychological and social effects experienced by women treated for advanced stages of cervical cancer. Gynaecologic Oncology 76:5–13

Klee M, Thranov I, Machin D 2000 The patients' perspective on physical symptoms after radiotherapy for cervical cancer. Gynaecologic Oncology 76:14–23

Kochhar R, Mehta S, Aggarwal R et al 1990 Sucralfate enema in ulcerative rectosigmoid lesions. Diseases of the Colon and Rectum 33:49–51

Krishnasamy M 2001 Nausea and vomiting. In: Corner J, Bailey C (eds) Cancer nursing: care in context. Blackwell Science, Oxford, 350–357

Levi S, Hodgson H 1990 Prevention of radiation enteritis. In: Galland R, Spencer J (eds) Radiation enteritis. Edward Arnold, London, p 121–135

Lodge N, Evans M L, Blake P, Fryatt I 1985 A randomised cross-over study of the efficacy of codeine phosphate versus ispaghuea husk in patients with gynaecological cancer experiencing diarrhoea during pelvic radiotherapy. European Journal of Cancer Care 4:8–10

Mennie A, Dalley V, Dinneen L et al 1975 Treatment of radiation-induced gastrointestinal distress with acetysalicylate. Lancet ii:942–943

Miller A, Martenson J, Nelson H et al 1999 The incidence and clincal consequences of treatment-related bowel injury. International Journal of Radiation Oncology, Biology, Physics 43:817–825

Nofthway M, Scobey M, Geisinger K 1988 Radiation proctitis in the rat: sequential changes and effects of anti-inflammatory agents. Cancer 62:1962–1969

Padilla G 1990 Gastrointestinal side effects and quality of life in patients receiving radiation therapy. Nutrition 6:367–370

Perez C, Lee H, Georgiou A et al 1994 Technical factors affecting morbidity in definitive irradiation for localized carcinoma of the prostate. International Journal of Radiation Oncology, Biology, Physics 28(4):811–819

Potish R 1990 Factors predisposing to injury. In: Galland R, Spencer J (eds) Radiation enteritis. Edward Arnold, London, p 103–119

Potish R, Jones T, Levitt S 1979 Factors predisposing to radiation-related small bowel damage. Oncology 132:479–482

Prentice T 1988 Radiation induced emesis. Clinician 6:40–43

Rhodes V, Johnson M, McDaniel R 1995 Nausea, vomiting and retching: the management of the symptom experience. Seminars in Oncology Nursing 11:256–265

Roberts J, Priestman T 1993 A review of ondansetron in the management of radiotherapy-induced emesis. Oncology 50:173–179

Roila F, Ciccarese G, Palladino M et al 1998 Prevention of radiotherapy-induced emesis. Tumori 84:274–278

Stryker J, Hepner G, Mortel R 1977 The effect of pelvic irradiation on ileal function. Radiology 124:213–216

Stryker J, Chung C, Layser J 1983 Colestipol hydrochloride prophylaxis of diarrhoea during pelvic radiotherapy. International Journal of Radiation Oncology, Biology, Physics 9:185–190

Sullivan M 1962 Dependence of radiation diarrhoea on the presence of bile in the small intestine. Nature 195:1217–1218

Tait D, Nahum A, Meyer L et al 1997 Acute toxicity in pelvic radiotherapy; randomised trial of conformal versus conventional treatment. Radiotherapy and Oncology 42:121–136

Tarnawski A 1984 Sucralfate: is it more than just a barrier? Current Concepts in Gastroententerology June/July:5–12

The Italian Group 1999 Radiation induced emesis: a prospective observational multicentre Italian trial. International Journal of Radiation Oncology, Biology, Physics 44:619–625

Wang C, Leung S, Chen H et al 1989 The correlation of acute toxicity and late rectal injury in radiotherapy for cervical carcinoma: evidence suggestive of consequential late effects. International Journal of Radiation Oncology, Biology, Physics 40:85–91

Waugh A, Grant A 2001 Ross and Wilson anatomy and physiology in health and illness, 9th edn. Churchill Livingstone, Edinburgh

Welch D 1980 Assessment of nausea and vomiting in cancer patients undergoing external beam radiotherapy. Cancer Nursing 3:365–371

Yeoh E, Horowitz M 1988 Radiation enteritis. British Journal of Hospital Medicine June: 498–504

Yeoh E, Lui D, Lee N 1984 The mechanism of diarrhoea resulting from pelvic and abdominal radiotherapy; a prospective study using selenium-75 labelled conjugated bile acid and cobalt-58 labelled cyanocobalamin. British Journal of Radiology 57:1131–1136

Yeoh E, Horowitz M, Russo A et al 1993 Effect of pelvic irradiation on gastrointestinal function: a prospective longitudinal study. The American Journal of Medicine 95:397–406

Yeoh E, Botten R, Russo A et al 2000 Chronic effects of therapeutic irradiation for localized prostatic carcinoma on anorectal function. International Journal of Radiation Oncology, Biology, Physics 47:915–924

Zimmermann F, Feldmann H 1998 Radiation proctitis. Strahlentherapie und Onkologie 174:85–89

14

Late toxicity: neurological and brachial plexus injury

Vincent Khoo   Sara Faithfull

INTRODUCTION

Neurological damage resulting from radiation therapy is classed as one of the most serious complications because of its potential to impact on the patient's quality of life significantly. Activities of day-to-day living are dependent on adequate neurological function. Any neurological damage resulting from radiation that causes difficulties with muscular power or coordination, sensory changes, organ and cerebral function will impact on an individual's quality of life. In addition, there may be other side effects related to surrounding tissues/organs, such as lymphoedema or muscle fibrosis, that can compound the clinical situation. This combination of side effects can be very distressing. Whilst it is valuable to consider each complication, it is more important to assess the contributions of each complication to evaluate properly the total effect on the patient's lifestyle. It is also vital to obtain the patient's perspective, as the needs of one person can be vastly different from that of another. Only in this manner can adequate management and treatment be organised.

The clinical spectrum of radiation-induced neurological damage is wide-ranging but, luckily, the incidence of severe neurological complications is rare. These are classified into delayed or late effects. Delayed side effects, occurring within a few weeks to months following irradiation, are usually limited and reversible. Late neurological complications occur from 6 months to several years after the initial radiation therapy, often developing insidiously, and may be inappropriately attributed to other causes. Late neurological complications are often unrelenting, progressive and irreversible. There has always been considerable awareness of the potential of radiation to cause neurological damage. In the modern radiotherapy era, prevention or minimisation of late damage is the basis of many radiotherapy techniques. The symptoms depend on the site of neurological damage. For example, irradiation of the spinal cord may lead to total or partial paralysis whilst excessive radiation to the cerebrum may result in neuropsychological dysfunction. The diagnosis of radiation-induced neurological damage can be difficult to make when the tumour is located close to neuronal structures. Uncontrolled growth of tumour or tumour recurrence following radiation can readily mimic the symptoms and signs of radiation damage, therefore it is crucial to exclude tumour recurrence as a cause of symptoms as this has implications for treatment.

The likelihood of any radiation-induced complication will depend on several factors, which include the location and extent of tumour, the patient's condition as well as radiotherapy factors such as the total dose delivered, the dose per fraction, the interval between fractions and volume treated. The importance and implications of these radiotherapy parameters, including the delivery method of radiation, radiation beam quality and energy, have been discussed in detail in Chapter 5. In this chapter, the pathophysiology and spectrum of radiation-induced neurological damage affecting both the central nervous system (CNS) and peripheral nervous system (PNS) will be reviewed, in particular the syndrome of spinal cord and brachial plexopathy. Whilst it is important to identify these syndromes, it is more important to prevent them from occurring. There is no substitute for poor radiation technique. Therefore, emphasis should be on prevention and these issues will be discussed in detail.

AETIOLOGY

The mechanism of radiation-induced neuronal damage is multifactorial. Radiation may cause direct damage to nerve cells or its supporting network such as myelin or vascular supply. The histological changes due to neurological damage have been mainly explored in animal models and characterised in human cases (Schulthesis et al 1988). Radiation-induced oedema or tissue swelling is thought to be responsible for most acute neurological side effects. This is particularly true of acute side effects resulting from CNS treatment because there is minimal room for expansion within the rigid confines of the bony skull. These acute effects are short lived and reversible and are commonly associated with large radiation treatment volumes and fraction sizes. Delayed CNS side effects are believed to be related to the temporary interference with the synthesis of myelin causing focal demyelination of the nerve cells (DeLattre et al 1988). Myelin is the white matter insulating the nerves and allows the conduction of nerve impulses. Radiation can also cause temporary changes in the permeability status of the vascular capillary beds supplying the nerves (DeLattre et al 1988). These vascular changes can adversely affect nerve function. Delayed neurological side effects are usually reversible but may take several weeks for recovery.

Permanent damage to nerve cells or to its vascular supply has been thought to be responsible for late radiation-induced neurological damage. Destruction of the nerve cell, myelin or its pathways results in necrosis. This necrosis of nerve tissue may be localised or widespread and symptoms will depend on the location and extent of damage. Extensive damage of crucial nerve networks can be potentially fatal. The function of the nerve cells can also be indirectly and permanently destroyed by inadequate blood supply or ischaemia as a result of the radiation damage to the microcirculation (Gerard et al 1989). The damage seen in irradiated blood vessels can range from telangiectasia with thickening and hardening of the blood vessel walls (endothelial proliferation and hyalinisation) to inflammation of the blood vessel walls leading to scarring (obliterative vasculitis), clot formation (vascular thrombosis), breakdown of the vessel wall and bleeding (fibrinoid necrosis and haemorrhage) (Alfonso et al 1997). Apart from direct radiation damage to the integrity of the nerve fibres, excessive radiation can also cause thickening or fibrosis of the surrounding soft tissue or muscles. The development of radiation fibrosis may cause compression of peripheral nerves, resulting in entrapment of nerves running within the muscle compartments.

CLINICAL MANIFESTATIONS AND IMPACT OF SYMPTOMS

The clinical picture and symptoms as a result of late toxicity depend on the neurological site irradiated and the function of the involved site. For example, injury to nerves of the brachial plexus in the axilla will cause difficulties with the function of the involved arm whereas damage to the optic nerves or chiasma can cause blindness. There are no clear distinctive clinical features of neurological injury related to radiation except that a previous history of radiation delivered to some part of the nerve plexus or pathway must exist. The type of radiation delivered, the dose and fractionation scheme and the volume treated must be considered as a possible cause of radiation damage to the nerves. For example, treatment of a superficial skin cancer overlying the axilla using superficial radiation, which only has a penetration depth of less than 5 mm, is not going to cause brachial plexus damage.

Careful assessment of individuals' presenting symptoms can sometimes be helpful in distinguishing between the possible differential diagnoses. In cancer patients suspected of developing any radiation-related complication it is crucial to exclude tumour progression or recurrence, as this occurrence is not uncommon. The diagnosis of any likely radiation-induced neurological damage often remains a diagnosis of exclusion. It is important to assess symptoms adequately, as the diagnosis will influence the person's subsequent management, rehabilitation and prognosis. The effects on the PNS and CNS are markedly different but there are some well-recognised neurological problems.

PNS neurological deficits

Radiation-induced myelopathy can present either as a delayed but reversible syndrome or a more serious late and permanent complication. A classic example of a delayed PNS syndrome is Lhermitte's sign, which can occur following irradiation of the upper thoracic/cervical cord such as in mantle irradiation for lymphoma or head and neck treatments. Patients describe symptoms of sharp electric-like numbness or paraesthesiae that radiate from the neck to the upper arms, lasting seconds to minutes. Bending the neck, walking on hard surfaces or other physical activities can precipitate these symptoms. Interestingly, neurological examination and imaging investigations (computed tomography (CT) and magnetic resonance imaging (MRI)) are usually normal. This syndrome is self-limiting, usually developing within 2–3 months following radiation treatment and resolves spontaneously in weeks or months. Lhermitte's sign does not appear to be related to the development of late spinal myelopathy (Sheline et al 1980).

Spinal cord myelopathy

Spinal cord myelopathy has been reported to occur bimodally at 12–14 months and 24–28 months following radiation treatment, although cases can occur many years later (Schultheiss et al 1995). Usually the initial symptoms are subtle, starting with paraesthesiae and/or sensory changes, becoming progressively worse. Severe acute myelopathy, characterised by loss of muscular power and reflexes, is less common and in this situation it is also important to exclude recurrence of cancer.

The pattern of neurological symptoms and signs depends on the level of spinal cord injury. Damage to sections of the spinal cord can cause segmental loss of muscle power and reflexes related to the supplied nerve supply. Impairment is seen below the involved spinal cord level with loss of sensation (numbness or paraesthesiae), impairment of pain, temperature and vibration perception. Muscular rigidity or spasticity and weakness of one side of the body (hemiparesis) can also develop. Varying degrees of bowel and bladder dysfunction can also occur, such as bladder retention, constipation or incontinence. In some patients, the functional loss may be partial, whilst in others the myelopathy may be progressive, resulting in complete paralysis over time. The extent of functional disability will depend not only on the level of myelopathy but also on the completeness of the neurological defect. These symptoms are usually irreversible if complete loss of a whole section of spinal cord or transection is present. If the cord transection is incomplete, there have been some encouraging case reports of partial recovery of function that can occur over several years (Esik et al 1999). Where damage is on one side of the spinal cord, this is called Brown-Séquard syndrome. This damage results in loss of muscular power and sensation on the same side of the body where the injury has occurred and loss of temperature and pain sensation on the opposite side of body to the spinal injury.

Brachial plexopathy

Brachial plexopathy can occur in patients who have received irradiation to the axillary and supraclavicular regions such as from breast radiotherapy or mantle fields used for Hodgkin's disease. Plexopathy can also occur in other sites, such as the lumbosacral plexus, but these are extremely rare. In a review of approximately 1600 breast cancer patients treated with conservative surgery and radiation, brachial plexopathy was reported to occur in 2% of patients (Pierce et al 1992). The onset of symptoms usually occurs at a median interval of 10–12 months following irradiation (Kori et al 1981, Pierce et al 1992). Patients suffering from this complication experience symptoms of paraesthesiae and numbness in the affected limb. The distribution of sensory change will depend on which branch of the brachial plexus was involved. Wasting of the small muscles of the hand will follow within months or years. Other symptoms include arm weakness, shoulder and arm pain, and these symptoms are influenced by the presence of other comorbid complications that can arise from irradiation of the region, such as lymphoedema, tissue fibrosis and bone complications. These additional complications can significantly compound the severity of the problem. Some investigators have suggested that lymphoedema is more common in the presence of radiation damage whilst Horner's syndrome is more often associated with metastatic involvement (Kori et al 1981). Similarly, upper motor branch involvement is more commonly reported with radiation damage whereas lower motor involvement is more commonly associated with tumour recurrence (Kori et al 1981). A rare complication of brachial plexopathy is diaphragmatic weakness secondary to phrenic neuropathy (Brander et al 1997).

Although this complication is rare, it can have distressing consequences. Of the many late radiation complications, brachial plexopathy is the most documented, as women who had experienced such symptoms formed a self-help group, Radiation Action Group Exposure (RAGE) to provide support for those with radiation side effects. There is little written about their experiences; however, documentary evidence exists describing how symptoms have impacted on patient's lives. One woman who had received radiotherapy for breast cancer told of how insidiously her symptoms occurred:

> It started with a pain in my arm ... it started to deteriorate badly, I used to have to put it [arm] in a pocket, I couldn't have it hanging any more it was just so painful. I started getting ulcers on the lower part of my arm. Then one day my arm went dead. You don't believe how much you need two arms. The pain just didn't stop, then I had phantom pains
>
> (The Big Story, Carlton TV, 4 November 1993).

The symptoms have devastating consequences and can lead to 1–4% of affected women requiring amputations of the arm.

CNS neurological deficits

Damage to the CNS can occur as a result of fractionated conventional external beam radiotherapy, commonly used for brain malignancies as well as from more specialised techniques such as stereotactic cranial radiotherapy. This damage can result in neurological deficits, impairment of mental processes (cognitive function) and neuroendocrine abnormalities. An important delayed irradiation symptom to recognise is the subacute encephalopathy or somnolence syndrome. Patients with this syndrome classically present 2–6 weeks following radiation therapy with a collection of symptoms that includes excessive drowsiness, fatigue and an inability to concentrate and sometimes exacerbation of focal neurological symptoms. Descriptive work by Faithfull & Brada (1998) mapping the pattern of symptoms of this syndrome, they found that patients considered somnolence as a sensation that was mentally disabling and disrupted their physical activity by an overwhelming feeling of exhaustion. The frequency and severity of somnolence syndrome may depend on the nature of the primary tumour, its location and the intensity and type of radiotherapy. Patients usually expect a rapid improvement in symptoms once treatment is completed, but somnolence creates anxiety and fear of disease recurrence at a time when clinical support is minimal. One individual describes how somnolence created anxiety:

I get worried that I am not recovering. The whole time you think, is it the tumour or is it the side effect?

(Faithfull 1991, p. 943).

Little is known about how best to alleviate somnolence symptoms, or identify those most at risk. It has been suggested that corticosteroids taken during treatment may reduce the symptoms. However, the benefit of steroids is uncertain and at present the best way to alleviate symptoms is through supportive measures until symptoms improve.

Focal CNS necrosis and nerve palsies

Focal CNS necrosis is a typical late neurological complication occurring in 0.1–5% of patients following doses of 50–60 Gy over 5–6 weeks to areas of the CNS (Halperin & Burger 1985). Focal necrosis can occur anywhere within the CNS: cerebral tissue, brainstem or cranial nerves. Patients present with symptoms and signs that can be non-specific, such as epileptic fits, and symptoms of raised intracranial pressure. Pain and headaches can also be a prominent feature. Cranial nerve palsies are a well-recognised complication of stereotactic radiotherapy treatment given for lesions located within the base of the skull. Loss of facial sensation and control of facial muscles can result from trigeminal and facial nerve neuropathy. The clinical symptoms relate to the function of the affected cranial nerve, for example, optic nerve and chiasma neuropathy resulting in partial vision or blindness is a drastic complication that will severely compromise a patient's quality of life. These two complications have been reported to occur in up to one-third of patients with acoustic schwannomas treated with stereotactic radiotherapy (Flickinger et al 1991). Most patients with cranial nerve palsies suffer partial dysfunction that usually gradually improves over 6 months to 2 years, except for rare cases, where complete dysfunction is initially present (Flickinger et al 1991).

Cognitive dysfunction

The development of cognitive dysfunction is a gradual process that can develop in adults and children treated with whole-brain irradiation. There is evidence that the immature developing brain, especially in children younger than 3 years of age, is more susceptible to irradiation damage (Roman & Sperduto 1995). A National Cancer Institute epidemiological study found that long-term survivors of CNS tumours treated before the age of 20 had experienced significant deterioration in quality of life. These survivors were more likely to be at risk for adverse outcomes such as having a health problem affecting their ability to work, higher probability of unemployment, inability to drive or describing their current health as poor (Mostow et al 1991). These late symptoms most commonly affect those treated with irradiation for supratentorial tumours.

Cognitive dysfunction has also been recorded in adults' postcranial irradiation. The extent of cognitive damage appears to depend on the volume of cerebrum treated, the dose/fractionation schedule and the use of other therapies such as chemotherapy or surgery (Johnson et al 1985). Irradiation of the whole brain or a substantial volume is more likely to be associated with changes in short-term memory, the ability for new task learning, abstraction and problem solving that may prevent return of the patient to premorbid social life and occupation (Maire et al 1987). Up to one-third of long-term survivors treated with radiation for gliomas have been reported to be unable to return to occupations comparable to those held prior to developing the cancer (Kleinberg et al 1993).

Neuroendocrine dysfunction can result from radiation damage to the hypothalamus–pituitary axis. Dysfunction of growth hormone production is the most common abnormality and its impact is greatest for children and adolescents where issues of growth and development are most important (Shalet et al 1976). Assessment and management details are outside the scope of this chapter. For further information, the reader is advised to peruse general radiotherapy/oncology or specific paediatric textbooks (Green & D'Angio 1992).

PREVENTION OF RADIATION-INDUCED NEUROLOGICAL DAMAGE

General principles

The aim of any radiation treatment is to achieve eradication of the tumour or a high probability of local control whilst ensuring that the likelihood of any treatment-related complication is as low as possible. Clinicians are acutely aware of the disastrous consequences of radiation-induced neurological damage. It is always a balance between providing a radical enough dose for tumour eradication and not exceeding the threshold for complications (Ch. 2). Often the presence of critical neurological structures close to the tumour, such as the optic chiasma or spinal cord, prevents the delivery of curative doses of radiation. In this situation, radiation treatment may reflect an attempt to control the tumour rather than to eradicate it. A conservative approach is often adopted to ensure that the total prescribed radiation dose is well below the threshold level required for the development of neurological complications. However, it is important to realise that uncontrolled cancer can also invade important neurological structures which are adjacent to it and cause the very complication that was hoped to be prevented by radiation. A balance exists between the need to prevent the cancer causing neurological complications, tumour invasion and the likelihood of radiation-related complications. These issues need to be discussed thoroughly so that the patient can make an informed decision.

The nature of late radiation complications is that development occurs at some time following completion of the radiation therapy. There is little opportunity to modify the radiation schedule during treatment. Therefore, knowledge of the three-dimensional relationship of the tumour to the surrounding organs or nerves, tolerance of tissues and/or organs, the impact of different dose/fractionation schedules and the consequences of uncontrolled disease are important factors in the decision-making process. Treatment decisions about technique and dose/fractionation schedules need to be made a priori based on an estimation of dose–complication probabilities. Reviews of published case reports are used to estimate the probability of radiotherapy complications, but the patient's CT and MRI can be useful in establishing potential areas of damage. However, the clinical data needed to establish the tolerance of various neurological tissues accurately are limited.

Fraction size is an important factor as large fractions are usually associated with an increased probability of late complications, especially if given with curative intent (Thames et al 1982). For example, most cases of focal neurological damage have been reported with fraction sizes of >2.2–2.5 Gy (Sheline et al 1980). The dose–complication relationship for spinal cord myelopathy has been reviewed by Schultheiss & Stephens (1992), who concluded that if conventional dose fraction sizes of 2 Gy are used it can be estimated that a threshold dose of around 57–61 Gy produces a 5% incidence of myelopathy at 5 years. Delivery of doses less than 50 Gy is associated with an extremely low risk of spinal cord myelopathy (Jeremic et al 1998, Wong et al 1994). Given that the spinal cord may possess a higher threshold level, for tumours that are perilously close to the spinal cord a higher dose may be delivered to achieve local control and avoid uncontrolled tumour extension into the spinal cord. In this situation, a small volume of spinal cord may receive a higher dose whilst still maintaining a low probability of myelopathy. In this clinical scenario, it is always important to discuss the risk–benefit ratio of such treatment options with the patient. Another important factor is the volume of irradiated tissue. Recent animal models suggest that the tolerance threshold for spinal cord myelopathy is reduced as the volume of spinal cord increases (van-de-Aardweg et al 1995). Therefore, reducing treatment volume in the high-dose region through methods such as intensity-modulated radiotherapy can potentially reduce a significant incidence of complications.

A short time interval between deliveries of radiotherapy fractions can also cause problems. A higher than expected incidence of myelopathy has been recorded using accelerated fractionation regimens, which involve more than one fraction given per day compared to conventional dose and fractionation schemes (Dische 1991, Wong et al 1994). The short time interval between fractions does not allow time for repair; this reduces the tolerance of the neurological tissue (Ch. 5). Radiobiological studies suggest that a minimal interval of at least 6–8 h is needed to maintain tolerance of normal tissue and avoid late neurological complications (Dutreix et al 1973).

Where tumour recurrence occurs, retreatment of a previously irradiated neurological site may be necessary. There is much concern about the tolerance of previously irradiated neurological tissue. Some animal studies and clinical cases have suggested that radiation-induced tissue changes or damage can be completely repaired if sufficient time is given. A recent case of reirradiation of the full cervical cord 17 years following initial radical radiotherapy has been reported (Ryu et al 2000). However, clinical reviews have suggested that neurological damage from irradiation is not fully repaired (Bentzen & Dische 2001), resulting in reduced tolerance, greater probability of myelopathy and a shorter latent time to myelopathy occurrence (Wong et al 1994).

The use of other agents with radiotherapy such as chemotherapy, biological modifiers or radiosensitisers can potentiate the effect of radiation. Some chemotherapeutic agents, such as platinum-based cytotoxic drugs, for example, are neurotoxic. Similarly, chemotherapeutic agents that cross the blood–brain barrier can also be neurotoxic. Case reports illustrate the interaction where spinal cord doses were well within accepted tolerance limits; however, the addition of chemotherapy was associated with spinal cord myelopathy (Chao et al 1998, Hirota et al 1993). There is potential that new radiotherapy treatment techniques such as intensity-modulated radiotherapy (IMRT) will reduce the need to treat the spinal cord at all. All these treatment factors need to be considered when planning radiotherapy treatment (Table 14.1).

Careful follow-up of patients and recording of late morbidity are essential to provide quality data to establish these tolerance ranges (Bentzen & Dische 2001). More recently, animal studies have been undertaken to understand better the parameters of neurological tolerance to therapeutic radiation. Together, these data provide insight into how radiotherapy technique, dose fraction delivered and tumour volume are correlated with the occurrence of side effects. These general principles will be discussed in relation to breast radiotherapy and brachial plexopathy.

In the case of brachial plexopathy, a range of factors are implicated – the total dose to the axilla, use of a third field and chemotherapy. For example, those women who had axillary doses of less than 50 Gy had a lower incidence of brachial plexopathy (1.3%) compared to those women who received doses over 50 Gy (5.6%) (Pierce et al 1992). One of the problems identified was overlapping treatment fields. Match line overlap of adjacent radiation fields is a serious problem that can result from poor radiotherapy planning and inaccurate treatment set-up of axilla and supraclavicular radiation fields (Bates & Evans 1995). In some cases this inadvertently irradiates the brachial plexus to doses beyond its range of tolerance. This is why it is so important that any errors related to the set-up of the patient for treatment and movement of the patient during treatment are minimised to prevent unintentional overlap of treatment fields and subsequent overdosage.

Table 14.1 Factors that influence the occurrence of radiation-induced neurological injury

Treatment-related factors	
Fraction size	Doses greater than 2.2–2.5 Gy per fraction have been associated with higher prevalence of focal neurological damage
Fractionation schedule	Short time intervals between fractions increase risk. A higher incidence of neurological injury has been recorded in accelerated regimes
Dose	A total dose of 57–61 Gy produces a 5% incidence of myelopathy at 5 years
Overlapping of treatment fields	Movement of the patient between treatment fields is associated with greater incidence of brachial plexopathy
Retreatment	Damage to tissues results in reduced tolerance to irradiation and greater probability of myelopathy
Site of radiotherapy field	Tumour or irradiation close to neurological structures carries greater risk of neurological late effects
Effect of adjuvant therapy	Chemotherapy, biological modifiers and radiosensitizers can potentiate the effect of radiation

Breast radiotherapy and brachial plexopathy

In the UK, as a result of an increased incidence of brachial plexopathy, attention was raised by a self-help group RAGE which led to two independent reports into brachial plexopathy commissioned by the Royal College of Radiologists (RCR). These reports (Bates & Evans 1995, Maher Committee 1995), funded by the Clinical Audit Unit of the NHS Executive, reviewed the possible causes of brachial plexopathy over a 14-year period from 1980 to 1993 in the UK and provided recommendations.

The incidence of brachial plexopathy was highest in the period 1980–1986, with 41 reported cases compared to seven cases in the period 1987–1993. The major factor appeared to be a treatment technique that allowed movement of the patient between treatment of the chest wall and subsequent treatment of the lymph nodes. This potentially produced accidental overlapping of treatment fields and subsequent overdosing at the level of the brachial plexus in the axilla. For cases where this movement was apparent, 72% (34/47 patients) developed brachial plexopathy compared to 24% (12/51 patients) where a restricted movement technique or static treatment position was adopted. Higher doses and large dose per fraction also appeared to predispose women to a higher incidence of brachial plexopathy, with 69% (25/36) developing brachial plexopathy. For the cases reviewed by the Commission report (Bates & Evans 1995), the greatest incidence occurred when potential for movement of the patient and higher dose per fraction were combined, with 21 of 23 patients (91%) suffering brachial plexopathy. The Commission report noted that the techniques described above were common in the period before 1987 and hence the incidence of brachial plexopathy was higher. Subsequently, most centres avoided the use of breast treatment techniques which allowed patient movements between treatment fields, treated all fields daily and used lower dose/fractionation schemes. This appeared to be associated with a lower incidence of brachial plexopathy.

This report clearly highlights the importance of careful attention to precise accurate techniques and dose/fractionation schemes. The Commission report (Bates & Evans 1995) provided the following recommendations for breast radiotherapy:

- Cervicoaxial radiation should *not* be given routinely.
- Breast radiotherapy requires static position techniques: this is particularly important if cervicoaxial radiation is to be given. The double arm pole used with the head straight was thought to provide reliable reproducibility and avoided patient set-up errors.
- The use of high-dose techniques with higher dose per fraction was associated with a greater risk.
- All fields should be treated daily and boosts to the base of the axilla should be avoided.
- Caution should be exercised for patients with collagen vascular diseases such as scleroderma, systemic lupus erythematosus and rheumatoid arthritis because these patients may have unusually severe early and late reactions.

The Commission report also documented that other late tissue sequelae were also likely to occur if brachial neuropathy was present. These other complications relate to the same radiotherapy factors responsible for the match line overdose to the deeper tissue. The list of possible late complications is listed below. They are fully discussed in the Commission report (Bates & Evans 1995, Maher Committee 1995) and in the other chapters in this book.

- Skin–skin telangiectasia and pigmentation changes
- Subcutaneous fibrosis with nerve and vascular entrapment syndromes (Ch. 19)
- Lymphoedema of the arm (Ch. 15)
- Shoulder stiffness
- Bone necrosis (Ch. 18)
- Lung fibrosis (Ch. 9)
- Psychosocial problems (Ch. 17).

GENERAL PRINCIPLES OF MANAGEMENT

Assessment for observed late neurological complications is important. Neurological problems as a result of radiation should reflect the involved nerve segment and these should be within the boundaries of the irradiated field. Otherwise, tumour recurrence or other non-radiation-related causes are more likely possibilities. It is important to exclude tumour recurrence as a possible cause, especially if the original tumour or related nodal regions are near the nerve complex. Assessment of patients' perceptions of symptoms, level of disability and distress is also important.

The range of dysfunction and disability experienced by patients is not only physical but also includes psychological and social difficulties. This is well illustrated by the reviews of brachial plexopathy in the UK and the foundation of the RAGE group where its members expressed considerable anguish and anger. Women felt that their problems were not taken seriously by healthcare professionals and that there was an attitude that, because their cancer was cured, they were fortunate to survive and should not complain. Therefore, integral to the management of any radiation complication is adequate patient information and education. A problem-solving approach, understanding the meaning of symptoms for the individual and using patient-centred care, is essential to deal with the multitude of problems faced. Identifying realistic goals which are set with the individual and regular evaluation of any management strategy should be agreed (Table 14.2). Although there is an absence of definitive treatment, symptom control

Table 14.2 Problem-solving approach for radiation-induced neurological injury

Initial assessment	Clinical and neurological examination. Physical, functional and psychological assessment
Goal-setting	Realistic goals that are achievable and negotiated with the patient. Optimise symptom control for both physical and psychological function
Implementation of treatment plan	Intervention requires a multifaceted approach. The simplest and least toxic treatment should be tried first
Reevaluation	Regular reassessment of progress

and optimising daily functioning can be addressed to maintain as good a quality of life as possible (Maher Committee 1995).

The multidisciplinary team approach

Neurological complications are best addressed by a collaborative multidisciplinary team approach. The RCR Maher Committee report suggested that a clinical oncologist or radiation oncologist would be the person best placed to recognise the condition, provide an honest explanation of the condition and its uncertainties, offer a realistic estimation of the prognosis and exclude or treat recurrent cases of cancer (Maher Committee 1995). Once late neurological complications are manifest, they are rarely reversible. In this situation, it is important not to provide unrealistic expectations that can hamper the patient's perception of functional gain and improvements in quality of life.

Specialist and experienced rehabilitation teams are needed to facilitate the return of the patient to functional and social independence. In order to provide complete treatment, the team should include the following healthcare professionals or units:

- Anaesthetist and psychologist/psychiatrist as part of the pain clinic
- Clinical nurse specialist with site specialisation, such as breast or spinal injuries
- General practitioner and district nurse
- Lymphoedema clinic
- Occupational therapists
- Physiotherapists
- Palliative care clinic
- Specialist rehabilitation physicians
- Surgeons.

Specialist teams are limited for the majority of women with breast cancer. Patients have reported difficulties in seeking a diagnosis or information about the condition and that this is reflected in poor pain management and rehabilitation. An update since the original report was written, identified that oncologists were not sufficiently interested, general practitioners lacked knowledge of radiotherapy-related problems, nurses were reluctant to give information on iatrogenic complications and most members of the specialised multidisciplinary team often provided inconsistent information (Maher 2000). It is clear that much work remains to establish standards and improve care for patients' experiencing late side effects.

Assessment of radiation-induced neurological damage

The diagnosis of radiation-induced neurological damage is often made by excluding other possibilities for the signs or symptoms. Early recognition is important. Once the condition is suspected, a thorough physical examination is warranted, followed by appropriate investigations (Box 14.1).

Imaging studies

Plain radiographic film will demonstrate gross bony changes but is unable to provide proper assessment of soft tissues. Evaluation using either CT and/or MRI

Box 14.1 Assessment strategies for neurological injury

- Assessment of neurological problems, pain complex and functional disability
- Plain X-rays of the relevant regions, such as chest, spine or bones
- Computed tomography and/or magnetic resonance imaging of the affected nerve complex or pathway. For example, for brachial plexopathy, the axilla, supraclavicular fossa and cervical spine should be imaged
- Biopsy of suspicious lesions
- Electrophysiological studies, for example nerve conduction

---

is more useful, however it can still be difficult to discriminate between tumour recurrence and radiation-induced damage. The imaging appearances of radiation damage, especially when necrosis is present, can be very difficult to distinguish from the necrosis due to tumour recurrence. Both have a degree of oedema. MRI is the gold standard for imaging of the brain and neurological system. Using MRI, contrast-enhancing lesions can be seen and have also been visualised in fibrosis (Wouter-van-Es et al 1997). In general, during the acute or early phase of myelopathy, abnormal signal intensity or focal enhancement can be seen with or without cord swelling (Melki et al 1994, Wang et al 1992). Subsequent imaging several months later often demonstrates cord atrophy without abnormal signal abnormality. Myelopathy has been reported to be associated with static neurological deficits and better survival rates compared to the presence of cord enlargement, which is more likely to result in progressive deficits and a poorer prognosis (Hirota et al 1993, Melki et al 1994).

Positron emission tomography (PET) scans have the potential to discriminate between necrosis and actively dividing tumour cells but its sensitivity and specificity remain to be confirmed (Ahmad et al 1999). PET has also been used to provide evidence of partial functional recovery of neurological function. In a recent case of established radiation-induced myelopathy, the increased metabolic activity in the irradiated spinal cord with lack of detectable protein synthesis suggested some restored neurological activity rather than tumour recurrence (Esik et al 1999). Even histology may not be able to confirm the diagnosis, as often viable tumour cells may coexist scattered between areas of tissue damage or necrosis (Harris & Adler 1996). Therefore, the diagnosis of radiation-induced neurological complication often remains a diagnosis of exclusion.

Pain management

Neuralgic pain is often present and proper management is vital. This type of pain is notoriously difficult to treat adequately as the intensity and nature of the pain, even for the same nerve regions, vary. Neuralgic pain is characterised by pain in the distribution of the nerve (Maher Committee 1995). The pain may be constant or intermittent. Patients describe sensations of burning, pins and needles, toothache-like, numbness, frostbite or tightness/cramping (Maher Committee 1995). In addition, neuropathic pain often coexists with pain from other radiation damage, such as bone pain and soft tissue/visceral pain, and this can complicate pain management. It is important to control pain early, even if the assessment for diagnosis is still ongoing. Again, this should be managed by an open collaborative multidisciplinary approach.

Neuropathic pain often requires narcotic analgesic control as it is relatively insensitive to non-narcotic analgesics, but even the effectiveness of narcotic analgesics has been questioned. However, non-narcotic analgesics such as non steroidal anti-inflammatory agents can be useful in managing pain from radiation damage to bone or soft tissue, which can contribute to the pain complex. Topical non-steroidal anti-inflammatory agents, local anaesthetics and capsaicin, a counterirritant, have been used for their direct effect on sensory cutaneous nerves (Portenoy 1993). Tricyclic antidepressants such as amitriptyline and dothiepin are often used as first-line therapy for neuropathic pain followed by anticonvulsants such as phenytoin, carbamazepine and sodium valproate. These agents can be used sequentially or in combination and the dose should be titrated to the individual patient (Davis 1995). Antiarrhythmic cardiac agents such as flecainide and mexiletine have been used for refractory pain but must be used cautiously in patients with poor or suspicious cardiac status. Baclofen, a skeletal muscle relaxant, has also been used to help pain from several different sources, especially if there has been an element of previous surgical damage such as intercostal/brachial nerve damage. Corticosteroids have also been used with some success for patients suffering from the effects of oedema secondary to radiation necrosis. Steroid therapy may last for several months depending on symptom response. However, protracted steroid treatment is associated with side effects such as muscle wasting, blood electrolyte imbalance and glucose intolerance. These side effects need to be carefully evaluated and monitored. The benefits of any treatment need to be balanced against the probability and severity of the side effects.

Non-pharmacological approaches include the local applications of heat or cold, gentle massage, transcutaneous electrical nerve stimulation (TENS) and acupuncture. TENS is a non-invasive method that can be effective (Thompson & Filshie 1993). This method is generally used for a minimum trial of 3 weeks with electrodes placed alongside the affected segments of the spine with or without additional peripheral electrodes placed on trigger points or proximal to the painful areas. The stimulation sites used and varying the treatment parameters such as continuous, bursts or modulated electrical outputs, may have to be adjusted for optimal effect and a physiotherapist performs this best.

When standard pharmacological and non-pharmacological approaches are inadequate to control the neuropathic pain complex, other approaches may be considered. Interventional approaches can be useful and include nerve blocks, sympathectomies and thermocoagulation procedures for nerve root ablation. These surgical approaches have variable results and require a specialised neurosurgical unit. In some cases, surgical decompression may be needed to provide symptom relief for mass compression caused by oedema from radiation necrosis. This situation applies mainly to space-restricted areas such as within the cranium. Other treatments, such as hyperbaric oxygen, surgery and antioxidants are rarely effective in reversing the neurological damage. Anticoagulation therapy has been hypothesised to arrest or reverse small-vessel endothelial injury, which may be responsible for some neurological damage. Using this therapy, partial neurological function recovery has been reported for myelopathy and cerebral radionecrosis (Glantz et al 1994).

Rehabilitation

Rehabilitation should be provided to improve patients' quality of life and reduce dependence (Dietz 1981). This includes taking into account the scale of the disability. The psychological impact of such disability can be devastating and requires substantial adjustment for the individual. Often counselling can be helpful. In general, the management of any radiation-induced late neurological complication needs to be directed at both the functional impairments faced by patients as well as the potential complications that can arise from their disabilities (Box 14.2). Physiotherapy is often needed to maintain muscular tone, range of movement and coordination and prevent spasticity that can result from the development of muscle fibrosis secondary to radiotherapy. Electrophysiological studies may provide semiquantification of motor impairment and allow monitoring of rehabilitation (Meyer & Zentner 1992). Occupational therapy intervention can minimise disability by providing assisted-mobility aids such as splints, limb braces, crutches and wheelchairs as well as adaptive equipment for the home (Cooper 1998).

Another important consideration is the loss of skin sensation with peripheral neuropathies. Patient education and instruction in prophylactic management are important. Patients need to be cautioned about the dangers of potential thermal and pressure injury. Daily skin inspection is important to detect early problems and avoid skin infection. Mobility and fine motor coordination may be difficult in patients with proprioceptive loss, especially if visual difficulties are also present. Preventive devices and aids can be helpful with these problems. For quadra- or paraplegic patients, close attention needs to be paid to bowel and bladder dysfunction. Constipation is a common bowel problem in these patients. Reduced bladder capacity, urinary retention and incontinence are some of the manifestations of neurogenic bladder that need proper urological assessment. Urinary tract infection, reflux nephropathy and hydronephrosis can complicate the neurogenic bladder. In addition, members of the UK's RAGE group have noted that aromatherapy massage, acupuncture and reflexology are helpful. Hypnotherapy and relaxation therapies have also been used. However, the RCR Maher Committee

---

Box 14.2 Guiding principles of management for neurological side effects

- Adequate information and sufficient explanation to empower patients to recognise the condition early if symptoms should arise. Those affected patients must have easy access to evaluation
- Thorough medical assessment and investigation to exclude recurrent cancer as a cause and establish a diagnosis
- Management by an experienced specialist multidisciplinary team
- Systematic management of pain
- Assistance with the functions of daily living with access to rehabilitation aids
- Psychological support, including access to a nurse counsellor, information on voluntary organisations and self-help groups
- Referral for social assistance such as mobility allowances or disability benefits
- Regular surveillance to detect recurrent cancer, particularly within the first 2 years after treatment

report was unable to make specific recommendations about the value of these therapies and suggested that further research is needed in these areas to assess their contribution.

SUMMARY OF KEY CLINICAL POINTS

- Neurological damage as a late side effect of irradiation can have a devastating effect on the individual.
- Factors implicated in the development of neurological complications are linked to radiotherapy treatment set-up, dose and fractionation schedules.
- Treatment techniques have improved over the past decade and the incidence of neurological complications has been decreasing.
- Recent advances in radiotherapy techniques have been instrumental in decreasing excessive dose to organs at risk and thereby reducing the probability of late tissue complications. Techniques such as conformal and intensity-modulated radiotherapy permit better shaping of the radiotherapy beams in three dimensions to the tumour profile and allow improved sparing of adjacent neurological structures.
- It is crucial to increase the level of awareness and knowledge about the benefits and risks of radiation treatment in healthcare professionals and to encourage better integration and coordination in patient management.
- Information of the possible long-term risks of radiotherapy should be discussed with patients when requiring informed consent for therapy.
- Assessment of neurological complications is required early so that further secondary damage is prevented and patients' distress is reduced. Diagnosis is through physical and functional assessment and imaging studies.
- Multidisciplinary intervention strategies are required to manage the complex problems associated with these neurological syndromes.
- Pain management requires both pharmacological and non-pharmacological approaches. Women suffering from brachial plexopathy have found complementary medicines helpful.
- Rehabilitation requires multidisciplinary team members for psychological, physical and functional support.

CONCLUSION

Whilst experimental radiobiology and animal studies have provided some estimates for the effect of treatment volumes, interfraction intervals and dose–complication curves for late complications related to radiotherapy, appropriate clinical data remain limited. Therefore, it remains difficult accurately to judge the likelihood of late damage for any particular radiotherapy regime. Thorough knowledge of patient- and treatment-related parameters influential in determining the probability of tumour control and normal tissue complication rates is needed in order to develop more rational and realistic therapeutic strategies. Elucidation of the pathogenesis of radiation-induced neurological injury may allow the development of strategies to modulate radiation damage and perhaps restore neurological damage. More research is also required in symptom control, establishment of care processes and managing psychosocial problems.

It is important for healthcare professionals to provide quality radiotherapy as well as to incorporate appropriate objective and consistent methods of recording the effects of radiation damage. This provides the basis for rational improvements in radiotherapy regimes and delivery. Just as important is the need to improve communication and understanding between patients and members of the health team. It is important to improve the evidence basis for intervention practices so that the efficacy of treatment approaches can be determined and subsequent guidelines will then have greater credibility. This will provide the necessary platform for assessment and quality assurance of current guidelines and permit quantifiable improvements in radiotherapy service and supportive care of those suffering with neurological complications.

FURTHER READING

Articles on complications related to breast radiotherapy and brachial plexus neuropathy have been produced by the Royal College of Radiologists, London:
- Maher Committee 1995 Management of adverse effects following radiotherapy. Royal College of Radiologists, London
- Bates T, Evans R G B 1995 Brachial plexus neuropathy following radiotherapy for breast carcinoma. Royal College of Radiologists, London
  http://www.rcr.ac.uk

A useful list of regional and hospital specialist teams for neurological complications in particular brachial plexopathy can be found in the RCR Maher Committee publication listed above.
- Clinical mangement of neuropathic pain: Beth Israel Medical Centre
  http://www.stoppain.org

REFERENCES

Ahmad A, Barrington S, Maisey M et al 1999 Use of positron emission tomography in evaluation of brachial plexopathy in breast cancer patients. British Journal of Cancer 79:478–482

Alfonso E R, De Gregorio M A, Mateo P et al 1997 Radiation myelopathy in over-irradiated patients: MR imaging findings. European Radiology 7:400–404

Bates T, Evans R G B 1995 Brachial plexus neuropathy following radiotherapy for breast carcinoma. Royal College of Radiologists, London

Bentzen S M, Dische S 2001 Late morbidity: the Damocles sword of radiotherapy? Radiotherapy Oncology 61:219–221

Brander P E Jarvinen V, Lohela P et al 1997 Bilateral diaphragmatic weakness: a late complication of radiotherapy. Thorax 52:829–831

Chao M W, Wirth A, Ryan G et al 1998 Radiation myelopathy following transplantation and radiotherapy for non-Hodgkin's lymphoma. International Journal of Radiation Oncology, Biology, Physics 41:1057–1061

Cooper J 1998 Occupational therapy intervention with radiation-induced brachial plexopathy. European Journal of Cancer Care 7:88–92

Davis C 1995 Symptomatic management of neuropathic pain. Royal College of Radiologists, London

DeLattre J Y, Rosenblum M K, Thaler H T et al 1988 A model of radiation myelopathy in the rat: pathology, regional capillary permiability changes and treatment with dexamethasone. Brain 111:1319–1336

Dietz J H 1981 Rehabilitation oncology. Wiley, New York

Dische S 1991 Accelerated treatment and radiation myelitis. Radiotherapy and Oncology 20:1–2

Dutreix J, Wambersie A, Bounik C 1973 Cellular recovery in human skin reactions: application to dose, fraction number, overall time relationship in radiotherapy. European Journal of Cancer 9:159–167

Esik O, Emri M, Csornai M et al 1999 Radiation myelopathy with partial functional recovery: PET evidence of long-term increased metabolic activity of the spinal cord. Journal of Neurological Science 163:39–43

Faithfull S 1991 Patients' experiences following cranial radiotherapy: a study of the somnolence syndrome. Journal of Advanced Nursing 16:936–946

Faithfull S, Brada M 1998 Somnolence syndrome in adults following cranial irradiation for primary brain tumours. Clinical Oncology (Royal College of Radiologists)10:250–254

Flickinger J C, Lunsford L D, Coffey R J et al 1991 Radiosurgery of acoustic neurinomas. Cancer 67:345–353

Gerard J M, Franck N, Moussa Z et al 1989 Acute ischemic brachial plexus neuropathy following radiation therapy. Neurology 39:450–451

Glantz M J, Burger P C, Friedman A H et al 1994 Treatment of radiation-induced nervous system injury with heparin and warfarin. Neurology 44:2020–2027

Green D M, D'Angio G J 1992 Late effects of treatment for childhood cancer. Wiley-Liss, New York

Halperin E C, Burger P C 1985 Conventional external beam radiotherapy for central nervous system malignancies. Neurologic Clinics 3:867–882

Harris O A, Adler J A 1996 Analysis of the proliferative potential of residual tumour after radiosurgery for intraparenchymal brain metastasis. Journal of Neurosurgery 85:667–671

Hirota S, Yoshida S, Soejima T et al 1993 Chronological observation in early radiation myelopathy of the cervical spinal cord: gadolinium-enhanced MRI findings in two cases. Radiation Medicine 1:154–159

Jeremic B, Shibamoto Y, Milicic B et al 1998 Absence of thoracic radiation myelitis after hyperfractionated radiation therapy with and without concurrent chemotherapy for stage III nonsmall-cell lung cancer. International Journal of Radiation Oncology, Biology, Physics 40:343–346

Johnson B E, Becker B, Goff W B et al 1985 Neurologic, neuropsychological and computed cranial tomographic scan abnormalities in 2- to 10-year survivors of small-cell lung cancer. Journal of Clinical Oncology 12:1657–1667

Kleinberg L, Wallner K, Makin M G 1993 Good performance status of long-term disease free survivors of intracranial gliomas. International Journal of Radiation Oncology, Biology, Physics 26:129–133

Kori S H, Foley K M, Posner J B 1981 Brachial plexus lesions in patients with cancer: 100 cases. Neurology 31:45–50

Maher E J 2000 Late radiation damage – whose point of view? Radiotherapy and Oncology 57:S1–S2

Maher Committee 1995 Management of adverse effects following radiotherapy. Royal College of Radiologists, London

Maire J, Coudin B, Guerin J et al 1987 Neuropyschologic impairment in adults with brain tumours. American Journal of Clinical Oncology 10:156–162

Melki P S, Halimi P, Wibault P et al 1994 MRI in chronic progressive radiation myelopathy. Journal of Computer Assisted Tomography 18:1–6

Meyer B, Zentner J 1992 Do motor evoked potentials allow quantitative assessment of motor function in patients with spinal cord lesions? European Archive of Psychiatry and Clinical Neuroscience 241:201–204

Mostow E N, Byrne J, Connelly R R et al 1991 Quality of life in long-term survivors of CNS tumors of childhood and adolescence. Journal of Clinical Oncology 9:592–599

Pierce S M, Recht A, Lingos T I et al 1992 Long-term complications following conservative surgery (CS) and radiation therapy (RT) in patients with breast cancer. International Journal of Radiation Oncology, Biology, Physics 23:915–923

Portenoy R 1993 Adjuvant analgesics in pain management. Oxford Medical Publications, Oxford

Roman D D, Sperduto P W 1995 Neuropsychological effects of cranial radiation: current knowledge and future direction. International Journal of Radiation Oncology, Biology, Physics 31:983–998

Ryu S, Gorty S, Kazee A M et al 2000 'Full dose' reirradiation of human cervical spinal cord. American Journal of Clinical Oncology 23:29–31

Schultheiss T E, Stephens L C 1992 Pathology of radiation myelopathy, widening the circle. International Journal of Radiation Oncology, Biology, Physics 23:1089–1091

Schulthesis T, Stephens L, Maor M 1988 Analysis of the histopathology of radiation myelopathy. International Journal of Radiation Oncology, Biology, Physics 14:27–32

Schultheiss T E, Kun L E, Ang K K et al 1995 Radiation response of the central nervous system. International Journal of Radiation Oncology, Biology, Physics 31:1093–1112

Shalet S M, Beardwell C G, Pearson D et al 1976 The effect of varying doses of cerebral irradiation on GH production in childhood. Clinical Endocrinology 5:287–290

Sheline G E, Wara W M, Smith V 1980 Therapeutic irradiation and brain injury. International Journal of Radiation Oncology, Biology, Physics 6:1215–1228

Thames H D, Withers H R, Peters L J et al 1982 Changes in early and late radiation responses with altered dose fractionation: implications for dose-survival relationships. International Journal of Radiation Oncology, Biology, Physics 8: 219–226

Thompson J W, Filshie J 1993 Transcutaneous electrical nerve stimulation (TENS) and acupuncture. Oxford Medical Publications, Oxford

van-de-Aardweg G J, Hopewell J W, Whitehouse E M 1995 The radiation response of the cervical spinal cord of the pig: effects of changing the irradiated volume. International Journal of Radiation Oncology, Biology, Physics 31:51–55

Wang P Y, Shen W C, Jan J S 1992 MR imaging in radiation myelopathy. American Journal of Neuroradiology 13:1049–1055

Wong C S, Van Dyk J, Milosevic M et al 1994 Radiation myelopathy following single courses of radiotherapy and retreatment. International Journal of Radiation Oncology, Biology, Physics 30:575–581

Wouter-van-Es H, Engelen A M, Witkamp T D et al 1997 Radiation-induced brachial plexopathy: MR imaging. Skeletal Radiology 26:284–288

15

Lymphoedema

Angela E Williams

INTRODUCTION

Lymphoedema is an incurable, progressive condition that manifests as chronic swelling. Although it can occur in any part of the body, it usually affects one or more limbs. Primary lymphoedema arises as a result of a congenitally determined abnormality of the lymph nodes or vessels, but it is secondary lymphoedema that is most relevant to patients with cancer. The principal causes of secondary lymphoedema are considered to be cancer and cancer therapy, with radiotherapy and surgery being the main treatment-related causes. Upper-limb lymphoedema related to breast cancer is probably the most well-recognised form, and it is generally agreed that it occurs in one in three or four cases, with consensus that surgery and radiotherapy to the axilla are associated with higher rates. The literature regarding cancer-related lymphoedema of the lower limb is limited, and even less information is available about lymphoedema of other parts of the body.

Lymphoedema causes considerable physical, emotional and social morbidity, yet patients consistently report that they were not given any information about the possibility of developing the symptom as a late side effect of cancer treatment. As recently as the mid-1980s lymphoedema was by and large regarded as untreatable as well as incurable. Although it is now recognised as a complex condition requiring a specialist team approach, it is still poorly acknowledged in practice. Lymphoedema specialists are few and far between, and as a result, many patients do not have access to appropriate support. Today it is generally agreed that lymphoedema is most successfully managed using a combination of physical treatment elements in two phases. However, there is disagreement in the published literature on what combinations of treatments are most effective and why.

WHAT IS LYMPHOEDEMA?

The lymph system is a one-way drainage system comprising lymph vessels and lymph nodes. It is responsible for regulating interstitial homeostasis, primarily by returning large molecules back to the vascular system. The removal of excess fluid from the interstitium by the lymphatics provides a 'safety-valve' system, as it ensures that any water, waste products and protein not removed by the vascular system can still be transported away from the tissues. Any damage to this important drainage system results in the build-up of protein-rich fluid, which then attracts further liquid into the tissues, provoking inflammation and fibrosis within them (Pain & Purushotham 2000). The protein-rich environment also provides an ideal focus for infection.

Foldi et al (1989) proposed that there are three discrete forms of oedema, only one of which is 'true' lymphoedema – that which occurs as a consequence of mechanical insufficiency (a reduction in the transport capacity of the lymphatic vessels). The second form of oedema, termed dynamic insufficiency, is seen in patients with chronic venous insufficiency, where the capacity of the normal lymphatic system is exceeded by a high lymphatic load. The combination of an abnormally high load and an already reduced transport capacity results in the third form of oedema, known as safety-valve insufficiency. This arises in patients with dependent limbs.

The International Society of Lymphology (ISL) agreed on four main features that characterise true lymphoedema:

- excess protein in the tissues
- excess oedema in the tissues
- chronic inflammation
- excess fibrosis (Casley-Smith 1985).

The excess tissue oedema is prominent in the early stages, with fibrosis becoming predominant as the condition progresses.

In the initial stages of lymphoedema, differential diagnosis is difficult, as the pitting which occurs with the application of pressure may reduce on elevation of the swollen limb. In mild cases, the clinician has to rely on clinical observation and the patient's medical history. In more advanced cases, lymphoedema can be distinguished by firm and non-pitting oedema, deepened natural skinfolds, hyperkeratosis with papillomatosis and Stemmer's sign, or the ability to pinch the thickened skin at the base of the digits (Harwood & Mortimer 1995).

CAUSES AND RISK FACTORS OF LYMPHOEDEMA

Cancer-related lymphoedema is attributed to obliteration, removal or obstruction of the lymphatic system. This may however be an oversimplification of the pathophysiology, since not all cancer patients develop lymphoedema despite being exposed to similar treatments that are potentially damaging to the lymphatic system, such as surgery and radiotherapy. Furthermore, lymphoedema can develop at any time, often many years after treatment, even where there is no sign of recurrent disease.

Studies of upper-limb swelling associated with treatment for breast cancer have implicated a variety of risk factors and risk markers, as shown in Table 15.1.

Halsted's (1921) classic paper was the first to conclude that impaired wound healing and infection play a major part in the development of upper-limb lymphoedema. In the following decades, several other authors suggested that

Table 15.1 Contributing factors in the development of upper-limb lymphoedema

Risk factor	Author	Year
(a) Radiotherapy and surgery factors associated with the development of lymphoedema		
Radiotherapy	Say & Donegan	1974
	Haagensen	1974
	Segerstrom et al	1992
Radiodermatitis associated with radiotherapy and/or surgery	Holman et al	1944
	Britton & Nelson	1962
	Mozes et al	1982
Fibrosis/benign scar formation secondary to radiotherapy causing obstruction to lymphatic flow and/or obstruction of the axillary and subclavian vein	Neumann & Conway	1948
	Britton & Nelson	1962
	Howell-Hughes & Patel	1966
Venous outflow obstruction or congestion (cause undefined in publication)	Svensson et al	1994a
Extent of removal of axillary lymph nodes	Britton & Nelson	1962
	Mozes et al	1982
Radical mastectomy compared with less radical surgery ± radiotherapy	Say & Donegan	1974
	Mozes et al	1982
Combination of axillary clearance plus axillary radiotherapy	Kissin et al	1986
(b) Other factors associated with the development of lymphoedema		
Impaired wound healing, e.g necrosis of skin edges, wound infection, seroma, prolonged and copious drainage, haematoma	Halsted	1921
	Britton & Nelson	1962
	Say & Donegan	1974
	Haagensen	1974
	Mozes et al	1982
	Segerstrom et al	1992
Thrombophlebitis with concomitant obstruction of the lymphatics in the vascular sheath	Smedal & Evans	1960
Excessive use of the arm	Zeissler et al	1972
Age (60 years or older)	Pezner et al	1986
Soft-tissue arm infections	Segerstrom et al	1992
Oblique skin incision	Segerstrom et al	1992
Increased arterial flow	Svensson et al	1994b

infection, radiodermatitis (skin reactions) and radiation fibrosis were causative factors (Holman et al 1944, Neumann & Conway 1948). In the 1960s, Britton & Nelson (1962) reached the conclusion that infection was the most important cause of upper-limb lymphoedema associated with breast cancer treatments, but they acknowledged that the susceptibility of the arm depended on the extent of removal of axillary lymphatics. They too recognised that radiodermatitis, late fibrosis in the axilla (due to radiation or surgery) and obstruction of the axillary vein appeared to play a part in the development of the symptom.

Two large retrospective reports then confirmed that damage resulting from a combination of surgery and radiotherapy was most likely to cause lymphoedema. Haagensen (1974) observed over 1000 women who had undergone radical mastectomy and found that oedema was most marked in women who received radiotherapy to the axilla and supraclavicular regions, those who were obese and those who had poor wound healing. Say & Donegan (1974) reviewed over 1500 women with breast cancer, the majority (77%) of whom had undergone radical mastectomy. The incidence of postoperative upper-limb lymphoedema was higher in patients who had undergone radical mastectomy (31.5%) or extended mastectomy (36.8%) compared with those who had undergone less radical surgery, such as simple mastectomy (9.1%). Furthermore, those who received radiotherapy as well as radical mastectomy had a higher incidence of lymphoedema.

Further work found that post-mastectomy patients who had experienced radiodermatitis or wound-healing complications were more likely to develop lymphoedema than matched controls who did not have such problems (Mozes et al 1982). Kissin et al (1986) confirmed that the combination of radiotherapy and surgery appeared to be the most significant risk factor for the development of upper-limb lymphoedema in breast cancer. Their retrospective study of 200 patients found similar incidences of late lymphoedema in those who had experienced axillary radiotherapy alone (8.3%), axillary sampling plus radiotherapy (9.1%) or axillary clearance alone (7.4%). However, the incidence after axillary clearance plus radiotherapy was significantly greater (38.3%).

Unfortunately, most of the published studies are retrospective, and their collective significance is limited by the fact that they use a variety of definitions and measurement techniques. However, there is still a consensus in the literature that a combination of axillary surgery and radiotherapy is associated with higher rates of upper-limb lymphoedema in patients with breast cancer. Other factors, such as obesity and age, remain controversial, although there is recent evidence to suggest that venous outflow obstruction and venous congestion may be implicated (Svensson et al 1994a) (Table 15.1b). Given the fact that studies have consistently shown that combination treatments are associated with lymphoedema, it is worrying that many breast cancer patients continue to report that they were not given any information on the possibility of developing lymphoedema as a late side-effect of cancer treatment (Woods 1993). If patients at risk of developing upper-limb lymphoedema are poorly informed, the likelihood is that those at risk of lymphoedema in the lower limb, genitalia, head and neck or breast are largely unaware of the possibility that they might be affected by the symptom.

THE INCIDENCE AND PREVALENCE OF LYMPHOEDEMA

Both the incidence and prevalence of lymphoedema in patients with cancer are difficult to estimate accurately, as studies use different definitions and measurement techniques, and treatment centres vary in their recognition and treatment of the problem. The incidence of upper-limb lymphoedema associated with the treatment of breast cancer has been quoted as ranging from 5.5% to 80% (Table 15.2). The high incidence rates reported in early studies probably reflect surgical or radiotherapeutic techniques which are now outdated. A recent review notes that the incidence of lymphoedema in patients with breast cancer is more likely to be around 24–28% (Pain & Purushotham 2000).

Table 15.2 Incidence of lymphoedema

Author	Cancer site	Year	Incidence figure (%)
(a) Upper-limb breast cancer-related lymphoedema			
Holman et al		1944	70
Neumann & Conway		1948	55
Lobb & Harkins		1949	80
Fitts et al		1953	49
Haagensen		1974	8
Golematis et al		1975	5.5
Markowski et al		1981	31
Kissin et al		1986	38
Segerstrom et al		1992	43
Thompson et al		1995	32
(b) Lower-limb cancer-related lymphoedema			
Martimbeau et al	Cervix	1978	23
Lampert et al	Soft-tissue sarcoma	1984	70
Soisson et al	Cervix	1990	9
Robinson et al	Soft-tissue sarcoma	1991	30
Werngren-Elgstrom & Lidman	Cervix	1994	22

As already described, several studies have found a higher incidence of lymphoedema in patients who were treated with surgery and radiotherapy. Segerstrom et al's (1992) study of 136 consecutive patients treated for breast cancer found the highest incidence of arm swelling (43%) to be among patients who had received radiotherapy. Those who had received radiotherapy to the axilla were at greater risk than those treated with parasternal or supraclavicular irradiation. A prospective study by Thompson et al (1995) reported an overall incidence of 32% amongst 121 consecutive patients who had been treated with various axillary procedures. The combination of axillary node dissection and radiotherapy carried the highest morbidity at 1 year following breast conservation surgery.

Follow-up studies of breast cancer patients illustrate that the prevalence of lymphoedema increases with time. A British study by Mortimer et al (1996) found that 302 (28%) of 1151 women surveyed had lymphoedema, with a mean interval since treatment of 9.5 years. Overall, arm swelling was nearly twice as common among women treated with radiotherapy or those treated by mastectomy as opposed to lumpectomy.

The literature on cancer-related lymphoedema of the *lower* limb is sparse and its interpretation remains problematic in view of the lack of precision and consistency in defining and measuring lymphoedema. Martimbeau et al's (1978) review of 402 patients with cervical cancer revealed that lymphoedema was the most frequent complication, affecting 94 (23%) patients over the 3-year period of investigation. The severity of lymphoedema ranged from mild (22 cases) to moderate (44 cases) to severe (20 cases), with eight remaining patients unranked because they were either dying or had developed lymphoedema secondary to pelvic recurrence. Further studies report an incidence of lymphoedema varying from 9% (Soisson et al 1990) to 22% (Werngren-Elgstrom & Lidman 1994) in patients with cancer of the cervix, identifying pelvic radiotherapy as a major contributory factor.

The risk of developing lymphoedema after treatment for soft-tissue sarcoma appears to be somewhat higher, although studies are small and less convincing (Lampert et al 1984, Robinson et al 1991).

Advanced disease in the pelvis, arising from cancers of the prostate, bladder, bowel and ovary, can also be responsible for lower-limb lymphoedema. Destruction of the lymphatics in the groin can result in genital lymphoedema (Haldar & Cranston 2000) and surgery and radiotherapy to the head and neck can cause facial lymphoedema, particularly if both sides of the neck are treated (Withey et al 2000).

THE IMPACT OF LYMPHOEDEMA

In 1969, Stillwell described post-mastectomy lymphoedema as merely 'the source of considerable annoyance' and 'occasionally the cause of disability'. Twenty years later, Mozes et al (1982) suggested that swelling of the arm should be generally accepted as an inevitable complication following mastectomy. The true impact of lymphoedema is becoming increasingly apparent, as studies continue to report the profound physical, emotional and social consequences of the condition. As early as 1966, Howell-Hughes & Patel described patients' experiences of breast cancer-related lymphoedema, finding that all 19 patients in their study complained of 'heaviness that rendered domestic work unduly tiring', and that seven described a dull ache in the region of the shoulder. Few studies have quantified the extent of physical symptoms, although heaviness, impaired mobility and pain are most frequently cited (Pain & Purushotham 2000). Badger & Twycross (1988) used visual analogue scores to assess tightness and pain, found to be two distinctive symptoms associated with lymphoedema. Piller et al (1988) found that patients reported feelings of 'bursting' (44%), 'tension' (54%), loss of mobility (72%) and 'loss of general well-being' (76%). In 1990, Rose et al reported that by far the commonest problem affecting patients with lymphoedema was finding clothes to fit.

Several studies of the psychosocial impact of lymphoedema have illustrated its far-reaching effects. Woods (1993) used semistructured interviews and the Psychological Adjustment to Illness Scale (PAIS) to gather information about patients' perceptions of their breast cancer-related lymphoedema. Woods found that confidence in appearance was one of the areas most affected by the presence of lymphoedema, and she concluded that the experience of lymphoedema is personal and unique to the individual. Tobin et al (1993) also used the PAIS questionnaire to elicit psychosocial morbidity in 50 patients with breast cancer-related lymphoedema and 50 matched controls. Patients with lymphoedema were found to have greater psychiatric morbidity and greater functional impairment. A loss of interest in dress and appearance and a loss of self-esteem were also reported, perhaps contributing to difficulties in sexual and interpersonal relationships. Patients also reported a loss of interest in social activities, thought to be associated with feelings of depression. Woods et al (1995) compared PAIS scores in the two above studies, finding that psychosocial difficulties were consistent over a 6-month period, even if the lymphoedema was being treated during this time.

It is clear that altered body image, reduced limb function, reduced mobility, sexual difficulties and social isolation can present significant problems for patients with lymphoedema. The wide range of psychological and physical impairments reported by patients was investigated in an Australian study by Mirolo et al (1995).

The quality of life of 25 post-mastectomy lymphoedema patients was recorded as high, using a lymphoedema subscale to the Functional Living Index – Cancer (FLIC). A second assessment, functional status, comprised a list of 20 activities of daily living. Although the need for assistance was not high, and many patients could perform all 20 activities independently, some difficulty or discomfort was experienced. The activities giving most difficulty were lifting/carrying, cleaning and reaching up or down. A third assessment demonstrated that patients perceived the image of their lymphoedematous limb on five dimensions to be poorer than their image of the rest of their body on a seven-point scale.

Physical and psychological morbidity, assessed by the Nottingham Health Profile Part 1 (NHP-1), was also the subject of a study by Sitzia & Sobrido (1997). Thirty-four patients (22 with cancer-related lymphoedema, of whom 17 had received radiotherapy) completed the baseline and 4-week follow-up NHP-1 along with clinical assessment, including limb volume measurement and skin condition. The overall follow-up NHP-1 scores were significantly lower than the overall baseline treatment scores, indicating an improvement in health-related quality of life (HRQOL) with treatment. The greatest change in a single dimension was in physical mobility. However, the change in limb volume was not associated with a change in any NHP-1 subscale.

It appears that significant predictors of distress and dysfunction in women with breast cancer-related lymphoedema include pain, lack of social support, avoidant coping and an affected dominant hand (Passik et al 1995). The degree of excess volume of the lymphoedematous limb seems not to be a major factor. As Pain & Purushotham (2000) point out, there are no studies showing any correlation between limb volume reduction and improved psychological morbidity, suggesting that limb size and volume alone are inappropriate measures of severity.

Further work on the objective measurement of morbidity is needed. The early development phase of a condition-specific HRQOL outcome measurement tool has been reported in the literature (Williams 1997). This tool has now been tested and is currently being compared with clinical measures and other HRQOL generic outcome measurements (Williams 1994). In developing the condition-specific HRQOL instrument, 40 patients were asked to list the five most important areas or activities of their life affected by the lymphoedema in the previous month. The 159 areas or activities identified were summarised into themes, later used to devise separate questionnaires for patients with upper- and lower-limb lymphoedema. The quotes below illustrate the broad spectrum of HRQOL issues raised by patients with upper- or lower-limb lymphoedema:

I am unable to get in and out of the bath.
I can no longer wash my hair.
Finding clothes to fit in high-street stores is very difficult.
I will not get undressed in front of anyone now as I feel so embarrassed.
I find it so difficult to have a good night's sleep.
Because I cannot sit down comfortably for long, I have stopped going to the theatre.

There is no published research to describe the impact of lymphoedema of the breast, genitalia or head and neck. Swelling of the breast following radiotherapy can be uncomfortable and distressing, particularly if it persists beyond the 3-month period in which acute reactions are expected to subside (Kirshbaum 2000).

Patients describe feelings of 'heaviness', 'tightness' and being 'lopsided'. Typically, the most marked swelling occurs in the lower part of the breast, where pooling of lymph is most likely. In male genital lymphoedema, patients can suffer significant debilitating functional, cosmetic and psychological sequelae in addition to pain and dysuria (Haldar & Cranston 2000). Head and neck lymphoedema in patients who undergo bilateral neck dissection and radiotherapy can be especially disfiguring, and can sometimes interfere with eating and speech. In extreme cases, the swelling gives rise to an appearance described as 'pumpkin-head oedema' (Withey et al 2000). Although most patients will not suffer this degree of swelling, many experience a collection of fluid in the submental area (so-called dewlap) following radiotherapy to the larynx or pharynx, and it is important that they are warned of this possibility.

MANAGEMENT OF LYMPHOEDEMA

The early diagnosis and treatment of lymphoedema are important if long-term control is to be achieved. Diagnosis is often slow because lymphoedema can be a late complication of cancer therapy, occurring years or even decades after the completion of treatment and routine follow-up.

At the time of cancer treatment it is vital that patients are given information on how to minimise the risk of developing lymphoedema as well as guidance on whom to contact if they are concerned that they may have developed the symptom at a later date (Regnard et al 1991). Patient information booklets and leaflets have been produced by Cancer British Association of Cancer United Patients (BACUP) and Breast Cancer Care, detailing preventive and self-care strategies to be used by patients at risk. The main features of these strategies are shown in Box 15.1.

Optimal management of lymphoedema is dependent on good assessment of the patient, including the characteristics of the oedema, associated symptoms, history of venous, arterial or inflammatory complications, movement of the affected part

---

Box 15.1 Preventive and self-care strategies advised in patient information leaflets

- Keep the skin as clean as possible, using warm rather than hot or cold water to wash, and making sure that the skin is dried properly afterwards
- Moisturise the skin every day to keep it supple and prevent cracking or drying
- Treat cuts and grazes quickly and see the doctor straight away if there are any signs of infection such as redness or inflammation – antibiotics may be necessary
- Wear gloves when doing housework or gardening so as to avoid injury, and wear a thimble when sewing
- Keep nails short using clippers rather than scissors
- Avoid constricting clothing, footwear and jewellery around affected limbs
- Avoid using a wet razor if shaving near to an affected area – electric razors are safer
- Use insect repellent and sunscreen when outside in hot weather
- Avoid injections, blood pressure readings and having blood taken from an affected limb
- Avoid excessive heat, i.e. hot weather, hot baths, sitting too close to a fire
- Take care with pets so as to avoid scratches, and wear gloves if handling cat litter

and skin condition (Jenns 2000). One of the problems with assessment is that there is a lack of consensus about the most appropriate method of measuring and defining the presence of lymphoedema. Although a change in the size of the limb provides an obvious method, there is no accepted gold standard for measuring or calculating limb volume. The two main methods are water displacement (Swedborg 1997) and calculation of limb volume based on surface circumferential measurements (Kuhnke 1976). Limb measurement is the outcome measure most frequently used, but there remain methodological inconsistencies with limb measurement across existing evaluative studies.

Approaches to the management of lymphoedema can be divided into three treatment categories: surgery, treatment with drugs and physical therapies, the latter being the most prominent today. However, as Badger (1997) noted, research in the field has largely concentrated on the structure and function of the lymphatic system as opposed to the effectiveness of these treatment options. Small studies have, however, concluded that treatment does have a beneficial effect on quality of life (Sitzia & Sobrido 1997).

Until fairly recently, the potential for treating lymphoedema was under-recognised. Although a reasoned, systematic approach to the management of lymphoedema had developed in Germany by the 1980s, the standard approaches to treatment in the UK were basic, consisting of elevation, pneumatic compression and Tubigrip. Very little attempt was being made to measure treatment effectiveness, treatment provision was notably haphazard and no one profession was taking responsibility for developing the field. In general, physiotherapists, nurses and occupational therapists managed problems which were considered appropriate for their profession in isolation (Williams & Badger 1996).

In 1989, Foldi et al reported the results of the programme developed in Germany, demonstrating that volume reduction of the lymphoedematous limb was achieved in 95% of the 399 patients who did not have active cancer. Enthused by their findings, a team of clinicians in Oxford adapted their two-phase treatment approach which consisted of an initial intensive phase (described by Foldi et al as complex decongestive physiotherapy) followed by a maintenance phase (described as conservation). Such treatment was initially only available in a few specialist centres in the UK, but funding for lymphoedema management has since improved and a greater number of treatment units do exist today, although they are by no means universal.

In general, patients who are referred for intensive treatment have to meet certain criteria for severe lymphoedema, as listed in Box 15.2. However, Badger (1997) has demonstrated that a period of intensive treatment before moving into the maintenance phase is more effective at reducing moderate as well as severe lymphoedema (> 20% excess limb volume) and is more likely to restore shape in the short and long term than the maintenance regimen alone. The intensive phase usually includes a 2–3-week course of outpatient treatment performed by a trained therapist. It comprises four components:

- skin hygiene
- lymphatic massage
- exercise
- multilayer bandaging.

> **Box 15.2** Indications for the two-phase treatment of lymphoedema
>
> • Long-standing or severe lymphoedema
> • An awkward-shaped limb
> • Oedema in the fingers
> • Lymphorrhoea
> • Damaged or fragile skin
> • Oedema of the trunk
> • Recurrent acute inflammatory episodes

(Badger & Twycross 1988)

The aims are to reduce the size of the limb, improve the condition of the skin and subcutaneous tissues and mould the shape of the limb to that of a normal one. The maintenance phase is designed to conserve and optimise the limb, and requires the patient to continue daily self-care as directed by the therapist. This phase depends on the patient wearing compression garments as well as performing skin care, exercise and lymphatic massage.

Skin hygiene

The aims of skin care are twofold:

• To improve the condition of the epidermis and dermis so that the skin is hydrated, intact and supple
• To eradicate and reduce the risk of bacterial and fungal infections.

Williams & Venables (1996) have described a daily skin care regimen for patients, detailing the most common skin complications that occur in this group of patients and summarising the management of skin problems in uncomplicated lymphoedema. It is particularly important that skin infections are treated promptly, and that risks to skin integrity are minimised using the strategies described in Box 15.1.

Lymphatic massage

In the UK the most widely used lymphatic massage is a simple form of skin surface massage following the principles of manual lymphatic drainage (MLD). It is taught to patients as a self-massage to be performed at least once a day. As with MLD, the self-massage technique aims to improve lymph drainage by increasing the activity of the lymphatics in the unaffected contralateral quadrant of the body and gently pushing fluid from the swollen quadrant into the 'prepared', cleared quadrant.

Exercise

Patients are encouraged to exercise while wearing bandages so as to use the muscle pumps to promote lymph flow. Exercises will also benefit joint movement and promote good posture. The optimum amount of exercise for an individual will vary; it should be sufficient to favour limb drainage but not excessive, so as to promote greater arterial inflow. Ideal activities include walking and swimming.

Multilayer bandaging

The application of bandages limits blood capillary filtration and provides high pressure during muscular contraction, thus improving the muscle pump efficiency. Only therapists with knowledge and training of its application should apply multilayer compression bandaging.

Maintenance therapy generally involves fitting an off-the-shelf high-compression (>40 mmHg) elastic garment, as opposed to the stronger, more rigorous, made-to-measure garment. A wide range of garments is available in the UK, but there is limited literature to guide the therapist towards the most appropriate selection. The results of a small study by Williams & Williams (1999) indicated that the apparently simple task of selecting a garment is in fact a complex endeavour.

The ongoing management of lymphoedema requires motivation and perseverance, since success is seen to be largely dependent on the degree of compliance patients show towards wearing hosiery, continuing lymphatic massage, caring for their skin and taking plenty of exercise. Rose et al (1990) have published the only study to assess compliance with long-term lymphoedema care, demonstrating that this is not always easy. The comments below reflect the problems patients face on a daily basis (Williams 1997):

> I have to get up nearly an hour earlier in the morning to allow time to put my stockings on after doing the massage and exercises.
> I can't be spontaneous as I have to fit in my self-management routine every day, even on holiday.

Compliance with therapy places considerable demands on patients, and failure to make appropriate adjustments to lifestyle commonly contributes to the reaccumulation of lymph and the deterioration of lymphoedema. The assessment and support of patients with lymphoedema by therapists and other healthcare professionals are critical for success.

Surgical techniques involving debulking or rerouting lymph drainage to reduce lymphoedema are rarely indicated (Carrell & Burnand 2000). Drug treatments also remain controversial, although some studies do indicate that benzopyrones (coumerols and flavonoids) can improve symptoms (Twycross 2000). Acute inflammatory episodes (such as cellulitis) are more frequent in patients with lymphoedema, and a combination of antibiotics and rest is usually indicated (Mortimer 2000). Pneumatic compression therapy is associated with a number of complications and is not widely used.

The management of breast, genital and head and neck lymphoedema requires the same early diagnosis, treatment, education and support of the patient. Advice and treatment include the fundamental elements of skin care, massage, compression/support and exercise. However, little is known about the most effective strategies for the management of non-limb lymphoedema and, as a result, patients often receive little help and advice. Although physical therapy has been adopted as the most appropriate management approach to lymphoedema in the UK, controversies still exist as to the most effective combination of physical therapies and the most important aspects of each one. Many questions persist, for example:

- To what extent is MLD more effective than a gentle self-massage technique when used as part of a combination approach to lymphoedema treatment?
- To what extent are the more expensive custom-made garments more effective than off-the-shelf garments used in the maintenance programme?
- What is the evidence for a two-phase approach to treatment as opposed to the patient being encouraged to undertake the same daily programme for a defined or continuous period?

Objective evaluation of physical treatment programmes is generally poor and further evidence for the effectiveness of therapy on limb volume and quality of life is urgently needed.

CONCLUSION

Lymphoedema is an extremely distressing consequence of cancer treatment, and is most likely to occur when lymph nodes are directly affected by radiotherapy and surgery in combination. Patients undergoing radiotherapy to the head and neck, axilla, breast and pelvis may be at risk of developing lymphoedema, yet many are unaware of the problem. Specialist lymphoedema services are not universally available and, as a result, many patients suffer the condition with little assistance. The physical, psychological, sexual and social impact of lymphoedema can be profound, but a comprehensive two-phase management approach can do much to improve patients' quality of life. Simply acknowledging the potential for lymphoedema to develop in patients undergoing radiotherapy is the first step towards improving the recognition and management of the problem. Self-care strategies are important as patients can be taught to minimise risks and improve symptoms. The assessment and measurement of lymphoedema are generally poor, and further research is required to ensure that the incidence of lymphoedema and its far-reaching consequences are widely realised amongst healthcare professionals caring for patients with cancer.

SUMMARY OF KEY CLINICAL POINTS

- The lymphatic system is largely responsible for regulating interstitial homeostasis, primarily by returning large molecules back to the vascular system.
- True lymphoedema as a consequence of a mechanical insufficiency occurs that is a reduction in the transport capacity of the lymphatic vessels due to some pathology.
- Lymphoedema is an incurable, progressive condition that manifests as chronic swelling, usually of one or more limbs.
- In the UK the commonest cause of secondary lymphoedema is cancer treatment; the combination of radiotherapy and surgery appears to be the most significant risk factor for cancer-related lymphoedema.

- Despite a lack of consensus on an objective method to measure and diagnose lymphoedema, it is generally agreed that the incidence of breast cancer-related lymphoedema is about one in three or four cases.
- A review of published literature on the morbidity associated with lymphoedema establishes that lymphoedema does have a wide range of physical and psychological implications for patients.
- Until recently, lymphoedema has not generally been seen as a complex condition requiring a specialist team approach.
- Today it is generally agreed that a combination of physical treatment elements used in a two-phase approach provides the best results but there is disagreement in the published literature on what combinations are most effective and why.
- There are still relatively few specialist lymphoedema services in the UK and, as a result, lymphoedema is still underrecognised and undertreated.

AREAS FOR FURTHER RESEARCH

Four important areas to note with regard to further research are aetiology, incidence and prevalence, management of lymphoedema and treatment outcomes.

- Aetiology: A variety of risk factors have been implicated but further research could clarify why not all cancer patients exposed to the causal agents of surgery and radiotherapy develop lymphoedema. Of those who do develop lymphoedema, why is there a delay of years in some cases? The multifactorial aetiology of breast cancer-related lymphoedema is widely accepted but more detailed investigation could help clinicians to target patients at greater risk of developing lymphoedema.
- Incidence and prevalence: Accurate and consistent data collection is needed to define the incidence and prevalence of lower-limb and other types of lymphoedema in cancer patients.
- Management of lymphoedema: Well-designed comparative studies should compare short- and long-term clinical and cost-effectiveness data of various combination physical therapies.
- Treatment outcomes: Having established that lymphoedema does have implications for patients' HRQOL, further work on the objective measurement of the physical and psychological impact is needed, e.g. condition-specific and generic HRQOL measures. Additional objective clinical measures could be developed to evaluate treatment outcomes such as skin condition and range of movement.

FURTHER INFORMATION

British Lymphology Society and Lymphoedema Support Network
www.lymphoedema.org

Information for patients and professionals
www.cancerbacup.org.uk

Information for patients and professionals
www.breastcancercare.org.uk

Patients' experiences of lymphoedema
www.dipex.org

REFERENCES

Badger C 1997 A study of the efficacy of multi-layer bandaging and elastic hosiery in the treatment of lymphoedema, and their effects on the swollen limb. PhD degree. University of London, London
Badger C, Twycross R G 1988 The management of lymphoedema: guidelines. Sobell Study Centre, Oxford
Badger C, Mortimer P S, Regnard C F B et al 1988 Pain in the chronically swollen limb. In: Partsch H (ed.) Progress in lymphology–XI. Excerpta Medica, Elsevier Science Publications, p 243–245
Britton R C, Nelson P A 1962 Causes and treatment of post-mastecomy lymphoedema of the arm: report of 114 cases. Journal of the American Medical Association 180(2):95–102
Carrell T, Burnand K 2000 Surgery and lymphoedema. In: Twycross R, Jenns K, Todd J (eds) Lymphoedema. Radcliffe Medical Press, Abingdon
Casley-Smith J R 1985 Discussion of the definition, diagnosis and treatment of lymphoedema (lymphostatic disorder). In: Casley-Smith J R, Piller N B (eds) Progress in lymphology. Proceedings on the Xth International Congress on Lymphology. University of Adelaide Press, South Australia, p 1–16
Fitts W T, Keuhnelian J G, Ravdin I S et al 1953 Swelling of the arm after radical mastectomy: a clinical study of its causes. Surgery 35(3):460–464
Foldi E, Foldi M, Clodius L 1989 The lymphoedema chaos: a lancet. Annals of Plastic Surgery 22:505–515
Golematis B C, Delikaris P G, Balarutsos C et al 1975 Lymphedema of the upper limb after surgery for breast cancer. American Journal of Surgery 129:286–288
Haagensen C D 1974 The choice of treatment for operable carcinoma of the breast. Surgery 76(5):685–714
Haldar N, Cranston D 2000 Male genital lymphoedema. In: Twycross R, Jenns K, Todd J (eds) Lymphoedema. Radcliffe Medical Press, Abingdon, p 331–337
Halsted W S 1921 The swelling of the arm after operations for cancer of the breast – elephantiasis chirurgica – its cause and prevention. Bulletin of the Johns Hopkins Hospital 32:309–313
Harwood C A, Mortimer P S 1995 Causes and clinical manifestations of lymphatic failure. In: Ryan T J, Mortimer P S (eds) Clinics in dermatology: cutaneous lymphatic system, vol. 13. Elsevier Science, p 459–471
Holman C, McSwain B, Beal J M 1944 Swelling of the upper extremity following radical mastectomy. Surgery 15:757–765
Howell-Hughes J, Patel A R 1966 Swelling of the arm following mastectomy. British Journal of Surgery 53(1):4–15
Jenns K 2000 Management strategies. In: Twycross R, Jenns K, Todd J (eds) Lymphoedema. Radcliffe Medical Press, Abingdon, p 97–117
Kirshbaum M 2000 Breast lymphoedema. In: Twycross R, Jenns K, Todd J (eds) Lymphoedema. Radcliffe Medical Press, Abingdon, p 321–330
Kissin M, Querci della Rovere G, Easton D et al 1986 Risk of lymphoedema following treatment for breast cancer. British Journal of Surgery 73:580–584
Kuhnke E 1976 Volumbestimmung as umfangmessungen. Folia Angiologica 24:228–232
Lampert M H, Gerber L H, Glatstein E et al 1984 Soft tissue sarcoma: functional outcome after wide local excision and radiation therapy. Archives of Physical Medicine and Rehabilitation 65:477–480
Lobb A, Harkins H N 1949 Post-mastectomy swelling of the arm with note on effect on segmental dissection of axillary vein at time of radical mastectomy. Western Journal of Surgery 57:550–557
Markowski J, Wilcox J P, Helm P A 1981 Lymphoedema incidence after specific post-mastectomy therapy Archives of Physical Rehabilitation 62:449–452

Martimbeau P W, Kjorstad K E, Kolstad P 1978 Stage 1B carcinoma of the cervix, the Norwegian Radium Hospital, 1968–1970: results of treatment and major complications. American Journal of Obstetrics and Gynecology 131:389–394

Mirolo B R, Bunce I H, Chapman M et al 1995 Psychological benefits of post-mastectomy lymphoedema therapy. Cancer Nursing 18(3):197–205

Mortimer P 2000 Acute inflammatory episodes. In: Twycross R, Jenns K, Todd J (eds) Lymphoedema. Radcliffe Medical Press, Abingdon, p 130–139

Mortimer P S, Bates D O, Brassington H et al 1996 The prevalence of arm oedema following treatment for breast cancer. Quarterly Journal of Medicine 89(5):377–380

Mozes M, Papa M Z, Karasik A et al 1982 The role of infection in post-mastectomy lymphoedema. Surgery Annals 14:73–83

Neumann C G, Conway H 1948 Evaluation of skin grafting in the technique of radical mastectomy in relation to function of the arm. Surgery 23:584–590

Pain S J, Purushotham A D 2000 Lymphoedema following surgery for breast cancer. British Journal of Surgery 87:1128–1141

Passik S D, Newman M L, Brennan M et al 1995 Predictors of psychological distress, sexual dysfunction and physical functioning among women with upper extremity lymphoedema related to breast cancer. Psycho-oncology 4:255–263

Pezner R D, Patterson M P, Hill L R et al 1986 Arm lymphoedema in patients treated conservatively for breast cancer: relationship to patient age and axillary node dissection technique. International Journal of Radiation, Oncology, Biology, Physics 12:2079–2083

Piller N B, Morgan R G, Casley-Smith J R 1988 A double-blind, cross-over trial of O-(beta-hydroxyethyl)-rutosides (benzo-pyrones) in the treatment of lymphoedema of the arms and legs. British Journal of Plastic Surgery 41:20–27

Regnard C, Badger C, Mortimer P 1991 Lymphoedema: advice on treatment, 2nd edn. Beaconsfield Publishers, Beaconsfield

Robinson M H, Spruce L, Eeles R et al 1991 Limb function following conservation treatment of adult soft tissue sarcoma. European Journal of Cancer 27(12):1567–1574

Rose K, Taylor H, Twycross R G 1990 Long-term compliance with treatment in obstructive arm lymphoedema in cancer. Palliative Medicine 4:75–78

Say C C, Donegan W 1974 A biostatistical evaluation of complications from mastectomy. Surgery Gynecology Obstetrics 138:370–376

Segerstrom K, Bjerle P, Graffman S et al 1992 Factors that influence the incidence of brachial oedema after treatment of breast cancer. Scandinavian Journal of Plastic and Reconstructive Hand Surgery 26:223–227

Sitzia J, Sobrido L 1997 Measurement of health-related quality of life in patients receiving conservative treatment for limb lymphoedema using the Nottingham Health Profile. Quality of Life Research 6:373–384

Smedal M I, Evans J A 1960 The cause and treatment of oedema of the arm following radical mastectomy. Surgery, Gynaecology and Obstetrics III:29–40

Soisson A P, Soper J T, Clarke-Pearson D L et al 1990 Adjuvant radiotherapy following radical hysterectomy for patients with stage IB and IIA cervical cancer. Gynaecologic Oncology 37:390–395

Stillwell G K 1969 Treatment of post-mastectomy lymphoedema. Modality of Treatment 6:396–412

Svensson W E, Mortimer P S, Tohno E et al 1994a Colour Doppler demonstrates venous flow abnormalities in breast cancer patients with chronic arm swelling. European Journal of Cancer 30A(5):657–660

Svensson W E, Mortimer P S, Tohno E et al 1994b Increased arterial inflow demonstrated by Doppler ultrasound in arm swelling following breast cancer treatment. European Journal of Cancer 30A(5):661–664

Swedborg I 1977 Voluminometric estimation of the degree of lymphoedema and its therapy by pneumatic compression. Scandinavian Journal of Rehabilitation 9:131–138

Thompson A M, Air M, Jack W J L et al 1995 Arm morbidity after breast conservation and axillary therapy. The Breast 4:273–276

Tobin M, Lacey H, Meyer L et al 1993 The psychological morbidity of breast cancer related arm swelling. Cancer 72(11):3148–3252

Twycross R (2000) Drug treatment for lymphoedema. In: Twycross R, Jenns K, Todd (eds) Lymphoedema. Radcliffe Medical Press, Abingdon, p 244–270

Werngren-Elgstrom M, Lidman D 1994 Lymphoedema of the lower extremities after surgery and radiotherapy for cancer of the cervix. Scandinavian Journal of Plastic Reconstructive Hand Surgery 28:289–293

Williams A E 1994 Clinical and quality of life outcome measurements: a case study of lymphoedema. Unpublished DPhil. University of York, York

Williams A E 1997 Developing a health-related quality of life outcome measure for patients with lymphoedema (research abstract). Quality of Life Research 6(7/8):743

Williams A E, Badger C 1996 The management of lymphoedema: a developing specialism for nursing? International Journal of Palliative Nursing 2(1):50–53

Williams A E, Venables J 1996 The management of skin problems in uncomplicated lymphoedema. Journal of Wound Care 5(5):223–226

Williams A F, Williams A E 1999 'Putting the pressure on': a study of compression sleeves used in breast cancer-related lymphoedema. Journal of Tissue Viability 9(3):89–94

Withey S, Pracy P, Rhys-Evans P 2000 Lymphoedema of the head and neck. In: Twycross R, Jenns K, Todd J (eds) Lymphoedema. Radcliffe Medical Press, Abingdon, p 306–320

Woods M 1993 Patient's perceptions of breast cancer-related lymphoedema European Journal of Cancer Care 2:125–128

Woods M, Tobin M, Mortimer P (1995) The psychosocial morbidity of breast cancer patients with lymphoedema. Cancer Nursing 18(6):467–471

Zeissler RH, Rose GB, Nelson PA (1972) Postmastectomy lymphedema: late results in 385 patients. Archive of Physical Medical Rehabilitation 53:159–166

16

Sexuality and fertility

Isabel White   Sara Faithfull

INTRODUCTION

Sexuality and fertility are distinct yet inexorably linked issues relevant to acute treatment and subsequent rehabilitation within radiotherapy practice. As survival prospects have continued to improve, and greater emphasis has been placed upon the quality of life of patients following completion of treatment, clinicians have increasingly begun to consider the impact of radiotherapy on these important facets of the patient's life. Despite this, contemporary healthcare literature indicates reluctance among practitioners to address these issues, particularly within the context of treatment for chronic or life-threatening illness (Guthrie 1999, Meerabeau 1999, Waterhouse 1996, Weijts et al 1993, White 2002).

There is often conflict in clinical practice concerning how appropriate it is to talk about sexual issues prior to treatment, particularly when patients' concerns are likely to be focused on the immediate side effects of treatment and how they will cope with the physical and psychological demands of radiotherapy. Sexual issues may not become a concern for patients and their partners until after therapy is completed, when clinical support may be more limited. In an interview study of men ($n = 33$) who were receiving or had completed pelvic radiotherapy for prostate or bladder cancer, sexual concerns such as lack of sexual desire or erectile dysfunction were often ranked last in priority. Urinary problems and diarrhoea were of more immediate concern both during and on immediate completion of treatment. However, at 6 months post-treatment, loss of interest in sex was third in priority after concerns about urinary problems and the efficacy of radiotherapy in controlling their disease (Faithfull 1995). The apparent dilemma is that, during periods of high symptom intensity and prevalence, sexual desire and function may not be seen as important by either the patient or healthcare professionals.

Not uncommonly, the question of impaired fertility or sexual function occurs after patients have recovered from the acute side effects of treatment. All too often, no pre-treatment counselling has been offered and infertility, loss of erectile function or vaginal dryness and stenosis come as a shock and bitter disappointment to the person with cancer and his or her partner. Difficulty can also arise when practical management of the sexual problem has been delayed, sometimes by up to 2–3 years following completion of radiotherapy. The organic dysfunction caused by cancer therapy is then accompanied by a significant psychogenic component. Accommodation to a loss or alteration in sexual activity by the individual or couple may have taken place, which often makes strategies to resolve the sexual difficulty more protracted or complex.

Although fertility and sexual expression may be recognised as distinct entities, a strategy frequently adopted in clinical practice is to use discussion of the impact of treatment upon fertility as an entrée to the more challenging consideration of sexual dysfunction caused by cancer therapy (White 1994). While this may be appropriate in clients where procreation remains a realistic goal, for a larger number of clients with cancer this strategy can become a barrier to the detailed discussion of specific concerns related to sexual expression. This may be the case where patients are postmenopausal, have completed their family, are elderly, have advanced disease or where the treatment field does not include the gonads but may still affect an aspect of sexual expression, for example radiotherapy to the head and neck region. While it is crucial to consider the impact of treatment upon reproductive potential, it remains equally important to address the systemic and local effects of radiotherapy upon sexual expression and sexual function. Where undue emphasis is placed upon the narrow association between sexuality and reproduction, more diverse and less traditional definitions of sexuality remain on the periphery of clinicians' awareness and thus on the margins of both professional acceptability and response. Thus, through such inherent heterosexism, couples in same-sex relationships continue to experience prejudice or ignorance of their sexual health needs within cancer care.

In this chapter the impact of radiotherapy upon fertility and on sexual health will be discussed separately, although it is acknowledged that disruption in fertility will often create disruption in the related domain of sexual expression (Irvine & Cawood 1996). This chapter recognises the fact that contemporary cancer treatment frequently involves a multimodal approach to therapy, thus the increased impact of combined modalities upon both reproductive and sexual function is acknowledged.

SUBFERTILITY, INFERTILITY AND FERTILITY PRESERVATION

Depending on the field of treatment, radiotherapy can cause damage to the entire reproductive system, including the hypothalamic–pituitary axis, gonads and the endometrium (Chatterjee & Goldstone 1996). The impact of radiotherapy upon reproductive function should be discussed with all adults of child-bearing age, including those in same-sex relationships. Such discussion should, where relevant, also include information regarding contraception during therapy and other periods of risk (Schover 1997). In general, it is advised that reproduction should be avoided within 12–18 months of any radiation to the gonads, as genetic damage may still be present. Specific information about fertility counselling is beyond the scope of this chapter but readers may find specialist texts on this subject helpful in their discussion of the emotional impact of infertility and fertility preservation options for people affected by cancer and their partners (Read 1995).

The counselling of children, adolescents and their parents requires particular sensitivity. With an increased number of adult survivors following childhood malignancy, there remains a need for clinicians with a specific interest in the late effects of cancer and cancer therapy in childhood, including the issues of future fertility, endocrine function and psychosexual development (Relander et al 2000, Waring & Wallace 2000).

In standard radiotherapy practice using 2 Gy per fraction, >60 Gy is usually given as a curative dose for epithelial tumours and >25–30 Gy for more sensitive tumours such as testicular malignancies. Both male and female reproductive function can be significantly affected by doses as low as 1–2 Gy. Reproductive organs are highly radiosensitive and it is important to be aware that a common source of damage to the tissues comes from the low doses of scattered internal radiation.

Ovarian effects

The ovary produces oocytes for reproduction and secretes a variety of steroid hormones responsible for sexual function, sexual maturity and other physiological effects, such as bone mineralisation. During fetal life, a maximum of around six million oocytes is produced which degenerates with time. At birth this number is reduced to around two million, with around 100 000 oocytes at puberty. Radiation destroys ovarian follicles/oocytes, impairs the maturation process of oocytes and produces fibrosis and atrophy of the ovary. Radiation tolerance of the ovary is lowered by older age, higher total dose and larger fraction size (see Table 16.1 for summary). Total body irradiation to doses of 8–12 Gy frequently results in ovarian failure. However, using fractionation to deliver 12 Gy over 6 days has allowed up to 24% of women under 26 years of age to recover ovarian function, compared to 6% among those receiving 10 Gy in a single fraction (Sanders et al 1988).

Women with ovarian failure not only have to adapt to the loss of their reproductive potential but also to the concept of long-term hormone replacement therapy to minimise the effects of a premature menopause. For some women these changes

Table 16.1 Radiation dose and its effect on ovarian function in women of reproductive age

Minimum ovarian dose (Gy)	Effect on ovarian function
0.6	No lasting damage
1.5	No lasting damage in most young women but some sterilisation risk in women >40 years
2.5–5.0	Variable effect depending on age 30–40% risk of permanent sterilisation in women 15–40 years >90% risk of permanent sterilisation in women > 40 years
5–8	Variable effect depending on age 50–70% risk of permanent sterilisation in women 15–40 years
>8	100% risk of permanent sterilisation

Adapted with permission from Ash (1980).

may be associated with feelings of reduced femininity and an alteration to both their gender identity and sexuality.

Testicular effects

The testis produces spermatozoa for reproduction and testosterone, responsible for sexual function and sexual maturity. Spermatogenesis is an exquisitely radiosensitive process and low doses of radiation will destroy the reproductive process. Leydig cells of the testes secrete testosterone and produce up to 75% of the total testosterone required by men. The tolerance of Leydig cells is much higher than that for spermatogenesis.

Doses of < 0.5 Gy often cause oligospermia with full recovery within 12–48 months following treatment. At fractionated doses between 0.5 and 2.0 Gy, azoospermia usually occurs after a lag period of 7 weeks and return of sperm counts may take up to 2–3.5 years (Kinsella et al 1989). In the human testis fractionated doses > 2.5 Gy will most likely produce sterility. Table 16.2 provides a summary of the impact of radiotherapy on spermatogenesis (Centola et al 1994). Older men treated with pelvic radiotherapy rarely have discussions about infertility as a result of radiotherapy, yet Schover et al (1987) found that this was a significant source of distress in 21% of patients. As Burke (1996) explains, many individuals

> … may find it difficult to separate the pleasurable from the reproductive aspects of sexual intercourse. Consequently, once the reproductive function has gone, the reason for having intercourse has disappeared as well (p. 240).

FERTILITY PRESERVATION APPROACHES

Ovarian shielding can sometimes maintain function, but despite this, many women lose ovarian function after pelvic irradiation. A small prospective study

Table 16.2 Radiation dose and its effect on spermatogenesis

Minimum testicular dose (Gy)	Spermatogenesis (effects compared with normal pre-treatment function)
< 0.1	No effect
0.1–0.3	Temporary oligospermia with full recovery by 12 months
0.3–0.5	Temporary oligo/azoospermia around 4–12 months following radiotherapy with full recovery by 48 months
0.5–1.0	> 90% temporary oligo/azoospermia for 3–17 months following radiotherapy with recovery around 8–26 months
1–2	100% azoospermia for 2–9 months following radiotherapy with return of sperm counts around 11–30 months
2–3	100% azoospermia beginning 1–2 months following radiotherapy. Some men will suffer permanent azoospermia and some will have recovery around 12–30 months
3–4	100% azoospermia. No recovery seen up to 40 months
12	Permanent azoospermia. Reduced testicular size and reduced testosterone production

Modified with permission from Centola et al (1994).

($n = 20$) evaluated the feasibility, morbidity and efficacy of unilateral ovarian transposition for female patients receiving pelvic radiation (external beam and brachytherapy) for the treatment of cervical cancer or Hodgkin's lymphoma (Clough et al 1996).

Laparoscopic ovarian transposition is translocation of the ovaries on a pedicle of the infundibulopelvic ligament to an area outside the treatment field, such as the paracolic gutter. In Clough et al's (1996) study this technique was capable of reducing the radiation dose to a mean of 1.75 and a maximum of 3.7 Gy, with 100% preservation of ovarian function at 2-year follow-up for women aged < 40 years. Ovarian transposition was considered an effective method of preserving reproductive function and avoiding the need for long-term hormone replacement therapy where the risk of subsequent ovarian metastasis was very low.

Embryo cryopreservation for use in subsequent in vitro fertilisation is only suitable for patients of reproductive age and it may take 4–6 weeks to obtain sufficient suitable oocytes, thus delaying the commencement of definitive cancer treatment. Furthermore, the ovarian hyperstimulation required to collect several oocytes may be contraindicated in the presence of steroid-dependent malignancies or, where there is no male partner, as donor sperm would then be required (Picton et al 2000). Patients who wish to consider this fertility preservation technique need to be given access to counselling by clinicians expert in this field. In vitro fertilisation remains a relatively unsuccessful procedure due to failure at the stage of embryo transfer, with only a 10–20% chance of implantation of the embryo in the uterus (Templeton 2000).

Where the patient has received a therapeutic dose of radiotherapy to the uterus there may be detrimental effects such as reduced uterine volume, decreased elasticity of the uterine musculature and impaired endometrial blood flow that can also compromise the successful outcome of any subsequent pregnancy (Chatterjee & Goldstone 1996, Waring & Wallace 2000).

Cryopreservation of ovarian tissue or germ cells and the use of culture technology to produce ripe gametes for assisted conception has become the most recent research imperative in this field (Picton et al 2000). Ovarian tissue banking is, at least in theory, a practical alternative to embryo storage that can be utilised for both adults and children. However, the technology associated with the autograft of ovarian tissue or the in vitro culture of oocytes from primordial follicles must, for the moment, be regarded as experimental (Picton et al 2000).

The conventional use of testicular shielding can reduce the dose of radiation to 1–2% of the total dose, but the adverse effects of even a small dose of scatter radiation have been mentioned previously (Frass et al 1985). Where the radiation field is restricted to the inguinopelvic region, and there are no disease-related contraindications, some clinicians have successfully used the technique of testicular transposition to preserve spermatogenesis through increasing the distance of the testicle from the radiation field (Deo et al 2001).

The use of gonadotrophin-releasing hormone agonists to create a protective hypogonadism has been advocated as a strategy for male and female patients; however, clinical evidence of its efficacy is inconclusive and animal studies have failed to show any protective effect against radiosensitivity (Gosden et al 1997). Further studies may be warranted.

Pre-treatment semen analysis and cryopreservation of sperm should be discussed with all men receiving abdominopelvic or total body irradiation and offered to those who wish to preserve their fertility potential. Many patients have suboptimal semen quality as a result of the disease or its treatment, but with the advent of intracytoplasmic sperm injection (ICSI), the criteria for semen cryopreservation in cancer patients have been revised. This technique injects the sperm directly into the cytoplasm of the oocyte, and requires very few sperm for successful fertilisation, therefore only azoospermic samples should be rejected (Chatterjee & Goldstone 1996). Where necessary, sperm can also be obtained through epididymal aspiration or testicular biopsy.

In the future, cryopreservation of testicular tissue may offer an opportunity to preserve the fertility of prepubertal boys but in current practice should still be regarded as experimental (Picton et al 2000, Waring & Wallace 2000). Long-term follow-up by reproductive endocrinologists is recommended for patients who have received treatment to the hypothalamic–pituitary axis (total body irradiation or cranial irradiation) or to the gonads and uterus. Unless contraindicated, hormone replacement therapy should be offered to all female patients with treatment-induced ovarian failure and testosterone replacement therapy offered to men where Leydig cell dysfunction is evident (Chatterjee & Goldstone 1996).

IMPACT OF RADIOTHERAPY ON SEXUAL EXPRESSION AND FUNCTION

It is often difficult to separate the physical effects of cancer and its treatment from the associated psychological and interpersonal responses that impact upon an individual's or couple's sexual expression. In addition, some people requiring cancer treatment will have pre-existing sexual difficulties that may or may not be attributed to their cancer diagnosis (Gerraughty 1994). Fear of cancer being caused by or transmitted through sexual intercourse can also lie behind a reduction in sexual activity or a failure to resume sexual intercourse following treatment (Cull et al 1993). Women with cervical cancer may consider the link between sexual activity and their illness as punishment for certain sexual behaviour or multiple partners. Other patients may fear that when cancer is still in the body it can spread to or damage their partners through sexual contact. A patient with bladder cancer undergoing pelvic radiotherapy believed that the epithelial debris he saw in his urine was the cancer seeding. He refrained from sex as he believed that these cancer cells would infect his partner and subsequently put her at risk of cancer (Faithfull 1995). Such beliefs and misunderstanding of how radiation affects such intimate aspects of people's lives are often left unexplored by clinicians and patients alike, contributing to sexual difficulties.

Sexual difficulties can contribute to relationship breakdown, and while there does not appear to be an increased incidence of divorce among couples whose lives have been affected by cancer, there is evidence that relationship difficulties may be exacerbated within couples who are already in conflict (Schover et al 1987). In the psychosocial oncology literature, partners of people with cancer have become an increasing focus of research in recent years (Carlson et al 2000). This growing number of studies has resulted in increased awareness among healthcare professionals of the partner's contribution to the adjustment and holistic rehabilitation of patients with cancer. What has also become evident is that the experience of cancer affects both members of a couple relationship, with partners frequently reporting higher levels of psychological distress, including psychosexual concerns, than patients (Carlson et al 2000).

It is important to explore both local and systemic effects of treatment on sexual function in order to understand the impact of radiotherapy upon each phase of the human sexual response cycle (Masters & Johnson 1966) and in turn to consider the most appropriate intervention. Figure 16.1 illustrates the impact of radiotherapy on each phase of the human sexual response cycle. The following section is structured to address treatment effects upon each individual phase, although such effects may create difficulties in more than one phase simultaneously. As the phases are interrelated, a detrimental effect on one phase is likely to impact on subsequent phases of the cycle and associated sexual behaviours and functions.

CLINICAL ASSESSMENT OF SEXUAL FUNCTION

It is helpful to conduct a systematic baseline assessment of sexual function prior to treatment, especially when sexual dysfunction is a known or anticipated side-effect of the proposed treatment plan, for example in pelvic radiotherapy or total body irradiation. Comprehensive assessment also ensures that clients without a diagnosis or treatment that directly affects the sexual organs are screened adequately for signs of sexual difficulties. Champion (1996) notes the relative

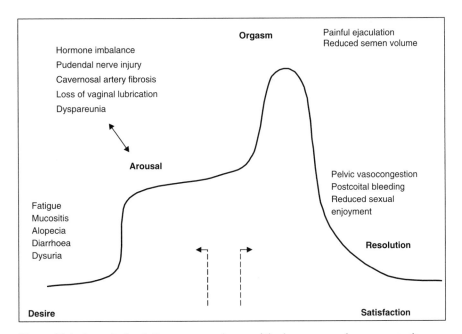

Figure 16.1   Impact of radiotherapy upon phases of the human sexual response cycle.

paucity of information about the sexual health repercussions for men and women who have malignancies with no obvious link to sexuality, for example those with leukaemia, cranial or oral tumours, whose treatment may well cause disruption. There are a number of sexual assessment schedules in use, although they are more commonly employed within the context of clinical trials as opposed to clinically regular use. Some schedules adopt a focus that is too narrow to be of use in diverse patient populations, for example the evaluation of erectile dysfunction. One comprehensive assessment framework in use adopts the acronym ALARM (Kelly 2002) and is summarised in Table 16.3. Such a framework can be used to conduct a baseline assessment of sexual function prior to treatment, although it is acknowledged that the physical and psychological impact of a cancer diagnosis may have already had an impact on sexual expression. This initial assessment can then be compared with both on-treatment and post-treatment evaluation of sexual expression and function in order to identify appropriate medical and/or psychosexual interventions to preserve or restore optimum sexual health for the individual or couple.

It is imperative that appropriate clinical and research evaluation of the validity and reliability of sexual assessments is conducted as an integral part of treatment toxicity monitoring and postradiotherapy rehabilitation studies.

Sexual desire/interest phase

Studies highlight the fact that physical changes postradiotherapy do not necessarily inhibit sexual desire, but that changes in body image, misconceptions or fears about spreading the cancer or hastening recurrence all have the capacity to impact on sexual function (Cartwright-Alcarese 1995). See Table 16.4 for a summary of the pathophysiological changes in the sexual organs caused by radiotherapy.

Table 16. 3 Sexual assessment model: ALARM

Activity	Range, mode(s) and frequency of sexual expression, form(s) of sexual relationships (heterosexual, same-sex, both)
Libido	Any change to normal level or change in pattern of sexual interest. How important is this to the individual/couple? How satisfied are they with the current situation?
Arousal	Any difficulties in achieving or maintaining erection or vaginal lubrication? Any pain or discomfort during sexual activity? Has this led to sexual difficulties?
Resolution	Is the nature/intensity of orgasm the same? Is the level of sexual satisfaction altered? Is there any pain or discomfort following sexual activity? If so, what is its nature and site?
Medical history	Are there any underlying physical or mental health problems contributing to sexual difficulties? Is the person taking medication (prescription or other drugs, including alcohol) which is likely to influence sexual function? Is he/she recovering from any concurrent illness or life disruption, e.g. bereavement?

Adapted with permission from Kelly (2002).

Table 16.4   Potential effects of radiotherapy on the sexual organs

Women	Men
Pelvic fibrosis	Pelvic fibrosis
Atrophy of the vaginal wall	Pudendal or sympathetic nerve injury
Thinning of vaginal/vulval epithelium	Decreased semen volume
Reduced tissue elasticity	Fibrosis of cavernosal arteries
Scarring	Reduction in penile blood pressure
Obliteration of small blood vessels	Decreased testosterone
Reduced vaginal lubrication	
Ulceration	
Decreased oestrogen	

The cause of reduced sexual desire in people affected by cancer is usually multifactorial, with social, cultural, psychological, physical and pharmacological components all affecting the complex interplay of sexual desire and expression. Loss of sexual desire may have physical causes such as a reduction in sexual hormones through ablative doses of radiotherapy (see sections on ovarian and testicular effects, above) or adjuvant hormone therapy as used in the management of breast or prostate cancer (Schover 1993). Concurrent medication may also contribute to loss of sexual desire (antidepressants, anxiolytics, antiemetics, strong opioids, antihypertensives, diuretics) and should be considered in the overall management of sexual difficulty. Psychological factors such as anxiety or depression often accompany the diagnosis and treatment of cancer and can have profound effects on sexual desire (Hawton 1985). As discussed in Chapter 17, altered self-concept as a result of cancer and its treatment can reduce self-esteem and lead to avoidance of social, intimate and thus sexual contact. For example, a person receiving radiotherapy for treatment of a malignancy of the head and neck region may not only experience significant disfigurement, but also related functional problems resulting in an inability to control salivation or to kiss normally (Roberts 2002). It is unclear whether clinicians really consider the sexual health needs of patients with radiation-induced symptoms beyond the pelvis.

Research findings indicate that sexual interest is at its lowest on completion of therapy, reflecting the direct impact of treatment side effects (Flay & Matthews 1995). Symptoms such as fatigue, pain, diarrhoea, dysuria, cystitis, nocturia and rectal bleeding can all contribute to a decrease in desire for sexual intimacy.

Symptom management and support should include information about how radiotherapy impacts on sexual interest and desire as well as taking steps to control side effects that are disrupting sexual interest, such as the control of dysuria or diarrhoea. Concurrent medication should be reviewed to see if alternative drugs can be substituted where loss of sexual desire is a known side-effect of the present medication regimen. Patients and their partners should be encouraged to maintain intimate contact during periods where intercourse is not feasible or desired due to treatment and disease effects. Alternative genital and non-genital forms of sexual expression can be explored with the couple, where acceptable to them, together with strategies to enhance existing couple communication. A consistent finding in a recent review of the psychosocial oncology literature by Carlson et al (2000) was the importance of the role of communication between partners in promoting adaptation to the negative consequences of both the cancer diagnosis and treatment for the patient and spouse. In addition, effective couple communication promoted successful role reallocation within the relationship (related to the impact of illness) and appeared to enhance the quality of the relationship. Within the context of the couple's sexual relationship, such role reallocation may include a change in who normally initiates sexual contact, together with where and when sexual expression takes place, in order to accommodate both illness and treatment effects. The promotion of effective couple communication is also important in dispelling myths associated with the illness, its treatment and related sexual difficulties, particularly where reduced sexual intimacy may be misinterpreted as rejection by the partner.

Where reduced sexual desire is directly related to ovarian or testicular failure, hormone replacement therapy should be offered unless there is a medical contraindication. Psychosexual therapy can also be of assistance in enabling couples to regain sexual interest within the constraints of their physical and psychological well-being, through provision of sexual growth and sensate focus programmes for individuals or couples (Bancroft 1989, Goodwin & Agronin 1997, Hawton 1985).

Sexual arousal and orgasm

In women being treated with radiotherapy for gynaecological cancer, the vaginal canal and ovaries are the areas most sensitive to radiation therapy and combined-modality treatment has a more profound effect on physical changes (Flay & Matthews 1995). Table 16.5 provides a summary of the radiotherapy-induced

Table 16.5 Radiation effects on female sexual expression and function

Symptoms/signs	Management strategies
Decreased sexual desire	Monitor oestrogen, FSH and LH levels Hormone replacement therapy (including topical oestrogen treatment for the vaginal cavity) Patient/couple education Psychosexual therapy
Vaginal dryness	Hormone replacement therapy (including topical oestrogen treatment for the vaginal cavity and vulva)
Vulvovaginitis	Use of vaginal lubricants
Burning sensation associated with semen	Use of barrier contraceptives (e.g. condom) Patient/couple education
Superficial or deep dyspareunia Vaginismus	Use of vaginal dilators and lubricants Alternative sexual positions to reduce depth of vaginal penetration (e.g. female superior or side-lying)
Pelvic pain Postcoital bleeding Pelvic vasocongestion	Psychosexual therapy Use of vaginal dilators Use of vaginal lubricants Hormone replacement therapy (including topical oestrogen treatment for the vaginal cavity) Patient/couple education

FSH, follicle-stimulating hormone; LH, luteinising hormone.

sexual difficulties experienced by women with cancer. If the radiation field includes vaginal tissue, women experience a decrease in both vaginal lubrication and sensation. The lining of the vagina undergoes rapid cell renewal as the epithelium is very sensitive to radiation damage. Depletion of cell supply, slow occlusion of blood vessels and gradual laying-down of fibrosis results in narrowing and lack of elasticity in the vaginal canal (Cartwright-Alcarese 1995). Stenosis and/or shortening of the vagina are late effects that occur progressively over time, with a consequent reduction in both length and diameter.

The common problem from these physiological changes is that patients complain of pain on intercourse (dyspareunia). As many as 43% of women considered pain on intercourse the main reason for their decreased enjoyment and frequency of sexual activity at 14 weeks following completion of radiotherapy (Flay & Matthews 1995). Patients were also frightened that sex would be painful and this reduced sexual pleasure (Cull et al 1993); in some women this can have the propensity to cause development of secondary vaginismus.

One of the most effective ways of preventing vaginal stenosis, adhesions and associated dyspareunia is the use of vaginal dilators as part of sexual rehabilitation following gynaecological radiotherapy. Dilators need to be used over a long time period unless the woman has regular sexual intercourse (Cartwright-Alcarese 1995). The initial use of dilators can be difficult as they may cause pain or discomfort. Assessment can create an opportunity to discuss a woman's fears that sexual intercourse may be painful (Burke 1996). The use of lubrication for a dry vagina reduces irritation and pain (Cartwright-Alcarese 1995). Decreased elasticity and scarring and associated vaginal shortening may make certain sexual positions uncomfortable, so suggesting different positions may increase comfort and satisfaction. For example, use of the female superior position gives the woman greater control over the depth and rate of vaginal penetration, thus reducing anxiety and potential dyspareunia.

In men, radiation to the pelvis for prostate, bladder, testicular or rectal malignancies has variable consequences for sexual functioning. Table 16.6 provides a summary of the radiotherapy-induced sexual difficulties experienced by men with cancer. External beam radiation therapy for prostate cancer can cause fibrosis of the pelvic vasculature and damage to the pudendal or sympathetic nerves, resulting in erectile dysfunction. In a study of the impact of external beam pelvic radiotherapy by Crook et al (1996), 35% of previously potent men considered their erections unsatisfactory for intercourse. Damage to the cavernosal arteries can result in reduced penile blood pressures, compounding arteriosclerotic changes in the pelvic arteries, particularly among older men, but also causing arterial insufficiency in younger men, for example those receiving total body irradiation for haematological malignancies (Chatterjee et al 2000). Fifty per cent of patients in one study developed erectile failure up to 7 years post-treatment as a direct result of vascular scarring (Kornblith et al 1994). Radiotherapy may accelerate pathological vascular and neural changes associated with concurrent illnesses such as diabetes, hypertension or increasing age. As discussed previously, decreased levels of testosterone and reduced sexual desire may also lead to erectile difficulties or anorgasmia in some men (Bancroft 1989).

The prevalence of erectile dysfunction associated with prostate cancer and its treatment varies considerably across studies reviewed, probably reflecting differences

Table 16.6 Radiation effects on male sexual expression and function

Symptoms/signs	Management strategies
Decreased sexual desire	Monitor testosterone, FSH and LH levels Testosterone replacement therapy Patient/couple education Psychosexual therapy
Erectile dysfunction: reduced number and quality of erections (early-morning and those associated with sexual stimulation)	Erectile dysfunction clinic: access to vacuum constriction devices, urethral administration of alprostadil, intracavernosal injections and oral/sublingual medication (sildenafil, apomorphine) Psychosexual therapy Penile prostheses (last resort)
Pain on orgasm/ejaculation Decrease in semen volume Pelvic vasocongestion	Patient/couple education Rule out and treat persistent organic cause, e.g. infection, inflammation Psychosexual therapy

FSH, follicle-stimulating hormone; LH, luteinising hormone.

in the precision with which erectile dysfunction is both defined and reported, among other factors. Estimates of erectile dysfunction range from 80% of men receiving antiandrogen therapy (Schover 1993) to 98% following radical and 79% following nerve-sparing prostatectomy (Walsh 1987, Yarbro & Ferrans 1998) and a range of 25–60% for radiotherapy (Schover 1993, Zelefsky et al 1999). Such figures are often difficult to interpret accurately as a substantial number of these men receive multimodal therapy.

Radiotherapy can result in pain on ejaculation, particularly when radiation urethritis or epididymitis is still present, together with a permanent decrease in semen volume, often referred to as 'dry ejaculation' (Schover 1987). Information about the changes in erectile function caused by cancer, surgery, radiotherapy or antiandrogen therapy, together with those associated with normal ageing, can assist the couple to create the most appropriate context within which pharmacological or physical interventions may be employed. Men in later life (over 65 years of age) may not only experience a reduction in desire for sexual activity but may find their erections are slower to develop and that they need greater genital or direct stimulation to achieve an erection sufficiently rigid to permit penetration (Crowe & Ridley 2000). Work with the couple can enable the partner to appreciate the mutual benefits of extended foreplay and the use of greater penile stimulation in encouraging the recovery of post-treatment erections where vascular and neurological mechanisms remain at least partially intact.

In a small-scale study ($n = 34$) of short-term (median follow-up 13 months) sexual function following prostate brachytherapy in low-risk prostate cancer, haematospermia (blood in the semen), painful orgasm and altered intensity of orgasm were reported by 26%, 15% and 38% of the men respectively (Merrick et al 2001a). At median follow-up, 65% of men studied had maintained their erectile function without the need for pharmacological intervention and, of the 12 men who developed erectile dysfunction, the four treated with oral sildenafil (Viagra) all achieved an erection sufficient for intercourse. Initial studies indicate that oral sildenafil appears to promote the resolution of erectile difficulties in the majority of men with radiotherapy-induced erectile dysfunction (Merrick et al 2001a, b Potters et al 2001). Sildenafil appears to be effective in 70% of men with radiotherapy-induced erectile failure, but appears less effective (40–50%) for those who have received surgical management (Vale 2000). However, it must be remembered that sildenafil is not normally successful when sexual desire is either reduced or absent. Sildenafil is also contraindicated in men with severe ischaemic heart disease and those receiving nitrate therapy (Goldstein et al 1998).

A new sublingual drug, apomorphine, is currently being evaluated for use and may enable greater sexual spontaneity due to its ease of administration and more rapid onset of action (Dula et al 2001). Other treatments, such as intraurethral or intracavernosal administration of alprostadil or use of a vacuum constriction device, may also be appropriate.

Penile implants are normally considered a treatment of last resort as it is necessary to remove the majority of erectile tissue in order to insert the implant and thus any subsequent implant failure results in permanent loss of natural erection. Insertion of an implant can also be more difficult after radiotherapy due to the presence of corporeal fibrosis; complication rates such as infection are also higher (Vale 2000).

Regardless of whether the cancer-related sexual difficulty originates with the male or female partner, it is important to consider the management of such issues within the context of the couple relationship. Where physical or pharmacological methods to restore erectile function are adopted, it remains important to ascertain their acceptability to both the man and his partner, otherwise compliance with such treatment may be adversely affected (McCarthy 2001). Furthermore, a number of studies confirmed the presence of erectile difficulties for up to 3 years prior to the man seeking treatment. Thus the recovery of erectile function may cause difficulties for a female partner (e.g. dyspareunia, postcoital bleeding), particularly where the partner is post-menopausal or where there has been prolonged abstinence. Increased sexual activity may alter the relationship dynamics and here an integrated management approach that includes couple therapy may be helpful in both providing information about the resumption of sexual activity and in restoring a new equilibrium for the couple (Hudson-Allez 1998).

An interesting finding from a study by Speckens et al (1995) was the relative reduction in sexual interest among the female partners of men with erectile dysfunction of organic origin ($n = 71$). The authors speculated that this reduction in sexual interest might have been a cognitive and behavioural adjustment to the likely permanence of erectile dysfunction in their partners. What is also important to acknowledge is that partner dynamics and sexuality may act as predisposing, precipitating or maintaining factors in sexual difficulties, even when that difficulty is of predominantly organic aetiology, as in people with cancer care. Thus it remains important to consider the intra- and interpersonal dynamics that contribute to the sexual satisfaction of the couple when considering the most appropriate intervention strategies for restoration of sexual expression and function (Barnes 1998). Radiotherapy treatment centres may therefore need to liaise with a variety of referral agencies (erectile dysfunction clinics, relationship or psychosexual therapy services, gynaecological or urology services) to optimise management of the sexual difficulties encountered among couples affected by cancer.

Resolution phase

This phase of the sexual response cycle is not well recognised by patients or healthcare professionals. It is during this phase that pelvic vasocongestion, penile, labial and clitoral engorgement and enlargement return to their prearousal state. Following pelvic radiotherapy, vascular changes caused by the treatment can result in delayed capillary drainage from the tissues. This may be experienced by the patient as a protracted sensation of fullness, aching or discomfort following intercourse or orgasm. There is no specific intervention recommended other than to explain the likely cause of this sensation and that it will diminish and is not harmful.

Postcoital vaginal bleeding may occur in up to 36% of woman receiving radiotherapy for gynaecological malignancy (Flay & Matthews 1995) and bleeding from the rectum may occur as a result of anal intercourse. Bleeding is usually related to radiation-induced damage to the epithelial mucosa and the impact of oestrogen depletion. Advice about the importance of adequate lubrication during sexual intercourse, together with a reduction in vigorous sexual intercourse until further healing has taken place, normally results in improvement. Use of a local oestrogen cream and hormone replacement therapy should alleviate postcoital bleeding where ovarian failure is implicated.

CONCLUSION

There remain both misconceptions and inconsistencies in the management of fertility and sexual difficulties associated with radiotherapy. Such inconsistencies may be understood in the light of inadequate knowledge of the effects of radiotherapy on fertility and sexual function, or, more importantly, of their specialised management. Inconsistencies may be as a result of the perception that such problems do not fall within the remit of the radiotherapy treatment team, or that adequate specialist personnel and resources are not readily available. Sexual difficulty following radiotherapy is clearly a multifaceted problem with both physical and psychological components that influence sexual desire and expression. Accurate and detailed information about potential sexual problems is often lacking and toxicity is rarely accurately monitored in this aspect of patient care.

Where sexual issues *are* addressed within the radiotherapy treatment centre, the focus of clinicians is often solely the provision of information about potential sexual difficulties. However, as we hope this chapter illustrates, practical management strategies and referral to specialist agencies as well as psychological or psychosexual insights need to be considered integral to any intervention. Providing cancer patients with information about the potential sexual and fertility problems they may experience during and after radiotherapy legitimises this as an area of care that can and should be discussed.

FURTHER INFORMATION

National Cancer Institute
http://www.nci.nih.gov/cancerinfo/pdq/supportive care/sexuality/health care professional

University of Iowa Health Care
http://www.vh.org/Patients/IHB/Cancer/Fertility/Fertility.html

Beth Israel Medical Centre
http://www.stoppain.org/services/featureprogs.html/ sexualhealth
http://www.cancernet.co.uk/sexuality-f.html

The Royal Marsden Hospital
http://royalmarsden.org.uk/patientinfo/booklets/feminine care/index.asp

REFERENCES

Ash P 1980 Influence of radiation on fertility in man. British Journal of Cancer 53:271–278
Bancroft J 1989 Human sexuality and its problems, 2nd edn. Churchill Livingstone, Edinburgh
Barnes T 1998 The female partner in the treatment of erectile dysfunction: what is her position? Sexual and Marital Therapy 13(3):233–239
Burke L M 1996 Sexual dysfunction following radiotherapy for cervical cancer. British Journal of Nursing 5(4):239–244
Carlson L E, Bultz B D, Speca M et al 2000 Partners of cancer patients: Part I. Impact, adjustment and coping across the illness trajectory. Journal of Psychosocial Oncology 18(2):39–63
Cartwright-Alcarese F 1995 Addressing sexual dysfunction following radiation therapy for a gynecologic malignancy. Oncology Nursing Forum 22:1227–1231
Centola G M, Keller J W, Henzler M et al 1994 Effect of low-dose testicular irradiation on sperm count and fertility in patients with testicular seminoma. Journal of Andrology 15:608–613
Champion A 1996 Male cancer and sexual function. Sexual and Marital Therapy 11(3):227–244
Chatterjee R, Goldstone A H 1996 Gonadal damage and effects on fertility in adult patients with haematological malignancy undergoing stem cell transplantation. Bone Marrow Transplantation 17:5–11
Chatterjee R, Andrews H O, McGarrigle H H et al 2000 Cavernosal arterial insufficiency is a major component of erectile dysfunction in some recipients of high-dose chemotherapy/chemo-radiotherapy for haematological malignancies. Bone Marrow Transplantation, 25:1185–1189
Clough K B, Goffinet F, Labib A et al 1996 Laparoscopic unilateral ovarian transposition prior to irradiation. Cancer 77(12):2638–2645
Crook J, Esche B, Futter N 1996 Effects of pelvic radiotherapy for prostate cancer on bowel, bladder and sexual function: the patient's perspective. Urology 47:387–394
Crowe M, Ridley J 2000 Therapy with couples: a behavioural-systems approach to relationship and sexual problems, 2nd edn. Blackwell Science, Oxford
Cull A, Cowie V J, Farquharson D I M et al 1993 Early stage cervical cancer: psychosocial and sexual outcomes of treatment. British Journal of Cancer 68:1216–1220
Deo S V S, Asthana S, Shukla N K et al 2001 Fertility preserving testicular transposition in patients undergoing inguino pelvic irradiation. Journal of Surgical Oncology 76:70–72
Dula E, Bukofzer S, Perdok R et al 2001 Double-blind, crossover comparison of 3 mg Apomorphine SL with placebo and with 4 mg Apomorphine SL in male erectile dysfunction. European Urology 39:558–564
Faithfull S 1995 'Just grin and bear it and hope that it will go away'. Coping with urinary symptoms from pelvic radiotherapy. European Journal of Cancer Care 4:158–165

Flay L D Matthews J H L 1995 The effects of radiotherapy and surgery on the sexual function of women treated for cervical cancer. International Journal of Radiation Oncology, Biology, Physics 31(2):399–404

Frass B A, Kinsella D J, Harrington P 1985 Peripheral dose to the testes: the design and clinical use of practical and effective gonadal shield. International Journal of Radiation Oncology, Biology, Physics 11:609–615

Gerraughty S M 1994 Sexual function in cancer patients. Physical Medicine and Rehabilitation 8(2):251–260

Goldstein I, Lue T F, Padma-Nathan H et al 1998 Oral Sildenafil in the treatment of erectile dysfunction. The New England Journal of Medicine 338(20):1397–1404

Goodwin A J, Agronin M E 1997 A woman's guide to overcoming sexual fear and pain. New Harbinger Publications Inc., Oakland

Gosden R G, Wade J C, Fraser H M et al 1997 Impact of congenital or experimental hypogonadotrophism on the radiation sensitivity of the mouse ovary. Human Reproduction 12:2483–2488

Guthrie C 1999 Nurses' perceptions of sexuality relating to patient care. Journal of Clinical Nursing 8:313–321

Hawton K 1985 Sex therapy: a practical guide. Oxford Medical Publications, Oxford University Press, Oxford

Hudson-Allez G 1998 The interface between psychogenic and organic difficulties in men with erectile dysfunction. Sexual and Marital Therapy 13(3):285–293

Irvine S, Cawood E 1996 Male infertility and its effect on male sexuality. Sexual and Marital Therapy 11(3):273–280

Kelly D 2002 Sexuality and people with acute illness. In: Heath H, White I (eds) The challenge of sexuality in health care. Blackwell Science, Oxford, p 204

Kinsella T J, Trivette G, Rowland J et al 1989 Long-term follow-up of testicular function following radiation therapy for early-stage Hodgkin's disease. Journal of Clinical Oncology 7:718–724

Kornblith A B, Herr H W, Ofman U S et al 1994 Quality of life of patients with prostate cancer and their spouses: the value of a database in clinical care. Cited in: Carlson L E, Bultz B D, Speca M et al 2000 Partners of cancer patients: part I. Impact, adjustment and coping across the illness trajectory. Journal of Psychosocial Oncology 18(2):39–63

Masters W, Johnson V 1966 Human sexual response. Little Brown, Boston

McCarthy B W 2001 Relapse prevention strategies and techniques with erectile dysfunction. Journal of Sex and Marital Therapy 27:1–8

Meerabeau L 1999 The management of embarrassment and sexuality in health care. Journal of Advanced Nursing 29(6):1507–1513

Merrick G S, Wallner K, Butler W M et al 2001a Short-term sexual function after prostate brachytherapy. International Journal of Cancer 96:313–319

Merrick G S, Wallner K, Butler W M et al 2001b A comparison of radiation dose to the bulb of the penis in men with and without prostate brachytherapy-induced erectile dysfunction. International Journal of Radiation Oncology, Biology, Physics 50(3):597–604

Picton H M, Kim S S, Gosden R G 2000 Cryopreservation of gonadal tissue and cells. British Medical Bulletin 56(3):603–615

Potters L, Torre T, Fearn P A et al 2001 Potency after permanent prostate brachytherapy for localized prostate cancer. International Journal of Radiation Oncology, Biology, Physics 50(5):1235–1242

Read J 1995 Counselling for fertility problems. Sage Publications Limited, London

Relander T, Cavallin-Stahl E, Garwicz S et al 2000 Gonadal and sexual function in men treated for childhood cancer. Medical and Pediatric Oncology 35(1):52–63

Roberts H 2002 Sexuality expression for people with disfigurement In: Heath H, White I (eds) The challenge of sexuality in health care. Blackwell Science, Oxford

Sanders J E, Buckner C D, Amos D 1988 Ovarian function following marrow transplantation for aplastic anaemia or leukemia. Journal of Clinical Oncology 6:813–820

Schover L R 1987 Sexuality and fertility in urologic cancer patients. Cancer 60:553–558

Schover L R 1993 Sexual rehabilitation after treatment for prostate cancer. Cancer 71(suppl.):1024–1030

Schover L R 1997 Safer sex after cancer: preventing disease and unwanted pregnancy In: Sexuality and fertility after cancer. John Wiley & Sons Inc., New York

Schover L R, Evans R B, von Eschenbach A C 1987 Sexual rehabilitation in a cancer centre: diagnosis and outcome in 384 consultations. Archives of Sexual Behaviour 17:445–461

Speckens A E, Hengeveld M W, Lycklama A et al 1995 Psychosexual functioning of partners with presumed non-organic erectile dysfunction: cause or consequence of the disorder? Cited in: Barnes T 1998 The female partner in the treatment of erectile dysfunction: what is her position? Sexual and Marital Therapy 13(3):233–239

Templeton A 2000 Infertility and the establishment of pregnancy – overview. British Medical Bulletin 56(3):577–587

Vale J 2000 Erectile dysfunction following radical therapy for prostate cancer. Radiotherapy and Oncology 57:301–305

Walsh P C 1987 Radical prostatectomy, preservation of sexual function, cancer control: the controversy. Urology Clinics of North America 14(4):663

Waring A B, Wallace W H 2000 Subfertility following treatment for childhood cancer. Hospital Medicine 61(8):550–557

Waterhouse J 1996 Nursing practice related to sexuality: a review and recommendations. Nursing Times Research 1(6):412–418

Weijts W, Houtkoop H, Mullen P 1993 Talking delicacy: speaking about sexuality during gynaecological consultations. Sociology of Health and Illness 15(3):295–314

White I D 1994 Nurses' social construction of sexuality within a cancer care context: an exploratory case study. Unpublished MSc thesis. City University, London

White I D 2002 Facilitating sexual expression: challenges for contemporary practice, In: Heath H, White I (eds) The challenge of sexuality in health care. Blackwell Science, Oxford, p 243–247

Yarbro C H, Ferrans C E 1998 Quality of life of patients with prostate cancer treated with surgery or radiation therapy. Oncology Nursing Forum 25(4):685–693

Zelefsky M J, Cowen D, Fuks Z et al 1999 Long term tolerance of high dose three-dimensional conformal radiotherapy in patients with localised prostate carcinoma. Cancer 85(11):2460–2468

17

Body image

Helen Dryden

INTRODUCTION

Perceptions of body image and self can be fundamentally challenged at any stage of the cancer trajectory. Patients receiving radiotherapy may commence treatment with an already altered body image, and many will experience further changes as a result of treatment. The effects of radiotherapy can produce symptoms, both visible and invisible, which threaten the integrity of the body and self. However, for those patients who are treated palliatively to improve symptoms, radiotherapy may result in real improvements in body image and quality of life.

As Wells discusses in Chapter 3, radiotherapy as a treatment modality cannot be viewed in isolation but must be considered in the context of the patient's entire cancer journey. It must also be remembered that the outward appearance of a patient undergoing radiotherapy may conceal the changes that have occurred in individuals' perceptions of themselves and their body. Sontag (1991, p. 3) comments that:

> *Illness is the night-side of life, a more onerous citizenship. Everyone who is born holds dual citizenship, in the kingdom of the well and in the kingdom of the sick. Although we all prefer to use only the good passport, sooner or later each of us is obliged, at least for a spell, to identify ourselves as citizens of that other place.*

Radiotherapy patients, perhaps more than others need to use both 'passports', as described above. A proportion may look and feel completely well before they commence cancer treatment, and for these patients the side effects of radiotherapy may be worse than the symptoms of cancer. As around 50% of radiotherapy is given with palliative intent (Richter & Coia 1985), significant numbers of patients may already have undergone surgery, chemotherapy or indeed have pre-existing health problems.

Attending for radiotherapy can be daunting, tiring and debilitating. Radiotherapy departments are often housed in the basement or away from the main body of the hospital, and the nature of the treatment necessitates that 'patients are left alone, lying under large frightening machines, often on uncomfortable couches, which can lead to feelings of loss of control and isolation' (Woodcock 1997, p. 140). In addition, the onset of side effects related to treatment can herald a sense of shock, bringing with it a realisation of the threat of diagnosis or changed prognosis, and an altered sense of security and well-being. Specific local reactions to radiotherapy treatment, such as skin reactions, mucositis and cystitis, are acknowledged to cause pain, discomfort and distress, and can contribute significantly to an already altered body image. Systemic effects, including anorexia, cachexia, fatigue, nausea and vomiting, can also produce unwelcome changes in body image as well as provide demonstrable evidence of serious illness to the world outside (Body et al 1997, Higginson & Winget 1996, Woodcock 1997). However, much of the experience of receiving radiotherapy and, in particular, its after-effects, can remain hidden from professionals' view (Wells 1998). As Price (1990, p. 40) points out, 'The fact that treatment is transitory doesn't mean that its effects are equally so'. Body image problems can persist for many months or years once treatment is over, and because they are often accompanied by embarrassment and secrecy, they can be particularly difficult to detect and alleviate.

This chapter aims to explore the complex concept of body image, by considering what constitutes normal body image and by discussing the potential impact that cancer and radiotherapy treatment can have on the individual. Strategies will be identified which promote the assessment and support of patients experiencing altered body image, so as to ensure that patients and families receive effective, compassionate care throughout radiotherapy treatment and beyond.

NORMAL BODY IMAGE

Authors have been attempting to define this complex concept since the 1930s. One of the first definitions emphasised the subjective and personal experience of body image, describing it as: 'the image of ourselves we form in our mind, that is to say the way in which our body appears to ourselves' Schilder (1935, p. 3). This concept was extended by psychoanalytical theorists, who suggested that body image is a learnt internalised representation of the body (Sandler & Rosenblatt 1962). Recently, Price's (1999) extensive work in the field of body image care has identified the central components of body image (Fig. 17.1). He stresses that 'body image is both private and public, it is dynamic and is of critical importance to our mental well-being' (Price 1999, p. 5).

More recently, Newell (2000) has criticised Price's model, instead proposing a model of body image care based on a cognitive-behaviourist approach to human experience and behaviour. This approach was principally developed with people who suffered from all types of facial disfigurement, but is not illness-specific. Newell does, however, acknowledge the value of disease-specific work, concerned not only with changes in appearance and function 'but also with many other issues such as the experience of being diagnosed with and living with a

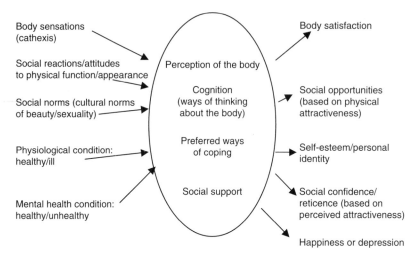

Figure 17. 1 Aspects of normal body image. (Reproduced with permission from Price B (1999) altered body image, Nursing Times Monagraphs no. 29. Emap Healthcare, London)

life-threatening illness, and the practical consequences of altered bodily functions' (Newell 2000, p. 3). Price's model, therefore, has particular relevance to issues of body image within the context of radiotherapy, as it relates specifically to a diagnosis of cancer.

STIGMA ASSOCIATED WITH THE DIAGNOSIS OF CANCER

One of the reasons why cancer fundamentally threatens a person's body image is that it remains a stigmatised condition (Mathieson & Stam 1995, Sontag 1991), particularly when compared to other chronic illnesses (Albrecht et al 1982). Stigma has been interpreted by society as a sign of personal or moral defect above and beyond any physical deformity (Goffman 1963), placing the person outside some socially acceptable standard for human attributes or performance (Bloom & Kessler 1994). Those who are stigmatised can never be sure when they are being related to honestly, and when they are being protected in some way (Goffman 1963). Griffiths (1989) suggests that the bearer of a stigma can be further alienated by feeling intense shame and self-hatred, leading to social withdrawal and even abject loneliness.

One of the many ways in which stigma is expressed is through the use of metaphor. As Czechmeister (1994) explains, cancer is 'mystical by definition, and transforming in a way that heart disease is not. Cancer is a metaphor for all things corrupt and unclean, retaining vestiges of fear and corruption'. Colyer (1996, p. 499) points out that the word cancer 'is synonymous with uncontrollable destruction. Unseen and unheard it represents the ultimate in alien invasion and complete loss of autonomy and control'. Cancer is treated as the enemy, an invader that must be destroyed. This military rhetoric persists when describing the impact of cancer and its treatments. Maguire & Murray-Parkes (1998) discuss how cancer 'invades' the family in a psychological sense, and Sontag (1991, p. 66) illustrates the way in which radiotherapy is described using 'the metaphors of aerial warfare; patients are "bombarded" with toxic rays'. The media also uses highly emotive terms whenever discussing cancer treatment and survival, whereas these are rarely used in relation to coronary heart disease, for example.

Corner (1997) proposes that the constant use of these terms serves to stigmatise those with a diagnosis of cancer further. Treatment is talked about in terms of mounting offensives, using a radical approach and aggressive chemotherapy. Even psychological therapy such as visual imagery makes use of terms such as 'mobilising defences' and 'attacking invaders'. This language depersonalises the body, and in a sense, converts it into a *recipient* of symptoms or therapy. It is perhaps not surprising that body image and the sense of self are damaged.

There is a need to emphasise aspects of care which focus on recovery, such as rehabilitation and pacing or resumption of activity. Numerous studies and specialist nursing posts concentrate on cardiac rehabilitation, yet we very rarely speak of *cancer* patients attending for rehabilitation. Corner (1997) suggests that we need to assist individuals to move towards healing and health in its broadest sense, and a positive body image is central to this notion. Care should be participative and empowering, not responsive only to problems. As previous chapters have emphasised, such an approach requires significant resources, as well as a shift in attitudes. Technical advances in treatment planning, delivery and verification put ever-increasing demands on the staff caring for patients undergoing radiotherapy, which, in addition to existing constraints, limit the extent to which these aspects of care can be addressed (Short & Griffiths 1996).

BODY IMAGE AND CANCER

It is well recognised that both the diagnosis of cancer and its treatment can have a profoundly negative effect on body image (Burt 1995, Dropkin 1999, Frank-Stromberg & Wright 1984, Hopwood 1993, Maguire & Murray-Parkes 1998, van der Molen 1999). If Price's (1990) interpretation of altered body image is adopted, then any physical or psychological change occurring as a result of cancer could cause a person's body image to suffer. Price defines altered body image as 'any significant alteration occurring outside the realms of expected human development' (Price 1990). The stigma and language of cancer, the physical and psychological impact of the disease and the resources (internal and external) available to patients, may influence their ability to cope with such alterations. The actual incidence of body image problems is, however, poorly researched and therefore largely unknown, except perhaps in the case of breast cancer patients. Maguire (1999) found, for example, that up to one-quarter of women who undergo mastectomy develop body image problems.

In a study conducted by Frank-Stromberg & Wright (1984), more than 50% of the 323 ambulatory cancer patients interviewed felt that the diagnosis of cancer and its treatment had changed their physical appearance. Of this group, nearly a quarter felt negatively about the imposed change in their body image. However, the impact of cancer on body image is not always negative. A comparative study found that young adults diagnosed with cancer had a more positive body image than those who were apparently healthy (Bello & McIntyre 1995). Individuals who had undergone more extensive surgery for cancer (including mastectomy, colostomy or amputation) were excluded on the grounds that these operations are known to affect body image. However, other patients (for instance, those with testicular cancer, vulval cancer and malignant melanoma) were included, despite the fact that they too had undergone surgery that could have profoundly altered their body image. It is possible that differences between the two groups could be partially explained by the age of the cancer patients (who were on average 4 years older than the healthy group) and the fact that the majority of them were married (compared to the 'healthy' group, who were mainly single). It may be that those diagnosed with cancer were able to put body image issues more into perspective compared with healthy young adults. Since social support has been implicated as a crucial factor in how people react to changes in their body image (Bloom & Kessler 1994, Price 1999), marital status may have also had a positive effect. However, the authors suggest that higher scores in those with cancer could indicate that health professionals can positively influence body image.

The degree to which changes in body image cause problems for cancer patients may be related to a series of risk factors, summarised in Fig. 17.2.

These risk factors provide a useful framework for the discussion of how patients undergoing radiotherapy are affected. It is important to recognise that these factors often overlap, and more than one may be relevant for an individual patient at a particular time.

VISIBILITY, LOCATION OF TUMOUR AND PROSTHETICS

The issues of visibility, tumour location and prosthetics are closely related, and are particularly relevant for patients with head and neck cancer, who may have a high risk of developing problems with body image. As Chapter 10 illustrates, these

Low risk ◄ -- ► High risk

Invisible or easily camouflaged	**Visibility**	Highly visible or unsightly
Little or no discomfort/transient	**Pain**	Discomfort severe/poorly controlled and chronic
Located in part of the body routinely ignored or not especially valued as part of personal identity	**Location of Tumour**	Located in a part of the body which is highly valued by the patient, e.g. face, sexual organs or limbs
Excellent prosthetics which blend with the patient's body/skin and which are hard to discern as artificial	**Prosthetics**	Prosthetics may be functional rather than aesthetic. May be considered unreliable
Control over body function and posture remains considerable	**Control**	Little or no control over body functions (e.g. incontinence)

Figure 17.2 Cancer-related risk factors that may influence body image. (Reproduced with permission from Price (1999) altered body image. Nursing Times Monographs no. 29. Emap Healthcare, London.)

patients may suffer considerable pain during and after treatment, in addition to having to adapt to visible changes in their appearance. Many individuals undergoing radiotherapy may already be coping with the effects of disfiguring surgery or prostheses. Changes in facial appearance can effect a double blow to the psyche, raising issues related to survival, as well as serving as an enormous threat to self-image, confidence and identity (Breibart & Holland 1988). I vividly remember a patient returning from theatre, after excision of a large maxillary tumour, who asked for a mirror to examine his new facial prosthesis. Still groggy from the anaesthetic, he sat up in bed, stared at his reflection and said, 'I look like something from Star Trek!' Despite several impressions being taken and adaptations made, this patient never wore his prosthesis and preferred to cover the defect by wearing a large triangular patch, which completely occluded one side of his face.

Radiotherapy can further damage a person's body image. During treatment it may become impossible to wear a usual prosthesis because of painful mucositis or moist desquamation. A patient having palliative radiotherapy to a breast lesion may find it extremely distressing to go without the bra and prosthesis that have become 'part' of her body. The discomfort associated with exposing parts of the body during radiotherapy planning and treatment may be particularly acute for those who have undergone previous mastectomy or indeed have scarring from any type of surgery. Even having to remove dentures to reduce the discomfort of oral symptoms can cause intense distress and embarrassment for some patients.

Specific visible effects of cancer treatment, such as alopecia, are recognised as having a significant effect on body image (Baxley et al 1984). It is estimated that over 46% of patients with cancer experience hair loss (Munstedt et al 1997), which not only diminishes a person's sense of attractiveness, but can be a stark reminder of the disease (Burt 1995, Webb 1985). Smith (1998, p. 78) suggests that it is 'symbolic of a future which is bleak and a visible manifestation of a progressive and unrelenting disease process within'.

Patients receiving radical brain irradiation are likely to experience patchy hair loss as well as skin reactions such as erythema and dry desquamation, any time from 10 to 14 days after commencing therapy (Guerrero 1998). Although patients receiving whole brain irradiation with palliative intent may not experience skin changes, they will suffer total alopecia, which can last for several months (Pinover & Coia 1998). Even patients receiving radiotherapy for some head and neck cancers can experience partial alopecia, in the form of square patches at the back of the head from radiotherapy exit sites, or loss of distinguishing features such as sideburns or moustaches. This can cause much distress, particularly if patients and their families have not been forewarned.

Studies have found that self-esteem is lower after treatment-induced alopecia than at the time of diagnosis of cancer (Carpenter & Brockopp 1994). The loss of body hair can be just as distressing as the loss of a full or partial head of hair. Men having radiotherapy to the tonsillar area, floor of mouth or larynx can mourn the loss of facial hair, and both men and women may find the loss of pubic hair following pelvic radiotherapy particularly difficult.

Chapter 11 highlights the fact that radiotherapy can contribute to significant problems with weight loss. The impact of cachexia on body image is often profound, but even a small degree of weight loss can alter the appearance of the face so that patients are self-conscious of the change. Skin changes such as increased pigmentation or erythema may also cause embarrassment and distress. Side effects such as these may not appear to healthcare professionals to be particularly severe, and thus little attention may be paid to their impact on body image.

Body image is not only threatened by the side effects of radiotherapy. Many cancer patients are on steroid therapy, which may lead to moonface, hirstuism and acne, all of which may negatively influence body image and sexuality (Fallowfield 1992). Others may have lymphoedema as a result of axillary or groin surgery, postoperative infections, intrapelvic, groin or axillary recurrence of cancer (Twycross 1997). Radiotherapy can cause as well as exacerbate lymphoedema, but healthcare professionals are not always quick to recognise or address this painful and visible condition, and specialist services are often lacking.

Not all changes in body image are clearly visible or immediately apparent. Evans (1997) suggests that any awareness of changes occurring within the body, such as disruption of the function and number of blood cells, can be just as upsetting as external, easily observed physical change. Patients receiving cranial radiotherapy may be disturbed by a degree of cognitive impairment or somnolence syndrome (Faithfull & Brada 1998, Guerrero 1998). These side effects are very distressing and can indicate to patients that treatment has not been effective or that cancer is recurring. All serve to remind patients that their body and self-image have been disrupted.

PAIN AND CONTROL

Price's categorization of risk factors (Fig. 17.2) also highlights the significance of pain and control in relation to body image. Recently I nursed a young woman with advanced cervical cancer who had excruciating pelvic pain. While receiving radiotherapy treatment and awaiting selectron therapy, she described how she felt 'no good to anyone, useless ... redundant as a wife, mother and lover', highlighting the fact that her self-image was inextricably linked with her perceived ability to function in her role and relationships.

The loss of privacy, dignity and control felt by patients who have to expose parts of their body for treatment each day must become familiar, but is no less distressing because of this. Loss of bodily control as a result of treatment-induced side effects can further affect body image (Price 1999). A recent study investigating patients' perceptions of physical symptoms after radiotherapy treatment for cervical cancer, found that the majority of patients had frequency of micturition and diarrhoea at the end of treatment and up to 3 months later (Klee et al 2000). Although these side effects may be hidden from view of others, they can significantly impact on quality of life, and may cause particular discomfort in social situations. Such symptoms may make it difficult for the individual to retain dignity and a positive self-concept (Evans 1997). Unpleasant smells from loss of bowel or bladder function or from discharging wounds can serve to isolate the individual further (Lawton 2000). Lawler (1991) explains that both cultural factors and personal notions ensure that we take for granted rules about how the body is to appear and be presented or controlled in our daily lives. The sense of being let down by our own body can persist in making the body something to distrust, fear and dislike (Bredin 2001).

Some patients and their families may feel that bodily changes and treatment-induced symptoms are a small price to pay if the treatment is to save their life, and patients may be reluctant to report these problems, as the following quotation illustrates:

> ... *it's only feeling sick, like a slight headache, so what, or you feel tired, so what, they're only minimal things ... the radiotherapy's dealing with the cancer, cancer's the big thing*

(Wells 1998, p. 845).

IMPACT OF BODY IMAGE CHANGES

Through the mass media we are constantly confronted with images of attractive healthy bodies (Price 1993, Salter 1997). These images can lead to people having unrealistic and unattainable expectations, making any perceived defect harder to bear (Burgess 1994). Physical attractiveness not only correlates with a positive self-concept (Lerner & Karabenick 1974), assertiveness and self-confidence (Dion & Stein 1978, Jackson & Huston 1975), but even good mental health (Adams 1981). As appearance, self-esteem and identity are so interrelated, patients coping with radical change in their body image can lose their sense of self (Bradbury 1996, Bredin 2001, Mathieson & Stam 1995, Wells 1998).

The journalist John Diamond movingly described the experience of his own changing body image following the diagnosis and treatment of his cancer, illustrating the point that the sense of self can be completely lost:

> *I had transcended the stage I hit during the first radiotherapy course where I became a person stuck at his proper weight; I had become a thin person. When I told people that I was not quite myself I meant it almost literally: in the mirror I was somebody else. Precisely I was a little old man whom I imagined to be called Albert or Norman or George*

(Diamond 1997, p. 191).

This perception of loss can lead to anxiety, depression and a grief response (Bradbury 1996, Cronan 1993, Dudas 1993, Evans 1997, Maguire & Murray-Parkes 1998). Patients can become socially withdrawn, seeking to manage their discomfort by limiting human contact or, at the very least, underplaying their distress (Price 1998, Wells 1998). Colyer's (1996) small study of three women's experience of cancer in a sexual organ revealed that there was a degree of *pretence* in the women's appearance of coping, mainly because it was felt that friends lacked understanding of the debility and pain involved in living with cancer.

ADAPTING TO CHANGES IN BODY IMAGE

Dewing (1989) suggests that those who experience alterations to their body through disease or treatment have four stages to negotiate, although these are not necessarily experienced in sequence:

- The initial *impact* of the diagnosis, resulting in shock, then anger, which may be directed at health professionals or the family, as well as depression and pessimism about their recovery.

- A period of *mourning* and yearning to return to the previous self. This may manifest through denial and severe withdrawal.
- *Acknowledgement* of the defect. This is a more adaptive response, with the person actively seeking information and trying out different coping strategies.
- The final stage is *reconstruction*. This is where the individual recognises the implications of the body image change, accepts the use of aids and dares to plan for the future.

This process of adaptation resembles grief theories put forward by other authors such as Kubler-Ross (1969), Marris (1974) and Worden (1991). Not everyone will reach the stage of reconstruction, and Price (1990) makes the pertinent point that we are unlikely to witness many of these reactions during a short hospital stay or course of radiotherapy. After radiotherapy, existing symptoms may persist or worsen and new symptoms may appear, which can indicate to patients that treatment has not been effective, causing further problems for adaptation (Eardley 1986, Faithfull & Brada 1998, Ward et al 1989).

The patient may in fact experience a 'flood' reaction to altered body image and self-concept several weeks after any initial change has occurred. Diamond (1997) clearly illustrated this point when describing his experience of being home from hospital.

I just couldn't bear the state I was in. And I couldn't. Somehow it seemed worse at home. In hospital being disabled seemed a reasonable state of affairs: at home it turned me into a disabled person, unable to eat or drink or speak properly

(Diamond 1997, p. 171).

The pattern of radiotherapy side effects and the reality of experiences like these have strong implications for discharge planning and continuity of care in particular, highlighting the importance of close liaison between hospital staff and the primary care team. Attending for treatment can be a time of intense activity, strict routine and close proximity with different health professionals. In contrast, the completion of treatment may be punctuated only by a single follow-up appointment one month later. It is, therefore, easy to understand how anxiety can resurface, making the end of treatment a time of uncertainty, loneliness and distress (Clinical Oncology Patients Liaison Group 1999).

THE POTENTIAL FOR RADIOTHERAPY TO IMPROVE BODY IMAGE

Previous discussion has centred on the ways in which radiotherapy can damage body image; however, it must be acknowledged that radiotherapy treatment can also improve body image problems related to local or metastatic disease. Potential benefits gained from palliative radiotherapy include pain relief, improvement in function and cosmesis, alleviation of obstruction and control of bleeding or haemorrhage (Pinover & Coia 1998). These are summarised in Table 17.1.

The example in Box 17.1 illustrates the value of palliative radiotherapy in controlling symptoms and alleviating body image problems.

Table 17.1   Potential positive effects of radiotherapy on body image

Symptom	Effect of radiotherapy
Bone metastases	Pain relief/improvement in mobility
Malignant cord compression	Improvement/prevention of further deterioration in function
Superior vena cava obstruction/facial tumours	Improvement in cosmesis and symptoms/reduction in oedema/tumour shrinkage
Oesophageal obstruction	Relief of obstruction, improvement in eating ability
Discharging/fungating wounds	Alleviation of discharge/tumour shrinkage
Haemoptysis/haematuria/rectal bleeding	Control of bleeding

Box 17.1   Example of how palliative care radiotherapy can improve body image

Bill, an active 72-year-old man, was devastated to discover that rectal cancer had recurred. He complained of tenesmus, a foul-smelling rectal discharge and severe pain on defecation. He was unable to leave the house to participate in his favourite sport of bowls and became withdrawn from family and friends.

After consultation with the radiation oncologist, Bill was prescribed a course of palliative radiotherapy. At the same time he was commenced on systemic antifungal antibiotics. After 24 h he noted that the smell became less offensive. The radiotherapy treatment improved the pain and alleviated the rectal discharge. Bill had previously not wished any input from the community nurses, however he subsequently agreed to the district nurse visiting him weekly at home to see how he responded to treatment. The reduction in his symptoms meant that he was once again able to bend over to play bowls, without fear of pain or embarrassment.

It also illustrates many of the factors in Price's (1999) model (Fig. 17.2), specifically how pain and loss of control lead to discomfort in social situations and self-imposed social isolation. Palliative radiotherapy, if given in few fractions, can cause minimal disruption to a patient's life, whilst having a major impact on *quality* of life by alleviating symptoms and improving physical, psychological and social functioning.

ASSESSMENT OF BODY IMAGE

The body image problems faced by individuals undergoing radiotherapy may be significant, and it is vital that healthcare professionals are sensitive to these issues and equipped to assess and manage actual and potential problems effectively. As Price's (1999) work illustrates, an altered body image is not an automatic sequela of the diagnosis of cancer and radical treatment, but is a complex interplay of the factors shown in Figures 17.1 and 17.2.

It has proven difficult to assess the incidence of body image problems because of the lack of a brief, systematic and rigorous measurement tool. Hopwood (1993) has, however, highlighted key areas that would need to be addressed in any assessment of body image in cancer patients. These include:

- Reluctance or avoidance to look at oneself naked
- Loss of femininity or masculinity
- Feeling less attractive or sexually attractive
- Adverse effects of treatment and loss of body integrity
- Feeling self-conscious about one's appearance
- Dissatisfaction with the scar or prosthesis.

These aspects concur with the general principles proposed by Price (1998), who also makes the point that healthcare professionals have a specific role to play in the assessment process. He suggests that staff need to observe how patients behave towards their body, listen to how patients refer to their body and explore how patients anticipate life beyond treatment, for instance, how others will react to their appearance or function.

Recently, Hopwood et al (2001) have developed a 10-item short scale to measure body image in cancer patients, which they suggest will be suitable for use in clinical trials. The items included on the scale are concerned with self-consciousness, physical attractiveness, dissatisfaction with appearance, femininity/masculinity, difficulty with nakedness, sexual attractiveness, avoidance of others, wholeness of the body, dissatisfaction with the body and appearance of scars (if relevant). The scale has been tested primarily with breast cancer patients, but could apply to other groups, and may help to assess the extent of body image problems in patients undergoing radiotherapy.

MANAGEMENT OF BODY IMAGE

The management of body image problems is dependent on an adequate assessment of the issues described above. It must be recognised that a single individual may be facing different challenges at different stages of treatment, and thus it is important that healthcare professionals consider how body image is affected prior to, during and after radiotherapy. There may be particularly stressful times for the patient, for instance, having a shell made, being tattooed or exposing a part of the body for the first time or to staff not met before. Patients' confidence and self-esteem may be especially challenged by exposure to the public gaze (Clinical Oncology Patients Liaison Group 1999). In addition, the sight of other patients who are frail and ill can be a distressing reminder of the impact of disease on the body.

Key strategies for the management of body image problems are summarised in Table 17.2. These strategies of assessment, tailored information and support must be based on an approach of courtesy, privacy and sensitivity. It is important that we regularly examine our own assumptions, challenging what we as healthcare professionals often take for granted about hospital practices. In a hectic department it is possible to lose sight of what the experience of radiotherapy is like for the individual. Routine occurrences such as taking medical photographs can seriously threaten a person's private body image. For instance, an elderly lady with a fungating chest wall recurrence of breast cancer recently described her absolute shock and embarrassment when asked for permission to be photographed prior to radiotherapy treatment.

Table 17.2 Strategies for minimising body image problems during radiotherapy treatment

	Pretreatment	During treatment	Post-treatment
Assessment	Preexisting health problems Risk factors (see Fig. 17.1) Prior surgery or chemoradiotherapy Expectations	Impact of treatment Any side effects/ concerns Mood/function/sleeping patterns Behaviours as described by Hopwood et al (2001)	Ask whether patient is resuming activities/ meeting friends, etc. Check symptoms are well managed
Tailored Information	Outline aims of treatment Expected side effects Written information What happens during planning/placement of permanent skin marks	Expected side effects Pacing of activity Importance of rest/diet/good oral hygiene/skin care Self-care strategies	Prepare for good days and bad days. Ensure clear information is given re fitting and wearing of prostheses
Support	Quiet confident attitude of staff Ask patients to identify their own social support network (practical and emotional support)	Weekly monitoring by same person if possible Allow expression of feeling Encourage self-care Provide practical support	Provide follow-up appointments and telephone contact. Liaise with primary care team. Refer on for future support. Warn that side effects may increase

Ensure courtesy, privacy and sensitivity throughout.

Staff working in radiotherapy have a duty to behave with sensitivity and tact and to maintain the dignity and privacy of patients. As a recent report on making radiotherapy services 'patient-friendly' points out, 'it is embarrassing, undignified and unnecessary to have to walk across a room partly naked' (Clinical Oncology Patients Clinical Liaison Group 1999, p. 14). Lay members of this group make several highly pertinent suggestions for improving practice from their unique vantage point of service users:

• Ensure that the patient is not left naked lying on the treatment couch
• Limit the time patients spend in gowns in public areas before and after treatment
• Where indicated, make use of a specially designed gown, e.g. for breast patients (Harris & Haas 1997)
• Ensure the minimum of staff are in treatment rooms
• Make sure patients are aware of the name and role of staff present.

If patients are treated by the same members of staff each day, feelings of vulnerability may be minimised.

INFORMATION AND SUPPORT

Communication skills are central to the sensitive management of body image 8 (Fallowfield 1992, Newell 1991, Slevin et al 1996). From the first appointment, all team members should be alert to potential problems, particularly if they notice either avoidance or excessive preoccupation with body changes or appearance. Professionals can help prepare the patient and family for losses to come, and reassure patients and families of the normality of a grief reaction. The perceived magnitude of the loss, the cumulative effect of several losses and the personal vulnerability of the patient may all affect the degree of anxiety, depression and sexual problems actually experienced. The evidence also suggests that a strong family support system enables patients to cope with the impact of disease and the physical and psychological stressors of cancer treatment (Feber 2000, Price 1998, 1999, Salter 1998). Health professionals should, therefore, assess available support at the first visit, helping the patient to identify and map social support networks (Price 1998). As carers are vital in providingcsupport, it is essential that they, too, feel well informed and supported.

Treatment radiographers or specialist cancer nurses can provide this support during weekly reviews and if possible by regular telephone contact after treatment is over (Wells 1998). Clear written information should be provided on the way in which the body is likely to change during or as a result of treatment. Early recognition of problems is essential. In addition to timely and regular liaison with multidisciplinary colleagues and the primary care team, staff should know how and when to refer for more specialised help. Local and national support agencies may offer invaluable advice, practical and emotional support to patients and their families. It is important that healthcare professionals are aware of these so that they can inform their patients (see Further Information section).

Health professionals must address the prevention and management of radiation-induced side effects which damage body appearance and function. All patients should be given skin care guidance as well as practical advice on the management of symptoms, so that self care and control can be maximised. Some may need help with camouflaging or minimising discrepancies in body shape or appearance, such as the selection and fitting of best available prostheses.

Addressing the psychosocial impact of body image change is as important as acknowledging symptoms, and recognising that disability and confinement contribute to distress (Worden 1989). Several authors comment on the efficacy of rehearsing coping strategies with patients so as to enable them to anticipate and deal with others' reactions, enquiries and even discomfort, and promote a sense of self-mastery (Feber 2000, Price 1998). Price (1999) also suggests that it is important to give space for grief. Chapter 3 highlights the significance of informational support during radiotherapy. There is a need for healthcare professionals to improve their skills in identifying patients who have particular needs for support. Interestingly, a recent Austrian study found that oncologists were unsuccessful in identifying patient distress, perceived social support and the need for psychosocial counselling during radiotherapy treatment (Sollner et al 2001). Oncologists correctly identified only 11 patients from a total of 30 who were severely distressed. The correct perception of distress was noted to be lower in patients with head and neck cancers, lung cancer and those from lower social classes. Given the risk factors already mentioned, it could be said that these patients are particularly vulnerable to body image problems.

It appears that healthcare professionals *can* make a difference to body image problems through awareness and sensitive management. One small study found that nursing interventions led to a clear reduction in symptoms in a population of ambulatory patients undergoing chemotherapy or radiotherapy. The greatest improvement was seen in psychosocial symptoms such as anxiety, sociability, body image and sexuality (Benor et al 1998).

CONCLUSION

The literature does not specifically associate body image changes with radiotherapy treatment, but it must be recognised that patients undergoing radiotherapy may experience altered body image in a number of different ways. There is no research to support the nature and extent of body image problems in this patient group, in particular how to assess body image and what strategies help patients cope with alterations imposed by cancer or its treatment. What is clear is that staff working in radiotherapy need to be aware of the potential for body image to be affected not only by cancer and the side effects of treatment, but also by the way in which care is organised and the approach of the staff. If radiotherapy care is to be truly supportive, body image issues must be acknowledged and given the attention they deserve.

SUMMARY OF KEY CLINICAL POINTS

- Body image is a complex, multifaceted problem.
- Radiotherapy treatment can have a positive or negative effect on body image.
- Factors affecting body image in cancer patients involve site of tumour, pain, visibility and prosthetics (Price 1999).
- Assessment of social support needs to be carried out at the first visit.
- Pre-treatment discussion can help reduce anxiety and promote the development of coping strategies, such as those used to combat fatigue, and to minimise skin reactions (Downing 1998).
- It is often at the end of radiotherapy that reactions are at their peak (Weintraub & Hagopian 1990, Wells 1998).
- Patients may experience disruption in body image soon after discharge. This can be sustained for many months, having a negative effect on quality of life and social functioning (Price 1998).
- Care cannot be prescriptive and individual patients need an individual approach (Price 1998).

FURTHER READING

Cohen M Z, Kahn D L, Steeves R H 1998 Beyond body image: the experience of breast cancer. Oncology Nursing Forum 25(5):835–841

Cook N F 1999 Self-concept and cancer: understanding the nursing role. British Journal of Nursing 8(5):318–324

D'haese S, Vinh-Hung V, Bijdekerke P et al 2000 The effect of timing of the provision of information on anxiety and satisfaction of cancer patients receiving radiotherapy. Journal of Cancer Education 15(4):223–237

Jenks J M, Morin K H, Tomaselli N 1997 The influence of ostomy surgery on body image in patients with cancer. Applied Nursing Research 10(4):174–180

Lawler J 1997 The body in nursing. Churchill Livingstone, South Melbourne, Australia

Luker K, Caress A L 1989 Rethinking patient education. Journal of Advanced Nursing 14:711–718

Meyer T J, Mark M M 1995 Effects of psychosocial interventions with adult cancer patients: a meta-analysis of randomised experiments. Health Psychology 14(2):101–108

Partridge J 1993 The psychological effects of facial disfigurement. Journal of Wound Care 2(3):168–171

Partridge J, Coutinho W, Robinson E et al 1994 Changing faces: two years on. Nursing Standard 8(3):54–58

Piff C 1998 Body image: a patient's perspective. British Journal of Theatre Nursing 8(1):13–14

Rushworth C 1994 Making a difference in cancer care. Souvenir Press, London

---

FURTHER INFORMATION

---

www.bacup.org
www.changingfaces.co.uk
www.dgc.org.uk
www.healthcentre.org.uk
www.nci.nih.gov

REFERENCES

Adams G R 1981 The effects of physical attractiveness on the socialisation process. In: Lucher G W, Ribbens K A, McNamara J A J R (eds) Psychological aspects of the facial form. Craniofacial growth series. University of Michigan, Ann Arbor

Albrecht G, Walker V, Levy J 1982 Distance from the stigmatised: a test of two theories. Science and Medicine 16:1319–1327

Baxley K O, Erdman L K, Henry E B et al 1984 Alopecia: effect on cancer patient's body image. Cancer Nursing 17(6):499–503

Bello L K, McIntyre S N 1995 Body image disturbances in young adults with cancer. Implications for the oncology clinical nurse specialist. Cancer Nursing 18(2):138–143

Benor D E, Delbar V, Krulik T 1998 Measuring impact of nursing intervention on cancer patients' ability to control symptoms. Cancer Nursing 21(5):320–334

Bloom J R, Kessler L 1994 Emotional support following cancer: a test of the stigma and social activity hypothesis. Journal of Health and Social Behaviour 35:118–133

Body J J, Lossignol D, Ronson A 1997 The concept of rehabilitation of cancer patients. Review Current Opinion in Oncology 9(4):332–340

Bradbury E 1996 Counselling people with disfigurement. British Psychological Society, Leicester

Bredin M. Altered self concept. In: Corner J, Bailey C (eds) 2001 Cancer nursing: care in context. Blackwell Scientific, Oxford

Breibart W, Holland J 1988 Psychosocial aspects of head and neck cancer. Seminars in Oncology 15(1):61–69

Burgess L 1994 Facing the reality of head and neck cancer. Nursing Standard 8(32):30–34

Burt K 1995 The effects of cancer on body image and sexuality. Nursing Times 91(7):36–37

Carpenter J S, Brockopp D Y 1994 Evaluation of self esteem of women with cancer receiving chemotherapy. Oncology Nurses Forum 21(4):451–457

Clinical Oncology Patients Liaison Group 1999 Making your radiotherapy service more patient-friendly. Royal College of Radiologists, London

Corner J 1997 Beyond survival rates and side effects: cancer nursing as therapy. Cancer Nursing 20(1):3–11

Colyer H 1996 Women's experience of living with cancer. Journal of Advanced Nursing 23(3):496–501

Cronan L 1993 Management of the patient with altered body image. British Journal of Nursing 2(5):257–261

Czechmeister C A 1994 Metaphor in illness and nursing: a two-edged sword. A discussion of the social use of metaphor in everyday language and implications for nursing and nurse education. Journal of Advanced Nursing 19(6):1226–1233

Dewing J 1989 Altered body image. Surgical Nurse 2(4):17–20

Diamond J 1997 Because cowards get cancer too. Vermilion, London

Dion K K, Stein S 1978 Physical attractiveness and interpersonal influence. Journal of Experimental Social Psychology 14:97–108

Downing J 1998 Radiotherapy nursing: understanding the nurses' role. Nursing Standard 12(25):42–43

Dropkin M J 1999 Body image and quality of life after head and neck cancer surgery. Cancer Practice 7(6):309–313

Dudas S 1993 Manifestations of cancer and its treatment: body image and sexuality. In: Groenwald S L, Hansen M, Goodman M et al (eds) Cancer nursing principles and practice, 3rd ed. Jones & Bartlett, Boston, MA, p 720–733

Eardley A 1986 Patients and radiotherapy 3. Patients' experiences after discharge 4. How patients can be helped. Radiography 52(601):17–22

Evans M 1997 Altered body image in teenagers with cancer. Journal of Cancer Nursing 1(4):177–182

Faithfull S, Brada M 1998 Somnolence syndrome in adults following cranial irradiation for primary brain tumours. Clinical Oncology (Royal College of Radiologists)10:250–254

Fallowfield L 1992 The quality of life, sexual functioning and body image following cancer therapy. Cancer Topics 9:20–21

Feber T 2000 Head and neck oncology nursing. Whurr, London

Frank-Stromberg M, Wright P 1984 Ambulatory cancer patients' perception of the physical and psychosocial changes in their lives since the diagnosis of cancer. Cancer Nursing 7:117–130

Goffman E 1963 Stigma: notes on the management of spoiled identity. Prentice Hall, New Jersey

Griffiths E 1989 More than skin deep. Nursing Times 85(4):34–36

Guerrero D 1998 Neuro-oncology for nurses. Whurr, London

Harris R, Haas A 1997 The use of a breast gown during radiotherapy by women with carcinoma of the breast. Radiography 3(4):287–291

Higginson I, Winget C 1996 Pyschological impact of cancer cachexia on the patient and family. In: Bruera E, Higginson I (eds) Cachexia and anorexia in cancer patients. Oxford University Press, Oxford, p 172–183

Hopwood P 1993 The assessment of body image in cancer patients. European Journal of Cancer 29A(2):276–281

Hopwood P, Fletcher I, Lee A et al 2001 A body image scale for use with cancer patients. European Journal of Cancer 37(2):189–197

Jackson D J, Huston T L 1975 Physical attractiveness and assertiveness. Journal of Social Psychology 96:79–84

Klee M, Thranov I, Machin D 2000 The patient's perspective on physical symptoms after radiotherapy for cervical cancer. Gynaecology Oncology 76(1):14–23

Kubler-Ross E 1969 On death and dying. Macmillan, New York

Lawler J 1991 Behind the screens: nursing, somology and the problem of the body. Churchill Livingstone, Melbourne

Lawton J 2000 The dying process: patients' experiences of palliative care. Routledge, London

Lerner R M, Karabenick S A 1974 Physical attractiveness. Body attitudes and self concept in late adolescents. Journal of Youth and Adolescence 3:307–316

Maguire P 1999 Late adverse psychological sequelae of breast cancer and its treatment. European Journal of Surgical Oncology 25(3):317–320

Maguire P, Murray-Parkes C 1998 Coping with loss: surgery and loss of body parts. British Medical Journal 316(7137):1086–1088

Marris P 1974 Loss and change. Routledge and Kegan Paul, London

Mathieson C M, Stam H J 1995 Renegotiating identity: cancer narratives. Sociology of Health and Illness 17(3):283–306

Munstedt K, Manthey N, Sachsse S et al 1997 Changes in self concept and body image during alopecia induced cancer chemotherapy. Supportive Cancer Care 5(2):139–143

Newell R 1991 Body-image disturbance: cognitive behavioural formation and intervention. Journal of Advanced Nursing 16:1400–1405

Newell B 2000 Body image and disfigurement care. Routledge, London

Pinover W H, Coia L R 1998 Palliative radiation therapy. In: Berger A M, Portenoy R K, Weissman D E (eds) Principles and practice of supportive oncology. Lippincott-Raven, Philadelphia

Price B 1990 A model for body image care. Journal of Advanced Nursing 15:585–593

Price B 1993 Dignity that must be respected. Body image and the surgical patient. Professional Nurse 8(10):670–672

Price B 1998 Explorations in body image care: Peplau and practice knowledge. Journal of Psychiatric and Mental Health Nursing 5(3):179–186

Price B 1999 Altered body image. Nursing Times Monographs no. 29. Emap Healthcare, London

Richter M P, Coia L R 1985 Palliative radiation therapy. Seminars in Oncology 12:375

Salter M (ed) 1997 Altered body image: the nurse's role, 2nd edn. Baillière Tindall, London

Sandler J, Rosenblatt B 1962 The concept of the representational world. Psychoanalytic Study of the Child 17:128–145

Schilder P 1935 Image and appearance of the human body. Kegan Paul, London

Short C, Griffiths S 1996 Radiotherapy: developments, contradictions and dilemmas. Radiography 2(3):177–189

Slevin M L, Nichols S E, Downer S M et al 1996 Emotional support for cancer patients: what do patients really want? British Journal of Cancer 74:1275–1279

Smith J 1998 Cultural issues associated with altered body image. In: Salter M (ed.) 1997 Altered body image:the nurse's role. Baillière Tindall, London, p 75–89

Sollner W, deVries A, Steixner E et al 2001 How successful are oncologists in identifying patient distress, perceived social support and need for psychosocial counselling? British Journal of Cancer 84(2):179–185

Sontag S 1991 Illness as metaphor, Aids and its metaphors. Penguin Books, London

Twycross R 1997 Introducing palliative care 2nd edn. Radcliffe Medical Press, Oxon

van der Molen B 1999 Relating information needs to the cancer experience: the perspectives of people with cancer. European Journal of Cancer 35 (suppl 4):18

Ward S, Viergutz G, Tomey D et al 1989 Patients' reactions to completion of adjuvant breast cancer therapy. Nursing Research 41(6):326–366

Webb C 1985 Sexuality, nursing and health. John Wiley, Chichester

Weintraub F N, Hagopian G A 1990 The effect of nursing consultation on anxiety, self care and side effects of patients receiving radiation therapy. Oncology Nursing Forum 17 (suppl 3):31–36

Wells M 1998 The hidden experience of radiotherapy to the head and neck: a qualitative study of patients after completion of treatment. Journal of Advanced Nursing 28(4):840–848

Woodcock J 1997 An oncological perspective. In: Salter M (ed.) 1997 Altered body image: the nurse's role. Baillière Tindall, London, p 133–148

Worden J W 1989 The experience of recurrent cancer. CA – Cancer Journal for Clinicians 39(5):305–310

Worden W J 1991 Grief counselling and grief therapy. A handbook for the mental health professional. Routledge, London

18

Late toxicity: bone problems

Vincent Khoo

INTRODUCTION

Late radiation damage can occur in any area of bone irradiated. Although this is a rare problem, it is of particular concern in some anatomical sites where the bone plays a vital function, such as the jaw bone (mandible) for chewing and in weight-bearing bones such as the femora. In these sites, bone complications will impact on the patient's quality of life by severely restricting eating and walking. In addition, bone complications can coexist with other late complications, for example, brachial plexopathy (Ch. 14). This chapter will review the general issues of late bone complications with particular attention to osteoradionecrosis of the mandible.

Whilst early detection of late radiation-induced bone damage and proper management of bone complications are important, the priority is to prevent or reduce their occurrence. Therefore, understanding of the predisposing factors and mechanisms underlying the development of this rare complication is essential.

Realistic treatment goals and the likely late side effects should be fully discussed with the patient in the planning stages of treatment. This will allow greater involvement in the decision-making and management process and will also reinforce the need, to the patient, for regular continued follow-up and proper assessment.

The radiation damage to underlying bony architecture is the same for bone in any anatomical site. However, the pathophysiological changes and clinical picture that develop are dependent on both the maturity and function of the bone. Disturbances in bone growth can result from irradiation of the immature skeleton and this can occur at doses lower than that required for damage to mature bone. This complication is pertinent for radiation delivered to children and adolescents. The magnitude of side effects depends on the age at irradiation, the dose delivered and the volume of bone treated. In general, growth abnormalities will become apparent within 6 months if radiotherapy is given to infants, and within 12 months in older children. Physical and functional disabilities depend on the type of bone. For example, craniofacial, mandibular and dental abnormalities can occur with radiotherapy to the head and neck region, joint dislocation can result from growth delays to irradiated joint fossa and scoliosis from vertebral irradiation (Pinkerton 1997).

For mature bones, osteitis, pathological fracture, osteoradionecrosis and radiation-induced second cancers are some of the possible late complications. The most serious and debilitating late complication of bone irradiation is osteoradionecrosis. This complication was recognised as early as 1926 (Phemister 1926). It can occur in any bone irradiated beyond its tolerance or with impaired repair processes. The development of osteoradionecrosis in the mandible is a well-known and debilitating clinical complication that is particularly challenging because of the complex functional arrangement between the facial bones and overlying soft tissues.

AETIOLOGY

Normal bone integrity is maintained by the interaction between the cellular components of the bone – osteocytes, osteoblasts and osteoclasts. Osteoblasts are bone cells that are involved in the synthesis and secretion of most of the organic matrix of the bone. Osteoblasts also regulate the mineralisation of bone. The organic matrix produced by the osteoblast surrounds it and is mineralised to form mature bone. The osteoblast trapped within the mineralised matrix then becomes an osteocyte. Osteoclasts are precursor cells related to macrophages and they are responsible for the removal of bone. Thus, growth and remodelling of bone are dynamic and result from an interaction between osteoblasts and osteoclasts.

High doses of radiation reduce the total number of the bone cells by causing death to bone cells. This results in enlarged empty bone spaces or lacunae, fatty degeneration and hypocellularity of the bone. Radiation can also affect bone microvasculature, causing a decrease in blood supply of the marrow and subsequent hypoxia. These physical insults on bone lead to devitalisation of the bone and diminish its capacity to replace normal collagen and cellular structure lost through routine wear, making it prone to any mechanical injury. Other risk factors such as osteopenia from advancing age and steroid use can also contribute to bone damage. Physical trauma can cause microfractures in bone. If normal bone repair processes are available, replacement and repair (or sequestration) of these bone fragments can occur and spontaneous healing of the bone is possible. If healing does not occur secondary to radiation damage then pathological fractures and osteoradionecrosis can develop.

A well-recognised site for the development of osteoradionecrosis is the jaw bone or mandible. Bone microfractures can occur as a result of the substantial mechanical stress from chewing. These microfractures usually heal spontaneously if normal tissue repair processes are available; however, irradiated bone tissue repairs are inadequate. Several microfractures may accumulate within a bony region and result in a pathological fracture.

The traditional sequence in the pathogenesis of osteoradionecrosis of the mandible was thought to be radiation, trauma and infection. However, Marx (1983b) challenged this process based on a review of 26 cases of osteoradionecrosis from which resection specimens were assessed for infection. Microorganisms were only cultured from the surface and all deep cultures were negative to infection. Marx (1983b) concluded that microorganisms played only a minor role in osteoradionecrosis and that trauma is only one mechanism of tissue breakdown leading to the condition. The sequence of osteoradionecrosis events is now considered to be:

1. Radiation
2. Hypoxic–hypocellular–hypovascular tissue
3. Tissue breakdown
4. Chronic non-healing wound.

CLINICAL MANIFESTATIONS

Often the diagnosis of osteoradionecrosis is made when patients present with a non-healing wound within a previously irradiated bone region (Costantino et al 1995). Symptoms may be slowly progressive over many months and often relate to the development of this ulcer. Pain is often one of the most prominent symptoms. The pain may be deep-seated and exacerbated by movement, may relate to the function of the surrounding muscles and nerves or be more superficial and relate to the subcutaneous tissues and/or the ulcer. For example, auditory difficulties or meningitis can be associated with osteoradionecrosis involving the temporal bone, whilst back pain and difficulty in mobility are often seen with osteoradionecrosis of the vertebrae or weight-bearing bones.

In the head and neck region, the mandible (95%) followed by the maxilla (5%) is the most common site for osteoradionecrosis. This usually occurs 1–2 years following radiotherapy (Curi & Dib 1997). Less commonly, temporal bones and the skull base can also be affected with radiotherapy for nasopharyngeal and anaplastic brain tumours. The bones of the extremities are rarely affected and usually problems here are associated with other precipitating factors. The majority of osteoradionecrotic lesions (89%) are triggered by trauma while 11% are spontaneous (Curi & Dib 1997). The reported incidence of mandibular osteoradionecrosis ranges from 0.4 to 8.6% with external beam irradiation (Dische et al 1997, Niewald et al 1996, Toljanic et al 1998, Turner et al 1996) and 2.1 to 40% with brachytherapy (Fujita et al 1996, Lozza et al 1997, Miura et al 1998). Early symptoms are toothache-like discomfort and pain, which may be present for some time before the development of any ulceration. Symptoms can also arise from the presence of pathological fractures, infection, abscess and fistulae formation. Other symptoms can occur as a result of irradiation on surrounding soft-tissue structures. For example, fibrosis of the temporomandibular joints or muscles of mastication will produce trismus or spasm when using the muscles to chew. Alterations in taste and saliva production can also occur from irradiation of the tongue and salivary glands (Ch. 19). Sensory changes can result from damage to the surrounding nerve complexes or pathways.

PREVENTION OF OSTEORADIONECROSIS

Osteoradionecrosis can be difficult to treat successfully, therefore prevention is important to minimise its occurrence. Bone regions remain at risk for many years following irradiation. Although spontaneous osteoradionecrosis can occur, predisposing causes include radiation, trauma, surgery, infection and prolonged steroid usage. Dental disease and dental surgery postirradiation are the major factors in the development of mandibular osteoradionecrosis (Morrish et al 1981). Radiotherapy risk factors include the total radiation dose, technique used, dose fraction size and tumour involvement of the bone (Dische et al 1997, Lozza et al 1997, Miura et al 1998, Niewald et al 1996, Withers et al 1995). The guiding principles for prevention of bone complications are outlined as follows:

- Awareness that osteoradionecrosis is a potential problem
- Full open communication and discussion with the patient and all members of the health team
- Written information for patients and general practitioners detailing the possible complications, early warning symptoms and signs, precautions and avoidance of precipitating factors
- Close review of predisposing tumour and patient factors for the bony site of irradiation and methods to minimise them. For example, in mandibular irradiation, a specialist dental review with appropriate dental planning prior to radiation
- Evaluation of radiotherapy fractionation, dose and treatment parameters.

Dental planning

Special attention to dental planning is crucial, especially when high-dose irradiation of the mandible is expected. The factors to consider include:

1. Anticipated dose to the bone
2. Pre-treatment dental status
3. Patient's dental hygiene and compliance with treatment
4. Retention of functional teeth exposed to irradiation.

Teeth extractions should be considered if the teeth are expected to be problematic following irradiation, such as with advanced peridontal disease, extensive caries or if there is expected chronic soft-tissue irritation such as from dentures. A period of at least 10–14 days should be allowed for adequate healing before commencing irradiation. Antibiotics should be used prior to extraction and in the healing period to minimise infection. If dental work or extractions are needed post-treatment, prophylactic hyperbaric oxygen has been reported to be successful in preventing the subsequent development of osteoradionecrosis in these susceptible bones (Vudiniabola et al 1999). Prophylactic fluoride applications can also reduce the incidence of dental caries. Regular 6-monthly dental checks are essential following irradiation.

Radiation parameters

The type of radiation technique can influence the risk of osteoradionecrosis. Brachytherapy or implantation of radioactive sources has been associated with a higher risk of osteoradionecrosis because of the dangers of implanting the radioactive sources too closely to the bone. Computed tomography (CT) planning techniques, which permit three-dimensional visualisation of the anatomy, and the use of spacers to increase the distance between radioactive sources and bone can reduce this. A retrospective study using low-dose-rate brachytherapy reported that the incidence of osteoradionecrosis was reduced from 40% (22/55 cases) *without* spacers to 2.1% *with* spacers, because the use of spacers allowed the dose near the bone surface to be reduced by 50% (Miura et al 1998).

Brachytherapy risk factors include higher dose rates, larger treatment volumes and the addition of external beam radiotherapy. One study of 100 consecutive patients with implants within the oral cavity revealed that 80% of bone necrosis cases occurred when the dose rate was > 50 cGy/h and the treatment volume was > 25 000 mm^3 (Lozza et al 1997). Another reported that total dose of > 90 Gy and an interstitial dose rate threshold of > 55 cGy/h were significant risk factors for bone necrosis (Fujita et al 1996). The addition of external irradiation also increases the risk, especially if the external beam and interstitial dose exceeds 30 and 60 Gy respectively (Fujita et al 1996).

The dose–complication curve for mandibular osteoradionecrosis using external beam irradiation is not clear. In the past many dose fractionation schemes have been used. Using conventional dose fractions of 2 Gy/day, the incidence of mandibular osteoradionecrosis has been reported to be as low as 2% with doses of up to 66 Gy (Dische et al 1997), rising to around 8–9% at 70 Gy (Niewald et al 1996). When the daily fraction size is increased to > 2 Gy, the incidence rises to around 6% with doses of 50–55 Gy (Turner et al 1996). Both total dose and fraction size appear to be important for the development of osteoradionecrosis of the mandible (Withers et al 1995). Poor fractionation techniques have resulted in a high and unacceptable incidence of osteoradionecrosis. Niewald et al (1996) utilised hyperfractionation with two daily fractions of 1.2 Gy separated by 4 h to a total dose of 82.8 Gy and reported a very high incidence of osteoradionecrosis at 23%. These data revealed that an interfraction interval of < 6 h is a significant risk factor for osteoradionecrosis and the authors subsequently discontinued this regime. Hyperfractionation can be given safely if adequate interfraction time and suitable total doses are used. Dische et al (1997) reported that hyperfractionation, when used appropriately, is associated with osteoradionecrosis in less than 1% of cases. The interrelationship total dose and fraction size still needs clarifying and this can be achieved by collection of radiotherapy data and late clinical effects.

All these parameters need to be carefully evaluated to ensure that tolerance limits are not exceeded, otherwise the risk of mandibular osteonecrosis rises substantially. Measures include restricting the total dose to < 70 Gy, using dose fraction sizes of < 2 Gy, careful correlation of doses and techniques, especially if combining interstitial brachytherapy with external beam radiotherapy, and thorough preirradiation dental assessment. In addition, organs at risk, such as major salivary glands that do not require treatment, should be spared as much as possible to minimise xerostomia which can exacerbate dental problems and increase the risk of bone complications.

GENERAL PRINCIPLES OF MANAGEMENT

The general principles of management for bone complications are similar to the model used for the management of late neurological complications described in

Table 18.1   Principles of management

Prevention	Awareness and recognition of potential problems by both clinician and patient, prior to radiotherapy
Assessment	Early reporting of symptoms Prompt and appropriate assessment by the oncology team Thorough physical examination, imaging investigations, microculture and biopsy of suspicious lesions Exclusion of recurrent cancer
Intervention	Hyperbaric oxygen and/or surgery
Rehabilitation	Multidisciplinary team approach, focusing on functional and symptom support

Chapter 14. The diagnosis of osteoradionecrosis needs to be early, when patients' symptoms are minimal, and intervention should be provided as part of a multidisciplinary team (Table 18.1). Regular follow-up and early reporting of symptoms to the clinician should be encouraged.

In general, treatment consists of assessment; minimisation of any aggravating factors such as infection; debridement of necrotic bone if necessary; systematic management of pain, psychological support, nutritional support, oral hygiene and aids to assist with functions of daily living. Intervention is therefore focused on managing any distress and complications. If further progression or difficulties occur for the patient, then more active management is needed. The specific case of osteoradionecrosis of the mandible will be discussed later.

Assessment

Appropriate investigations are needed to determine the aetiology of the osteonecrotic lesion, the predisposing factors for the individual and to assess the severity of the complication. As with many late complications, tumour recurrence or new disease can easily mimic the symptoms and signs of osteoradionecrosis and this needs to be excluded. This is particularly important if the necrotic bone lesion is situated in the vicinity of the original tumour site. Histological assessment of any recurrent disease may be necessary. Infection may also be present and can impede healing. The site of ulceration should always be cultured for microorganisms and, where appropriate, antibiotics should be used.

Imaging is useful to evaluate the extent of the complication and may provide an indication of the probable aetiology. It also provides a useful baseline for comparison and follow-up. CT can define better than plain radiology the presence of microfractures and alterations in bone architecture (Store & Larheim 1999). CT of the affected regions may reveal abnormal soft-tissue or nodal masses near the fracture or resorption site and this is more likely to represent recurrent tumour.

Magnetic resonance imaging (MRI) may provide further definition of the abnormal changes in late bone damage. The intensity patterns from MRI may be enhanced with contrast agents such as gadolinium (Bachmann et al 1996). Bone scanning may also be useful if acute osteomyelitis is present. Typical signs, such as hyperperfusion, high blood pool activity and increased bone metabolism, are seen in acute infection and inflammation. Immunoscintigraphy using technetium-labelled antigranulocyte Fab fragment has shown some promise in diagnosing infective processes compared to standard bone scanning (Kampen et al 1999). This may a useful non-invasive method of distinguishing the presence of subacute chronic inflammation from malignant or postoperative changes.

Multidisciplinary team

The need for specialist multidisciplinary care mirrors that of late neurological damage. Management requires specialist nursing and medical care, pain control, dental and nutritional care, assessment by an oral facial maxillary surgeon, occupational therapy and physiotherapy. Further team members may include the general practitioner and community nurses in supporting the patient at home.

Management of osteoradionecrosis of the mandible

The management of any radiation complication involves addressing the holistic needs of the patient through the provision of information and support. Goals of treatment are to obtain pain control, establish a diagnosis and provide a coordinated plan of management and follow-up. Once recurrent tumour has been excluded, imaging studies are needed to establish the baseline condition. Radiographic studies of the mandible can confirm the presence of pathological fractures or identify sequestrum formation. If X-ray films are used, panoramic radiography (panorex) is a cost-effective radiographic technique to evaluate osteoradionecrosis of the mandible (Costantino et al 1995). Compared to panorex radiographic imaging, CT has been reported to provide better visualisation of the anterior–posterior extent of osteoradionecrosis, cortical destruction, central necrosis and sequestration (Store & Larheim 1999).

With conservative measures, the majority of osteoradionecrosis lesions (42–48%) will resolve, 14–33% will stabilise and approximately 25–36% will progress (Curi & Dib 1997, Wong et al 1997). Prevention of recurrent trauma and infection is an important consideration and can allow healing in up to 70% of cases (Morrish et al 1981, Wong et al 1997). It is important to avoid postirradiation dental extraction and mucosal irritants such as ill-fitting dentures, alcohol and smoking. Oral antibiotics should be used if infection is present. Appropriate wound and abscess management may include gentle debridement, saline irrigation and antiseptic/antibiotic packing of any abscess.

Specific therapies such as hyperbaric oxygen are available to promote healing of osteoradionecrotic lesions. Hyperbaric oxygen at two to three times the atmospheric pressure at sea level causes transient high increases in tissue oxygen tension. In turn, this stimulates fibroblast proliferation, collagen synthesis and vascular capillary formation. This can reduce further damage and promote healing of the late radiation damage. Hyperbaric oxygen has been used in the management of osteoradionecrosis with good results. Resolution of symptoms was reported in 53–100% and new bone growth in osteoradionecrotic lesions was noted in up to 50% of cases treated with hyperbaric oxygen (Aitasalo et al 1995, Feldmeier et al 1995, London et al 1998, van-Merkesteyn et al 1995). There have been successful case reports of symptom resolution for osteoradionecrosis using hyperbaric oxygen in the sacrum (Ashamalla et al 1996, Videtic & Venkatesan 1999), mastoid (Ashamalla et al 1996), temporal bone (Ashamalla et al 1996) and chest wall (Feldmeier et al 1995). However, hyperbaric oxygen alone is often inadequate to resolve extensive osteoradionecrotic lesions and it may need to be combined with appropriate surgery to ensure successful outcomes.

If there is progression of the lesion or symptoms despite conservative treatment, then surgery is required. The aim of surgery is to resect necrotic and scar tissue, remove the focus for continued infection and allow replacement with normal vascularised tissue using bone grafts. An important consideration with surgery is cosmetic result and function. Continuity of the mandible should be maintained if possible. Small segmental or lateral defects of the mandible may be left unreconstructed without any significant functional or cosmetic consequences.

In general, extensive osteoradionecrosis with multiple fistulas and large exposed areas of necrotic bone with or without coexistent fracture should be treated with radical and aggressive surgery with or without the use of hyperbaric oxygen. In these situations, primary sequestrectomy/mandibular resection and reconstruction using microvascular free flaps is currently the method of choice (Cordeiro et al 1999). Osseous free flaps from the fibula have been preferred for primary reconstruction of segmental mandibular defects (Anthony et al 1997, Cordeiro et al 1999). These have been used with a high success rate and good-to-excellent functional and aesthetic results (Cronje 1998). The combination of treatment approaches, surgery and hyperbaric oxygen has been used with mandibular osteonecrosis, improving resolution rates (Cronje 1998, Marx 1983a).

SECONDARY MALIGNANCIES

Another important but rare complication of irradiation on the mature skeleton is the development of a radiation-induced malignancy. The most common type of radiation-induced malignancy is soft-tissue sarcoma. This incidence is less than 1% (Brady 1979, Lee et al 1992); however, patients need to be informed of this risk when considering radiotherapy. Criteria for the development of radiation-induced sarcoma in bone were initially categorised by Cahan et al (1948) and later refined by Brady (1979) (Table 18.2). Treatment of these second malignancies should be considered individually.

Table 18.2 Criteria for defining postirradiation sarcomas

Cahan et al 1948	Brady 1979
Histological or radiological evidence of non-malignant nature of initial bone problem	No histological or radiological evidence of abnormality in bone at the time of radiotherapy
Lesion must arise in irradiated area	Significant radiation dose delivered
Five-year latency period required	Relatively long symptom-free latent period (median of 11 years)
Histological proof of sarcoma	Microscopic evidence of sarcoma
	No exposure to other known carcinogens

SUMMARY OF KEY CLINICAL POINTS

- Osteoradionecrosis is a serious, debilitating late complication of irradiation of bone that can be difficult to treat.
- Prevention should be the primary goal, followed by minimisation of the probability of late damage.
- Avoidance of predisposing factors and careful consideration of radiotherapy dose/fractionation schemes and techniques are essential.
- Thorough assessment and investigation are needed to exclude recurrent tumour as a cause. A persistent lesion despite comprehensive therapy should raise the suspicion of tumour recurrence.
- Patients should be managed by a multidisciplinary team that will address the specialist needs of the patient.
- Hyperbaric oxygen is usually successful in resolving symptoms in 53–100% of cases.
- Surgical intervention is necessary in cases that do not respond or progress with bone loss or functional deformity. The principles of surgery include removal of necrotic tissue, maintenance of function and cosmesis, with restoration of any deficits with non-irradiated vascularised flap where appropriate.
- Symptom management, such as pain control, and specialist support, including nutritional and dental care, are required.

CONCLUSION

More careful and complete compilation of radiation data is crucial in developing better strategies to prevent or minimise this complication. This will enable the development of radiobiological modelling algorithms that may permit more reliable predictions of late tissue complications and will subsequently allow the adjustment and refinement of current radiation schemes that include bone as part of their target volume.

Much work is still needed to define the optimum use of hyperbaric oxygen, its integration with surgery and the timing of surgery. New techniques to enhance bone growth have been explored recently. Promising animal studies have shown that transplanted human recombinant bone morphogenic proteins are capable of allowing new bone formation in irradiated bone defects (Wurzler et al 1998). This concept of bone regeneration by bone morphogenic proteins has immense potential for transforming impaired bone repair processes that result from irradiation and methods of reconstructive surgery in irradiated bone. However, the onus remains on prevention if possible and minimisation of its occurrence if not.

REFERENCES

Aitasalo K, Grenman R, Virolainen E et al 1995 A modified protocol to treat early osteoradionecrosis of the mandible. Undersea Hyperbaric Medicine 22:161–170
Anthony J P, Foster R D, Pogrel M A 1997 The free fibula bone graft for salvaging failed mandibular reconstructions. Journal of Oral Maxillofacial Surgery 55:1417–1421
Ashamalla H L, Thom S R, Goldwein J W 1996 Hyperbaric oxygen therapy for the treatment of radiation-induced sequelae in children. The University of Pennsylvania experience. Cancer 77:2407–2412

Bachmann G, Rossler R, Klett R et al 1996 The role of magnetic resonance imaging and scintigraphy in the diagnosis of pathologic changes of the mandible after radiation therapy. International Journal of Oral Maxillofacial Surgery 25:189–195

Brady L W 1979 Radiation-induced sarcomas of bone. Skeletal Radiology 4:72–78

Cahan W G, Woodward H Q, Higinbotham N L et al 1948 Sarcoma arising in irradiated bone: report of eleven cases. Cancer 1:3–29

Cordeiro P G, Disa J J, Hidalgo D A et al 1999 Reconstruction of the mandible with osseous free flaps: a 10-year experience with 150 consecutive patients. Plastic Reconstructive Surgery 104:1314–1320

Costantino P D, Friedman C D, Steinberg M J 1995 Irradiated bone and its management. Otolaryngology Clinics of North America 28:1021–1038

Cronje F J 1998 A review of the Marx protocols: prevention and management of osteoradionecrosis by combining surgery and hyperbaric oxygen therapy. South Africa Dental Journal 53:469–471

Curi M M, Dib L L 1997 Osteoradionecrosis of the jaws: a retrospective study of the background factors and treatment in 104 cases. Journal of Oral Maxillofacial Surgery 55:540–544

Dische S, Saunders M, Barrett A et al 1997 A randomised multicentre trial of CHART versus conventional radiotherapy in head and neck cancer. Radiotherapy and Oncology 44:123–136

Feldmeier J J, Heimbach R D, Davolt D A et al 1995 Hyperbaric oxygen as an adjunctive treatment for delayed radiation injury of the chest wall: a retrospective review of twenty-three cases. Undersea Hyperbaric Medicine 22:383–393

Fujita M, Hirokawa Y, Kashiwado K et al 1996 An analysis of mandibular bone complications in radiotherapy for T1 and T2 carcinoma of the oral tongue. International Journal of Radiation Oncology, Biology, Physics 34:333–339

Kampen W U, Brenner W, Terheyden H et al 1999 Decisive diagnosis of infected mandibular osteoradionecrosis with a Tc-99m-labelled anti-granulocyte Fab'-fragment. Nuklearmedizin 38:309–311

Lee A W M, Law S C K, Ng S H et al 1992 Retrospective analysis of nasopharyngeal carcinoma treated during 1976–1985: late complications following megavoltage irradiation. British Journal of Radiology 65:918–928

London S D, Park S S, Gampper T J et al 1998 Hyperbaric oxygen for the management of radionecrosis of bone and cartilage. Laryngoscope 108:1291–1296

Lozza L, Cerrotta A, Gardani G et al 1997 Analysis of risk factors for mandibular bone radionecrosis after exclusive low dose-rate brachytherapy for oral cancer. Radiotherapy and Oncology 44:143–147

Marx R E 1983a A new concept in the treatment of osteoradionecrosis. Journal of Oral Maxillofacial Surgery 41:351–357

Marx R E 1983b Osteoradionecrosis: a new concept of its pathophysiology. Journal of Oral Maxillofacial Surgery 41:283–288

Miura M, Takeda M, Sasaki T et al 1998 Factors affecting mandibular complications in low dose rate brachytherapy for oral tongue carcinoma with special reference to spacer. International Journal of Radiation Oncology, Biology, Physics 41:763–770

Morrish R B, Chan E, Silverman S et al 1981 Osteonecrosis in patients irradiated for head and neck carcinoma. Cancer 47:1980–1983

Niewald M, Barbie O, Schnabel K et al 1996 Risk factors and dose–effect relationship for osteoradionecrosis after hyperfractionated and conventionally fractionated radiotherapy for oral cancer. British Journal of Radiology 69:847–851

Phemister D 1926 Radium necrosis of bone. American Journal of Radiology 16:340

Pinkerton C R 1997 Paediatric oncology: clinical practice and controversies, 2nd ed. Chapman & Hall, London

Store G, Larheim T A 1999 Mandibular osteoradionecrosis: a comparison of computed tomography with panoramic radiography. Dentomaxillofacial Radiology 28:295–300

Toljanic J A, Ali M, Haraf D J et al 1998 Osteoradionecrosis of the jaws as a risk factor in radiotherapy: a report of an eight-year retrospective review. Oncology Reports 5:345–349

Turner S L, Slevin N J, Gupta N K et al 1996 Radical external beam radiotherapy for 333 squamous carcinomas of the oral cavity – evaluation of late morbidity and a watch policy for the clinically negative neck. Radiotherapy and Oncology 41:21–29 van-Merkesteyn J P, Bakker D J, Borgmeijer-Hoelen A M 1995 Hyperbaric oxygen treatment of osteoradionecrosis of the mandible. Experience in 29 patients. Oral Surgery Oral Medicine Oral Pathology Oral Radiology Endodontics 80:12–16

Videtic G M, Venkatesan V M 1999 Hyperbaric oxygen corrects sacral plexopathy due to osteoradionecrosis appearing 15 years after pelvic irradiation. Clinical Oncology 11:198–199

Vudiniabola S, Pirone C, Williamson J et al 1999 Hyperbaric oxygen in the prevention of osteoradionecrosis of the jaws. Australasian Dental Journal 44:243–247

Withers H R, Peters L J, Taylor J M et al 1995 Late normal tissue sequelae from radiation therapy for carcinoma of the tonsil: patterns of fractionation study of radiobiology. International Journal of Radiation Oncology, Biology, Physics 33:563–568

Wong J K, Wood R E, McLean M 1997 Conservative management of osteoradionecrosis. Oral Surgery Oral Medicine Oral Pathology Oral Radiology Endodontics 84:16–21

Wurzler K K, DeWeese T L, Sebald W et al 1998 Radiation-induced impairment of bone healing can be overcome by recombinant human bone morphogenetic protein-2. Journal of Craniofacial Surgery 9:131–137

19

Other late effects

Vincent Khoo

INTRODUCTION

Radiation is a localised therapy affecting tissues mainly within the confines of the radiation field. It is crucial to be aware of all possible normal organs that lie inside as well as near the region of any radiotherapy field, as they are all at some risk. This probability increases with high doses or if the organ tolerance to radiation is exceeded. Advances in radiotherapy such as three-dimensional planning have reduced late toxicity by evaluation of the spatial relationship between the treatment volume and organs at risk.

Organs outside the radiation field can also sometimes be affected by treatment: one example is severe and late damage to blood vessels within the radiation field. If these blood vessels are an important supplier to organs outside the radiation field, then the function of these organs may be compromised. Another example is when the tolerance threshold of the organ is very low, such as with reproductive organs. In this situation, even if the testis is located at some distance from the radiation field, scattered low doses of radiation to the testis in the order of 1 Gy can severely impair spermatogenesis.

The principles of managing late radiation-related morbidity remain the same for most sites. It is important for the clinician to recognise the risk factors involved in the development of radiation complications. Prevention and minimisation of the risk factors for late radiation damage must be foremost in the clinical decision-making process. The issues of controlling or curing patients of their cancer must always be balanced against the likelihood of late complications arising from treatment and patients should be informed of these risks. In some cases, late radiation damage may be unavoidable if cure is to be achieved and this needs to be discussed with the patient when seeking informed consent. It is therefore important to evaluate possible risk factors:

- Evaluation of the cancer type, its extent and its influence on the function of nearby organs (for example, is the cancer close to important adjacent organs or does it surround/invade normal organs or lymph nodes? If this is the case, then the use of radiation may include a significant portion of normal organs, in which case, the chance of delivering a high dose for cure is limited by the high probability of causing late damage)
- The baseline function of the organs at risk for example lung, heart, liver and kidney function. This provides an important reference point on which to measure and assess the rate of deterioration if another non-malignant disease process is already present or future late damage is relevant
- The tolerance of the normal tissues or organs at risk of late radiation damage
- The radiation dose, fractionation scheme and technique used
- The contributory effect of other risk factors, such as chemotherapy
- The patient's general condition and other illnesses that may contribute to risk.

Furthermore, the tolerance of different soft tissues and organs varies widely. Therefore the incidence and magnitude of any radiation-induced complications will depend on the type of tissue treated, volume of tissue irradiated, dose/fractionation scheme used, as well as the baseline function of the organ at risk. Patient and treatment parameters have already been discussed in previous chapters but the concept of tissue or organ tolerance is worthy of further discussion. In radiation therapy, tolerance ranges are used to allow a more objective method of assessing the likelihood of late radiation damage using a particular radiation regime. There are three important factors implicit in assessment of tolerance ranges for radiation damage:

- The radiosensitivity of the organ. (For example, reproductive organs can be sterilised at doses of around 1–5 Gy compared to late damage to bones with doses of 60 Gy)
- The arrangement of the organ into functional subunits, i.e. parallel or series. (The spinal cord is considered a classic example of a series organ. If only one segment of spinal cord is destroyed, this also damages the rest of the spinal cord below the lesion. The liver and kidney can be considered parallel organs because they consist of complete subunits, each capable of functioning individually. Therefore, there is no critical chain or series effect. Up to two-thirds of the organ/tissue can be damaged and the remaining one-third still provides normal function)
- The volume of organ irradiated. This is also dependent on the functional subunit arrangement of the organ, as described above.

These tolerance ranges have been summarised by Emami et al (1991) in Table 19.1 and relate to the likelihood of late damage to the volume of organ treated and the total dose delivered. These tolerance ranges are based on the small amount of known published data and thus, this table remains a 'guesstimation'. The prediction of

Table 19.1 Normal tissue/organ volume and tolerance to therapeutic irradiation

Organ volume	$TD_{5/5}$			$TD_{50/5}$			
	1/3	2/3	3/3	1/3	2/3	3/3	
Brain	60	50	45	75	65	60	Necrosis; infarction
Brainstem	60	53	50			65	Necrosis; infarction
Spinal cord	50	50	47	70	70		Myelitis; necrosis
Eye (lens)			10			18	Cataract requiring treatment
Eye (retina)			45			65	Blindness
Optic nerve			50			65	Blindness
Optic chiasma			50			65	Blindness
Parotid gland		32	32		46	46	Xerostomia
Lung	45	30	17.5	65	40	24.5	Pneumonitis
Heart	60	45	40	70	55	50	Pericarditis
Oesophagus	60	58	55	72	70	68	Stricture; ulceration; perforation
Stomach	60	55	50	70	67	65	Ulceration; perforation
Small intestine	50		40	60		55	Obstruction; ulceration; perforation ;fistula
Large intestine	55		45	65		55	Obstruction; ulceration; perforation; fistula
Rectum			60			80	Severe proctitis; necrosis; fistula
Kidney	50	30	23		40	28	Clinical nephritis
Liver	50	35	30	55	45	40	Liver failure

$TD_{5/5}$, the tolerance dose for the probability of a 5% complication rate within 5 years; $TD_{50/5}$, the tolerance dose for the probability of a 50% complication rate within 5 years. The TD rates are approximate for the volume of organ treated. Note that the tolerance ranges are described for a dose/fractionation scheme using daily fraction sizes of 2 Gy given five times a week. It also assumes uniform irradiation of all or part of an organ, normal base-line organ function, no influence from chemotherapy or surgery and has been derived from data related to adults. Note also that both $TD_{5/5}$ and $TD_{50/5}$ are defined for severe endpoints or those complications that are classified as $\geq$ Radiation Therapy Oncology Group Grade 3. Modified from Emami et al (1991).

late complications is classified as the likelihood of either 5% ($TD_{5/5}$) or 50% ($TD_{50/5}$) chance of complications at 5 years. The probability of developing complications will also depend on the length of survival following radiotherapy treatment. Patients cured of their original cancer or with long disease-free intervals have the greatest chance of experiencing late complications of radiotherapy and this continues to be a lifelong risk.

Comprehensive collection of late treatment-related morbidity data is an important means of validating tolerance ranges. This provides evidence-based thresholds, which in turn allow for refinement and better design of radiotherapy schedules. It is essential that a standard grading system is utilised so that results from different centres and in different time periods can be reliably correlated (see Ch. 6, Appendix 1). In this chapter, other late radiation-induced complications that have not been previously discussed will be briefly reviewed.

VASCULAR COMPLICATIONS

Vascular structures within organs are often irradiated and contribute substantially to the late complications of the irradiated organs. Vascular damage from irradiation can cause secondary effects to organs outside the radiation field, especially if the damaged blood vessels are important suppliers of blood to the organ. Radiation damage can occur at the level of capillaries, venules, arterioles or larger blood vessels. The end result is altered blood flow to the organ, resulting in hypoxia of the tissues and reduced capacity of the tissues to repair damage.

The aetiology of capillary damage is a result of changes to the endothelial cell. This can result in cellular swelling, with obstruction of capillary blood flow, leading to alteration in vascular permeability, obliterative vasculitis, thrombosis and death of the endothelial cells. Subsequent repair processes along the course of the blood vessel are often non-uniform and this results in an irregular 'sausage segment' effect (Hopewell 1986). For venules and arterioles, degenerative change, hyperplasia and fibrosis can occur within the vessel wall. Atherosclerosis can accumulate in the altered blood vessel lumen, causing thrombosis and blood flow obstruction. In larger blood vessels, late damage to the media and adventitia can produce thickening or replacement of the wall by fibrous tissue. Degeneration of the wall results in hyalinisation of the blood vessels with intimal thickening, collagen deposition, fibrinoid necrosis, ulceration and plaque formation (Fajardo & Berthrong 1988). Subsequent effects are occlusive thrombosis or rupture of the blood vessel with ischaemia of the supplied tissue or organ.

The result of these changes is dependent on the tissue or organ supplied by the damaged blood vessel or vascular system. For example, telangiectasia of blood vessels can be visible on skin, bladder or rectal mucosa, leading to easy bleeding. More seriously, obliterative vasculitis can occur within the renal tissues, causing renal impairment, or within the liver, leading to venoocclusive thrombosis. Ischaemic necrosis can also occur in cerebral tissues, myocardium or bowel, leading to functional neurological or cardiac damage, bowel ulceration and infarction. The impact of these complications can be very traumatic and severely influence patients' quality of life.

Interventions to improve vascular supply relate to enhancing soft-tissue healing (Dion et al 1990). Oxpentifylline, a peripheral vasodilator, has been used to alter defective microcirculation. This drug may allow healing of radiation damage related to poor vascular supply and symptom relief of radiation fibrosis (Werner-Wasik & Madoc-Jones 1993). Radiation-induced vascular changes also contribute to other complications and affect other structures.

EYE AND PERIORBITAL COMPLICATIONS

Eye injuries from irradiation depend on which structures of the eye are treated. Damage can occur to the lacrimal ducts, eyelids, lens, retina and optic nerves. These different structures vary in radiosensitivity and tolerance thresholds and cause distinct clinical syndromes (Table 19.2).

Table 19.2 Late radiation effects on the eye

Late effects	Factors	Symptoms/signs	Management
Lacrimal glands	RT > 35 Gy	Dry-eye syndrome (dry, red, irritated itchy eye)	Ophthalmic and orbital (eyelid) examination Eye education (avoid rubbing, trauma) Artificial tears
	RT > 55 Gy	Severe dry-eye syndrome Photophobia Lacrimal duct fibrosis (blepharitis, infection, bleeding) Eyelid telangiectasia, bleeding, ulceration	Ophthalmic and orbital (eyelid) examination Eye education (avoid rubbing, trauma, chemicals) Artificial tears Topical antibiotics (for infection) Duct dilatation for duct fibrosis Topical steroids Pain control medications Enucleation (rare)
Lens	RT ($TD_{5/5}$) > 10 Gy	Cataract (progressive visual impairment to blindness) Opaque lens	Ophthalmic examination Lens replacement
Retinopathy	RT ($TD_{5/5}$) > 45 Gy	Painless visual impairment (blurred vision, decreased visual fields, visual spots) Retinal telangiectasia, neovascularisation, infarction, haemorrhage, exudates, macular oedema	Ophthalmic examination Eye education Topical steriod, beta-blocker, atropine or Diamox drops Photocoagulation and laser therapy
Optic neuropathy	RT ($TD_{5/5}$) > 50 Gy	Blindness, pale optic disc	Ophthalmic examination Visual aids

Lacrimal gland, duct and eyelid complications

Tears are necessary for lubrication and cleansing of the cornea and originate from the lacrimal gland. These glands are located in the upper and lower eyelids. When all the lacrimal glands are irradiated to a dose around 36 Gy, a dry-eye syndrome can occur as a result of decreased tear production. Incidence of this syndrome increases to 100% with doses around 55–60 Gy (Parsons et al 1994b). Symptoms develop within a few months following irradiation. Patients complain of severe eye pain; this can be as a result of telangiectasia, ulceration and lacrimal duct fibrosis, which can cause blockage of the duct and secondary infection. Avoiding excessive dose and irradiation of all the lacrimal glands can prevent such complications. This can be achieved by careful treatment planning and appropriate shielding of the lacrimal glands during treatment.

Lens complications

Tolerance of the lens to radiation is low; it can cause a cataract at doses of < 6.5 Gy and up to one-third of patients will experience some opacification of the lens following treatment. The incidence and severity of radiation-induced cataracts depend on the dose per fraction and the total dose delivered (Henk et al 1993). At fractionated doses of 6.5–11.5 Gy, approximately one-third of patients will have stationary opacities that will result in visual defects. Cataract formation is universal with doses >16.5 Gy. A cataract may remain static and cause little visual impairment or it may be progressive and result in blindness. The latent period to the development of cataracts is 8–9 years with doses <6.5 Gy, and 4–5 years with doses between 6.5 and 11.5 Gy. Keeping radiation doses to below these thresholds can avoid cataract development. The management of cataracts will depend on the severity of the visual impairment, the rate of progression and the presence of other eye complications, such as dry-lens syndrome, retinopathy or optic neuropathy. If there are no other potential ocular complications, cataract removal and intraocular implant is a relatively effective and safe procedure to improve vision.

Retinal complications

Radiation-induced retinopathy is similar to diabetic retinopathy and can occur 1.5–3 years after radiotherapy. Patients complain of blurred irregular light spots or a visual field defect. They can be progressive, leading to complete blindness. These symptoms are usually painless unless glaucoma develops. An ophthalmologist should see patients at risk of optic retinopathy regularly. If problems occur, treatment with panretinal laser therapy may prevent progressive visual loss. The eye should be preserved at all times, even if vision is lost, because eye prostheses are poorly tolerated following high-dose irradiation to the orbit.

Optic neuropathy

Optic neuropathy is a disastrous complication for patients and prevention is the best management as there is no proven therapy. Radiation-induced optic neuropathy usually affects only one optic nerve. Symptoms described are those of an acute painless monocular visual loss (Roden et al 1990). The optic nerve is sensitive to the fraction dose, with a tolerance of around 65 Gy using fraction sizes of < 1.9 and 55 Gy with fraction sizes of > 1.9 Gy (Parsons et al 1994a). Tolerance is reduced in patients with diabetes or in patients having neoadjuvant or concurrent chemotherapy. Cases of optic neuropathy have been reported at doses of 40–49 Gy using 2 Gy per fraction when delivered in conjunction with chemotherapy (Choi et al 1991, Wilson et al 1987).

SALIVARY GLAND COMPLICATIONS

The salivary glands have an important role in oral hygiene and digestion. They produce saliva that moistens food, aids digestion through the enzymes contained

Table 19.3 Late radiation effects on the salivary glands

Late effects	Factors	Symptoms/signs	Management
Xerostomia	Radiotherapy > 30 Gy	Decreased saliva production (dry mouth, difficulties in swallowing and speech, altered taste, dental caries, oral *Candida*)	Dental examination and regular checks with attention to early peridontal disease Dental and diet education, good oral hygiene Prophylactic fluoride Artificial saliva Pilocarpine Antibiotics/antifungals

within it and protects against the formation of dental caries by its antimicrobial activity. Irradiation of the salivary glands to doses above 30 Gy causes destruction and atrophy of the salivary acinar cells, fatty degeneration of the salivary glands and fibrosis (Table 19.3). Patients complain of decreased production of saliva and xerostomia (dry mouth, altered taste, difficulties in speech and swallowing, oral *Candida*). The severity of xerostomia is partially related to the dose and volume of salivary gland treated (Table 19.1). Recovery of salivary function can occur in up to 6–12 months but in some patients xerostomia may persist indefinitely. Secondary problems can occur, giving rise to caries and other dental problems.

Management of symptoms involves maintaining saliva production or providing a substitute. The reduction in saliva production can be partially overcome by sips of water and water rinses. Some patients find sugarless chewing gum or citrus-flavoured confectionery helpful in promoting saliva production. Artificial salivary substitutes such as carboxymethocellulose-based saliva or mucin-based saliva have been used for symptomatic relief with some success. Pilocarpine, a muscarinic cholinergic agonist, has been used with some success to stimulate remaining salivary gland function (Reike et al 1995). As emphasised in Chapter 10, it is important to provide dental prophylaxis, maintain regular dental checks and treat dental caries promptly if salivary function is reduced. For further advice on the management of xerostomia, see Chapter 10.

CARDIAC COMPLICATIONS

Irradiation to the heart can affect all three cardiac tissue layers (pericardium, myocardium and endocardium), coronary arteries, heart valves and the conducting system of the heart. The factors that need to be considered in evaluating risk include the radiation fractionation and dose delivered to the different layers, structures and volume of the heart treated and assessment of any adjuvant cardiotoxic agents such as anthracycline chemotherapy. Other cardiac risk factors that need to be evaluated are a family history of cardiac disease, obesity, high blood pressure, high cholesterol and smoking. One of the histological features of radiation damage to the heart is the presence of diffuse fibroblasts in the cardiac muscle with relatively normal-looking cardiac cells (myocytes) and evidence of vascular damage affecting the capillaries and arteries (Stewart et al 1995). Pericardial damage is most common, followed by myocardial damage, coronary artery disease and, rarely, valvular or conducting defects (Table 19.4).

Pericardial complications

Complications of the pericardium are common in patients undergoing radiation to the chest. Late side effects include pericarditis, pericardial effusion with or without

Table 19.4   Late radiation effects on the heart

Late effects	Factors	Symptoms/signs	Management
Pericardial damage	RT > 35 Gy	Breathlessness, pleuritic chest pain, friction rub, pulsus paradoxus, decreased heart sounds	ECG, CXR and echocardiogram Diuretic therapy Pericardiostomy Pericardiectomy
Cardiomyopathy	RT > 35 Gy Anthracyclines	Fatigue, breathlessness, palpitations, syncope, left heart failure (exertional dyspnoea, orthopnoea, paroxysmal nocturnal dyspnoea, wheeze, cough, haemoptysis), right heart failure (right upper abdominal discomfort, nausea, fatigue, peripheral oedema), arrhythmias, hypertension, cardiomegaly	ECG, CXR and echocardiogram Holter monitor (for arrhythmias) Exercise stress testing Cardiac education and decrease risk factors (smoking, diet, cholesterol, obesity, alcohol) Heart failure drug therapy (diuretics, vasodilators, inotropes) Antiarrhythmic drug therapy Heart replacement
Coronary artery damage	RT > 35 Gy	Severe central chest pain (radiating to neck, jaw and/or arm on exertion, anxiety, cold weather, after heavy meals), dizziness, breathlessness, sweating, hypotension, arrhythmias, myocardial infarction	ECG and CXR Exercise stress testing Coronary catheterisation Cardiac perfusion scan Ambulatory ECG monitoring Cardiac education and decrease risk factors Antianginal drug therapy Coronary artery dilatation and bypass grafts
Valvular damage	RT > 40 Gy	Breathlessness, syncope, fatigue, murmur, hepatomegaly, arrhythmias	ECG, CXR and echocardiogram Coronary catheterisation Antibiotic prophylaxis for surgery and dental procedures to prevent bacterial infestation of the heart valves Heart valve replacement

RT, radiotherapy; ECG, electrocardiogram; CXR, chest X-ray.

cardiac compression (tamponade) and pericardial constriction. Pericarditis can be asymptomatic or of sudden onset. Patients complain of pleuritic chest pain, shortness of breath, friction rub and fever, but rarely have cardiac failure. This can occur 6 months following radiation and may be complicated by pericardial effusion. Pericarditis has been reported in up to 30% of Hodgkin's disease patients and those receiving a mean cardiac dose of 46 Gy (Green et al 1987). If the cardiac dose is reduced to below 35 Gy, the incidence decreases to 2.5%. Treatment is aimed at reducing symptoms through the use of aspirin or non-steroidal antiinflammatory agents. Steroids are reserved for severe and persistent symptoms.

Pericardial effusion is usually asymptomatic in patients and is often discovered incidentally on routine follow-up chest X-ray. The majority of cases develop within 12 months of radiotherapy. It usually resolves within 1–10 months of diagnosis. Chronic effusion may occur in 10–15% of cases. Up to 40% may develop some degree of cardiac tamponade. An echocardiogram is useful in establishing the diagnosis, assessing the severity of tamponade and providing a baseline measurement. Monitoring and assessing symptoms is the preferred option for management unless the patient's symptoms warrant intervention, in which case guided needle pericardiocentesis is the initial treatment. Recurrent pericardial fluid accumulation requires a pericardial window (pericardiostomy) or pericardial stripping (pericardiectomy).

Symptoms of breathlessness on exertion are usually indicative of constrictive pericarditis and right heart failure. A computed tomography (CT) scan is diagnostic in demonstrating thickening of the pericardium; cardiac catheterisation will also confirm altered ventricular pressures. Fluid retention from heart failure may respond to diuretic therapy but pericardiectomy is the only definitive therapy. Surgery needs to be carefully considered in radiation patients, taking into account the current status of the cancer, pulmonary and other cardiac conditions that may minimise the potential benefit. This is a serious complication that can substantially impact on patients' well-being.

Myo- and endocardial complications

Cardiomyopathy as a result of irradiation usually presents as congestive cardiac failure (Table 19.4). The incidence of clinically symptomatic cardiomyopathy is relatively low, especially if the cardiac doses are < 40 Gy (Stewart et al 1995). However, up to 57% of patients who have been investigated sometimes after radiotherapy to the cardiac region have some abnormal ventricular function (Burns et al 1983, Perrault et al 1985). Changes in radiotherapy techniques, with appropriate cardiac shielding, mean that this incidence is unlikely to be representative of late complications for current patients (Constine et al 1997). Cardiotoxic chemotherapy such as anthracyclines can exacerbate cardiomyopathy and other factors such as dose, age, coexisting cardiac disorders or other predisposing cardiac factors such as obesity, hypertension, small-vessel disease and smoking, all contribute to occurrence. Pancarditis is rare but if it occurs is severe. Patients experience severe congestive cardiac failure that responds poorly to conventional cardiac medications. This complication is usually associated with radiation doses of > 60 Gy (Stewart et al 1995).

Coronary artery complications

Cardiac irradiation can cause small and large blood vessel damage. The proximal coronary artery branches are usually affected and this may be because these sites are difficult to shield with routine cardiac blocking. Symptoms and signs are similar to those for non-radiation-related ischaemic heart symptoms (Table 19.4).

Contributing factors can be coronary artery disease which can lead to ischaemic heart disease and death from myocardial infarction (Boivin et al 1992). Patients most at risk of this are long-term survivors of cancer treatment. In breast cancer survivors, postoperative irradiation to the left breast or chest has been reported to increase the incidence of coronary artery disease, with a subsequent increase in relative risk by 3.2 times, of dying of a myocardial infarction (Cuzick et al 1994). Data from a randomised trial have also supported this finding (Rutqvist et al 1992). Excess cardiac mortality, especially with coronary artery disease, has been recorded in patients receiving mantle irradiation for Hodgkin's disease (Eriksson et al 2000, Hancock & Hoppe 1996, King et al 1996). This relative risk is substantially higher (44.7 times) when patients are irradiated at a younger age (10–19 years) and this risk increases the longer the patients are followed (Hancock & Hoppe 1996). Thus, it would be appropriate to ensure that the cardiac dose was ≤ 30 Gy since this dose range has not been associated with an increased relative risk (King et al 1996). It is therefore important to inform patients of this possible long-term effect and relative risk.

The management of coronary artery disease is dependent on the severity of symptoms and the risk of myocardial infarction. Investigations such as exercise stress testing of the heart and coronary angiography are needed to establish the severity of any arterial disease. Patients at risk should also be advised about additional cardiac risk factors such as smoking, diet and lifestyle and be advised of health-promoting behaviours. Cardiac medications and specific treatments such as coronary artery dilatation or grafting can be used depending on the extent of the damage.

Valvular and conductive complications

Valvular disease is a less common late toxicity, although thickening and fibrosis of the cardiac valves could be found in up to 70% of autopsy cases of patients who had received radiotherapy to the chest (Perrault et al 1985). The mitral, aortic and tricuspid valves are frequently affected. The management of valvular damage is outlined in Table 19.4. Conductive abnormalities are rare and usually involve the atrioventricular node (Stewart et al 1995). These changes are usually associated with high doses of cardiac radiation.

RESPIRATORY COMPLICATIONS

Irradiation of the lung damages the cells lining the alveolus (pneumocytes), vascular endothelial vessels, fibroblasts and macrophages. Radiation causes injury of the alveolar type 2 pneumocyte cells and alveolar capillary endothelial cells, which alters the surfactant system (Burger et al 1998). Surfactants are important respiratory substances that allow the alveolus to remain open with less pressure. The damaged vascular endothelial cells, which are important in respiratory gas exchange, release inflammatory chemicals. These allow protein leakage into the alveolar spaces. Patients complain of breathlessness, fever, pleuritic pain and cough (Table 19.5). In the acute phase, the release of cytokines, including transforming growth factor-alpha (TGF-α) and -beta (TGF-β), can influence the production of collagen formation and stimulation of fibroblasts, which in turn contribute to the development of longer-term pulmonary fibrosis (Burger et al 1998). Exacerbation of lung damage can also occur with the use of chemotherapy or biological agents such as actinomycin D, bleomycin, BCNU, doxorubicin and interferon therapy (Roach et al 1995). It is important to exclude other causes of symptoms such as infection, pulmonary embolism, hypersensitivity or, more importantly, tumour recurrence. The management of pneumonitis is discussed in Chapter 9.

Pulmonary fibrosis

Pulmonary fibrosis is a late side effect occurring several months to years postirradiation; however, radiographic changes can be apparent within 1–2 years, with symptoms. Chronic respiratory impairment can occur in patients resulting in a restrictive clinical pulmonary picture (Movsas et al 1997). Chronic respiratory symptoms include breathlessness on exertion, orthopnoea and cyanosis, with severe cases progressing to right heart failure. Often, there are other exacerbating factors for the patient such as chronic airways disease or emphysema from smoking and specific bronchodilators or steroid therapy may be required. Infections can often complicate the diagnosis.

Table 19.5 Late radiation effects on the lungs

Late effects	Factors	Symptoms/signs	Management
Pneumonitis	RT dose and volume effects (Table 19.1) Bleomycin	Fever, congestion, pleuritic pain, breathlessness, cough, pleural rub	CXR, lung function tests Sputum culture (if productive) Bronchodilators, steroid therapy Antibiotics (for infections) Avoid smoking
Pulmonary fibrosis	RT dose and volume effects (Table 19.1) Bleomyoin	Breathlessness, orthopnoea, cyanosis, cor pulmonale (right heart failure secondary to pulmonary hypertension)	CXR, CT scan, lung function tests (restrictive ventilation pattern) Respiratory education and decrease risk factors (smoking, obesity) Bronchodilators, steroid therapy Antibiotics (for infections) Avoid smoking

RT, radiotherapy; CXR, chest X-ray; CT, computerised tomography.

Exclusion of recurrent tumour or other treatable medical and infective diseases is important. In contrast to the non-specific radiological changes of pneumonitis, plain chest X-ray and CT scanning can be useful in pulmonary fibrosis. Pleural thickening and contraction of the lung lobes, with retraction of the hilum and tenting of the diaphragm caused by the fibrosis, may be seen on chest X-ray. The presence of pulmonary opacification or consolidation that resembles the straight edges of the radiotherapy treatment portal is suggestive of late radiation fibrosis. Lung function tests reveal a restrictive pulmonary pattern but these need to be compared to baseline lung function tests. These tests can also be used to monitor the severity and progression of the condition. Studies have suggested that selective inhibition of TGF-β (Border & Noble 1994) or antigen receptor CD40 production (Fries et al 1995) can potentially reduce fibroblast proliferation and subsequent pulmonary fibrosis. These methods appear promising for future treatment.

GASTROINTESTINAL COMPLICATIONS

The gastrointestinal tract is responsible for digestion, absorption of nutrients and removal of waste products. Complications can occur from the oesophagus to the anal canal. Irradiation of the gastrointestinal tract damages the rapid mucosal cellular regenerating system and the bowel vascular supply. Progressive vascular damage reduces gastrointestinal mucosal repair and regeneration. Incomplete repair of mucosa and hyperplasia of blood capillaries can result in thinned friable mucosal epithelium and telangiectasia that can be fragile to contact trauma. Obliteration of supplying blood vessels and increasing fibrosis of the gastrointestinal tract walls can result in strictures, ulceration and necrosis. Late bowel ulceration is often focal, resulting in loss of specific segments of mucosa that may lead to perforation or allow the formation of fistulas.

The effects of radiation are dependent on the volume of tissue treated, together with the total dose delivered and fraction size used (Table 19.1). For most of the gastrointestinal tract, tolerance is around 50–60 Gy using conventional radiotherapy fractionation, with 2 Gy per fraction given daily (Coia et al 1995, Emami et al 1991). The small bowel appears to have a lower tolerance of around 45–50 Gy (Coia et al 1995, Emami et al 1991). Predicting the extent of bowel within an abdominal or pelvic field is difficult, as peristaltic bowel activity may allow sections of bowel to move in and out of the radiotherapy field on a day-to-day basis. This minimises the chance that the same section of bowel will be irradiated beyond its tolerance but also, the presence of adhesions from previous surgery may restrict normal bowel movement and increase the risk of damage. The use of concurrent chemotherapy may also reduce the tolerance of the bowel and result in a higher incidence of late complications (Danjoux & Catton 1979). The severity of acute gastrointestinal effects does not appear to predict for the development of late sequelae (Coia et al 1995). Prevention is the key – assessing patients' risk factors and reducing the amount of subsequent bowel irradiated.

Oesophageal complications

Surgery and high radiation doses increase the incidence of late oesophageal damage. A Radiation Therapy Oncology Group (RTOG) study reported a 6% incidence of late effects with 60 Gy given postoperatively compared to 1% with 50 Gy delivered preoperatively (Kramer et al 1987). The $TD_{5/5}$ (see Table 19.1) for strictures or ulceration is 60 Gy for one-third of the oesophagus and 55 Gy for the whole oesophagus (Emami et al 1991). The most common late radiation-induced oesophageal symptom is dysphagia. Patients complain of symptoms of pain or difficulty in swallowing, which occur 3–6 months following irradiation. This is caused by oesophageal muscle incoordination as a result of fibrosis and stricture formation of the wall. Ulceration and perforation are possible, especially after the use of intraluminal brachytherapy (Hishikawa et al 1991). Perforation can allow aspiration of the oesophageal contents into the lung, causing aspiration pneumonia.

During radiation, unless the oesophagus is the radiation target, the oesophagus may be excluded from radiation fields by simple positioning of the patient (supine vs prone). This procedure can reduce the dose to the oesophagus. Management of symptoms depends on the impact for the patient on quality of life (Table 19.6). Promoting nutritional status is important; soft food may be preferred for ease of swallowing, but referral to a dietician is essential (see Ch. 11). Topical anaesthetics and analgesia are valuable in reducing discomfort (see Ch. 9). Oesophageal stricture formation can respond well to periodic dilatation. Proton pump inhibition therapy may prevent further oesophagitis, reflux difficulties and mucosal ulceration. Severe cases of stricture formation may require a stent or feeding by other mechanisms such as a percutaneous tube into the stomach (see Ch. 11).

Small-bowel complications

There is a steep dose–complication curve for small-bowel complications. Doses to the small bowel of 45–50 Gy are associated with < 5% complications (Pilepich et al 1987) compared to 15–25% incidence with doses of 50–55 Gy (Tewfik et al 1982). Late small-bowel side effects include malabsorption syndromes, hypermotility, diarrhoea, pain from recurrent episodes of subacute bowel obstruction and, less frequently, ulceration, fistulas, perforation and ischaemia (Table 19.6). Symptoms occur 6–24 months following the completion of radiotherapy. Contributing factors include previous abdominal surgery, chemotherapy, especially vinca alkaloids, and poor general health.

Avoidance of the small bowel is the most useful method of preventing these complications. Careful radiotherapy planning is required to exclude as much normal bowel as possible from the radiation field. Various methods are available to separate the bowel from the radiation fields, such as volume spacers, compression gadgets to push the bowel out of the way and cut-away table tops (belly-boards) that allow the abdomen to fall into a space distant to the radiation fields. As with all late side effects, tumour recurrence must always be excluded as a cause of symptoms. Subacute bowel obstruction often settles with conservative treatment. Conservative measures using antidiarrhoeal, antispasmodic or antiemetic medications and lactose-free diets are often helpful for altered bowel function. Dietary management and enzyme supplementation may be needed for malabsorption syndromes. Symptoms of bleeding need to be promptly investigated to elucidate the site and cause of bleeding. Rarely, surgery may be required to resect unresolved obstruction or necrotic segments of bowel.

Table 19.6   Late radiation effects on the gastrointestinal tract

Late effects	Factors	Symptoms/signs	Management
Stricture	(See text for separate sites)	Difficulty swallowing (dysphagia) for the oesophagus Altered bowel habits, especially constipation for the rectum Pain	Education Soft diet (oesophagus) Stool softeners (rectum) Topical anaesthetic lotions and analgesia Proton pump inhibition therapy Dilatation Stent Bypass feeding methods (oesophagus)
Bowel obstruction (subacute)	(See text for separate sites)	Colic (spasmodic abdominal pain), restlessness, altered bowel habits, loss of appetite, nausea, vomiting, weight loss, abdominal distension, tinkling bowel sounds	Plain abdominal erect and supine X-rays, barium studies, endoscopy Education Diet Conservative treatment for subacute bowel obstruction Decompression surgery for complete bowel obstruction
Perforation, fistula	(See text for separate sites)	Peritonitis (severe abdominal pain, tenderness, guarding, rebound tenderness) shock, prostration, rigid abdomen, absent bowel sounds	Thorough assessment Abdominal X-ray, U&E, FBC, blood cultures Hospital admission, nil by mouth, treatment of shock (intravenous fluids or blood), pain relief Surgery if required
Bleeding	(See text for separate sites)	Haematemesis (vomiting of blood), melaena (altered blood)	Endoscopy to elucidate site and cause of bleeding Assessment of severity of bleed Replacement of blood loss if required Treatment directed to the cause of bleeding

U & E, urea and electrolytes; FBC, full blood count.

Large-bowel and rectal complications

Large-bowel toxicity includes the development of colitis, strictures, bowel obstruction (often subacute), ulceration, fistulas, perforation and ischaemia (Table 19.6). Patients present with abdominal pain but the pattern of the pain can differ and will depend on the underlying cause. Altered bowel function is also common. Late rectal side effects also include tenesmus, bleeding and rectal strictures.

The tolerance for irradiation of colorectal regions is higher than that for small bowel. Studies show that the incidence of colorectal side effects, from a total of 1000 men irradiated for prostate cancer, is between 6 and 19% for moderate side effects and 1–3% for severe side effects requiring surgery (Aristizabel et al 1984, Forman et al 1985, Zagars et al 1987). The commonest late rectal side-effect is proctitis with or without rectal bleeding (grade 2): this occurs in 3–15% of cases. Severe late rectal complications requiring colostomy are < 1% (Hanks 1988, Shipley et al 1994). Incidence of side effects appears to increase from 6% to 11% when patients received more than 65 Gy using conventional radiation techniques (Hanks et al 1988). However, other investigators have not noted an increase in rectal complications with doses up to 70 Gy (Pilepich et al 1987, Smit et al 1990, Zagars et al 1987). New treatment techniques such as conformal radiotherapy can significantly reduce rectal side effects and allow dose escalation with acceptable morbidity (Dearnaley et al 1999).

Prevention of excessive radiation dose to the rectum is the main method of reducing the probability of late colorectal damage. This is usually performed by selecting appropriate treatment beam angles to minimise dose to the bowel, optimal patient positioning and the use of volume spacers, omental slings or absorbable mesh to prevent the movement of bowel into the radiation fields. Colorectal management of late radiation symptoms is similar to the management described for small bowel (Table 19.6). Rectal proctitis or anal discomfort may require steroid suppositories, topical anaesthetics and regular analgesia. Selective laser therapy, electrocautery, silver nitrate or formalin rectum instillations may be used for persistent rectal bleeding. In rare cases, surgical resection of damaged or obstructed bowel may be needed.

LIVER COMPLICATIONS

Damage by radiation to the liver occurs as a result of changes to the venous system. Central vein occlusive disease causes a characteristic lesion which is easily distinguished from tumour recurrence. Thrombosis occurs in the central veins of the liver lobules causing congestion which results in secondary haemorrhage and necrosis of the surrounding hepatocytes (Lewin & Millis 1973). This can eventually give rise to progressive fibrosis and cirrhosis with liver failure.

Late radiation-induced liver complications can manifest as obstructive liver disease that can be either asymptomatic or symptomatic hepatitis with jaundice. Patients complain of right upper quadrant abdominal pain, hepatomegaly, ascites and, occasionally, hepatic encephalopathy. This usually occurs within 3–5 months following irradiation but occurs earlier with total body irradiation, over 1–4 weeks. This is because radiation combined with chemotherapy for bone marrow transplantation enhances the reaction (Ganem et al 1988, Lawrence et al 1995). A marked elevation of liver enzymes is seen on liver function tests with a modest rise in bilirubin levels.

The dose–volume relationship of organ tolerance is well demonstrated by the liver (Table 19.1). This tolerance is lowered by the use of concurrent chemotherapeutic agents such as doxorubicin, Mitomycin C and 5-fluorouracil (Lawrence et al 1995). Using estimations from late complication probability models, a good correlation between dose/volume and clinical data has been demonstrated (Lawrence et al 1992). Careful treatment planning with three-dimensional techniques permits proper assessment of the critical dose/volume interrelationship so that tolerance ranges are respected and high doses of radiation can be safely delivered to portions of the liver. However, there is no effective therapy to reverse the radiation-induced damage. Management initially involves the exclusion of other causes of liver dysfunction and obstruction, including hepatotoxic drugs, infective hepatitis and malignant involvement (Table 19.7). Treatment of symptoms is the mainstay of therapy. Using diuretics, anticoagulation, avoidance of potentially hepatotoxic drugs and, in severe cases, steroids (Lawrence et al 1995).

RENAL COMPLICATIONS

In renal complications, the main radiation damage occurs at the level of the functional subunit of the kidney, which includes the glomerulus and its microvasculature (Hoopes et al 1985, Krochak & Baker 1986). Radiation causes progressive loss and fibrosis of the glomerulus, nephron tubules and the surrounding capillaries, leading to the development of glomerulosclerosis. This results in both loss of the nephron subunits and impaired renal function.

Late renal damage manifests as chronic nephritis or renal failure, depending on the extent of damage on the pair of kidneys (Table 19.8). Clinical effects are usually seen 12–18 months following radiotherapy but mild symptoms may not appear

Table 19.7 Late radiation effects on the liver

Late effects	Factors	Symptoms/signs	Management
Hepatitis	RT > 30 Gy (whole liver)	Jaundice, itching, bruising	Liver function tests, plasma biochemistry and renal function, full blood count; Liver imaging (ultrasound, CT scan); Assessment of disease severity; Determination of the aetiology; Liver disease education and decrease risk factors
Cirrhosis	RT > 30 Gy (whole liver)	Lethargy, chronic liver disease (spider naevi, liver palms, gynaecomastia, small testes, jaundice, ascites, oedema), encephalopathy, hypoglycaemia, bleeding, infection; Portal hypertension (severe and chronic hepatitis), bleeding	Liver function tests, plasma biochemistry and renal function, full blood count; Liver imaging (ultrasound, CT scan); Assessment of disease severity; Determination of the aetiology; Treatment of the specific complication, e.g., bleeding, infection, ascites, hypoglycaemia; Liver disease education and decrease risk factors

RT, radiotherapy; CT, computed tomography.

Table 19.8 Late radiation effects on the kidney

Late effects	Factors	Symptoms/signs	Management
Nephrotic syndrome, nephritis	Chemotherapy RT	Peripheral oedema, ascites Proteinuria, hypoalbuminaemia	Plasma biochemistry, renal function, full blood tests Urine specimen for creatinine clearance and protein excretion Urine microscopy for casts Renal imaging Bed rest, protein- and calorie-rich diet, diuretics
Chronic renal failure	Chemotherapy RT	Lethargy, nausea, itch, nocturia, impotence, oedema, breathlessness, vomiting, hiccups, confusion	Plasma biochemistry, renal function, full blood tests Urine specimen for creatinine clearance and protein excretion Urine microscopy for casts Renal imaging Medications for specific renal problems Renal education re diet, fluid intake and avoidance of exacerbating drugs Dialysis and renal transplantation if appropriate

RT, radiotherapy.

until many years later. Symptoms vary depending on the severity of the damage. In its mildest form, there may be hypertension with minimal proteinuria – some granular and red blood cell casts seen in the urine (Krochak & Baker 1986). Irradiation can produce a small scarred and encapsulated kidney, which results in the development of hypertension. If nephritis progresses to nephropathy and both kidneys are compromised, then chronic uraemia will develop with a clinical picture of anaemia, hypertension, ventricular failure and pleural effusion as well as moderate to large amounts of albuminuria and proteinuria. Patients describe symptoms of fatigue, ankle swelling and breathlessness on exertion. In contrast, renal damage from chemotherapeutic drugs such as platinum agents is more likely to produce renal failure with decrease in creatinine clearance rather than hypertension and proteinuria, which are more commonly associated with radiation-induced damage (Cohen et al 1995, Schilsky 1982).

With localised treatment such as radiotherapy, a substantial portion of both kidneys needs to be damaged before clinical manifestations are observed. In most cases, one kidney can be spared from any substantial radiation dose, thus preserving adequate renal function. This is in contrast to chemotherapy, which usually affects both kidneys equally. Careful evaluation is needed to ensure that there are no congenital defects or absence of one kidney. The advantage of a pair of kidneys is that if one kidney needs to be sacrificed in order to treat the malignancy adequately, then there is another kidney that can maintain adequate renal function.

It is therefore important that the function of the remaining kidney is adequate and preserved through meticulous radiotherapy planning. Assessment of renal function prior to treatment is vital and any chemotherapeutic agents used should be documented. Prior damage may affect the function of the kidneys and lower the renal tolerance to irradiation (Schilsky 1982).

The severity of any damage depends on both the volume and dose received and whether one or both kidneys are irradiated. The tolerance ranges for a single kidney are shown in Table 19.1. If the whole of one kidney is to be irradiated, the dose should not exceed 20–23 Gy if some renal function is to remain. It has been suggested that a minimum of one-third of the renal volume of one kidney needs to be excluded from any radiation in order to maintain adequate renal function (Krochak & Baker 1986). When both kidneys are irradiated, the $TD_{5/5}$ for renal failure is approximately 20 Gy (Cassady 1995).

Management of symptoms will depend on the severity of the damage. This will need to be assessed initially by renal function tests such as blood electrolytes, urea and creatinine, urinalysis and creatinine clearance. Blood flow renograms have correlated well with biochemical and clearance thresholds. Mild hypertension may be controlled by a low-protein diet and fluid and salt restrictions. Antihypertensive medications such as angiotensin-converting enzyme inhibitors have been reported to be useful in animal studies in the setting of radiation-induced renal damage (Juncos et al 1993, Moulder et al 1993). Anaemia can be treated with iron therapy, blood transfusion or erythropoietin. Progressive uraemia will eventually require dialysis, to replace the function of the kidneys. If patients are considered to be cured of their initial cancer then consideration can be given to renal transplantation.

UROLOGICAL COMPLICATIONS

Urological complications can result from radiotherapy to the pelvis with external beam, brachytherapy or a combination of both treatment approaches. Damage can occur to any portion of the lower urinary system (ureter, bladder and urethra) depending on where the radiation is delivered. The origin of such damage is in the epithelium and its microvasculature. Loss of the epithelial cells, poor repair of damaged cells and telangiectasia give rise to fragile linings that are susceptible to easy trauma, bleeding, scarring and fibrosis. Neurovascular bundles may also be affected and cause altered urinary function. The major urological complications include haemorrhagic cystitis, urinary incontinence, urethral dysfunction and erectile dysfunction (Table 19.9). The most frequent late urinary side effects are cystitis, sometimes with haematuria (2–11%), urethral stricture (2–11%) and incontinence (1–2%) (Hanks 1988, Lawton et al 1991, Pilepich et al 1987, Shipley et al 1994).

Haemorrhagic cystitis

Haemorrhagic cystitis is inflammation of the bladder lining causing symptoms of frequency and dysuria. There may also be bleeding from the bladder mucosa resulting in a need for transfusions. Management is dependent on its severity

Table 19.9 Late radiation effects on the urinary system

Late effects	Factors	Symptoms/signs	Management
Bleeding	Chemotherapy RT (see text)	Haematuria, pain	Plasma biochemistry, renal function, full blood tests Urine specimen for creatinine clearance and protein excretion Urine microscopy for casts Renal imaging Cystoscopy Treatment for specific site of bleeding and surgery if appropriate
Stricture	RT > 55 Gy	Stricture compression along the urinary tract from ureter to urethra may cause urinary blockage and present as renal failure	Renal imaging Cystoscopy Treatment for specific site of obstruction and surgery if appropriate

RT, radiotherapy.

and conservative measures are often successful. Tumour involvement or recurrence of bladder cancer should always be excluded as a cause of symptoms. Urine should be cultured as urinary tract infection can cause similar symptoms and antibiotics should be prescribed if indicated. Minor bleeding episodes may respond to aminocaproic acid, which prevents fibrinolysis by inhibiting plasminogen-activating substances. Maximal response can be expected within 8–12 h. Clot formation may require a bladder catheter for evacuation and irrigation. Diffuse uncontrolled haemorrhagic cystitis may require bladder instillation of silver nitrate or formalin solution to fix the bladder mucosa. Focal bleeding may be effectively controlled by electrocautery or Nd:YAG laser therapy.

Urinary strictures and incontinence

The main predisposing factor for the development of urinary strictures and urinary incontinence is previous transurethral resections (Hanks et al 1988, Lawton et al 1991, Pilepich et al 1987, Shipley et al 1994). The main treatment for symptomatic urinary strictures is periodic urethral dilatation. Extensive bladder surgery or repeated transurethral resections can also predispose to significant bladder wall contracture, resulting in a small bladder capacity. Urinary incontinence requires full urodynamic and flow assessment, with therapy directed to the problems that cause patients most distress. Behavioural approaches, such as exercises to increase bladder capacity and bladder-retaining techniques, have been found to be helpful for managing urinary incontinence (see Ch. 12). Antispasmodic or muscle-relaxing medication may be useful for unstable urinary incontinence.

SECONDARY MALIGNANCIES

There is an increased risk of developing a second malignancy with irradiation. However, other factors, such as the use of chemotherapeutic agents, genetic predisposition of the individual patient and carcinogenic environmental factors, can also influence its development. Carcinogenesis or the transformation of normal cells to cancer cells is a detailed subject in its own right. It is a multistep process, which will be covered briefly here. The classic description of carcinogenesis involves a process of initiation, promotion and progression. Put simply, initiation occurs when an agent (i.e. radiation, viruses, toxic chemical or environmental agents, genetic factors) initiates the injury of the DNA of a cell, giving rise to either a mutant cell or damaged normal DNA repair proteins. Following this, repeated injury of a second agent causes promotion. Progression occurs when the mutant cell evolves and exhibits malignant behaviour. Contemporary models of carcinogenesis involve the complex interaction of multiple genes whereby tumour-suppressor genes are inactivated and growth-stimulating oncogenes are activated.

The review of atomic bomb survivors provides an excellent illustration and a model of the long-term effects of radiation exposure. The time interval between irradiation and the appearance of a cancer is referred to as the latent period. There is a dose-related increase for leukaemia as well as cancers of the oesophagus, stomach, colon, lung, breast, ovary, thyroid, urinary tract and multiple myeloma (Boice 1988). Compared to leukaemia, the excess risk associated with secondary solid cancers only develops after the exposed individual reaches the age when the cancer is prone to develop. Long-term Hodgkin's disease follow-up studies revealed that young patients who were less than 20 years when irradiated with mantle fields were likely to have up to a 40-fold increased risk of breast cancer (Bhatia et al 1996, Hancock & Hoppe 1996, van-Leeuwen et al 2000). This implies that there is an age-related factor important in the expression of the cancer. Furthermore, the relative risk is greater for those exposed at younger ages. Other factors include long-term follow-up or cure following radiation therapy and therapeutic parameters including type of organ, volume of organ treated and dose received, as well as other carcinogens such as smoking. Patients with Hodgkin's disease who continued to smoke during or following irradiation were noted to be at a higher risk of subsequent lung cancer than patients who did not (van-Leeuwen et al 1994). The clinical effects of a secondary cancer are no different from that of a primary malignancy and are dependent on the site of origin.

SUMMARY OF KEY CLINICAL POINTS

- The aetiology of late radiation-induced damage is multifactorial.
- Late effects can occur months to years following irradiation.
- Treatment effects may be directly as a result of damage to the tissues within the treatment field or indirectly as a result of damaged blood supply to the region.
- Awareness and assessment of influencing factors leading to the development of radiation-induced complications are essential.
- Informing patients of the risk of long-term complications is part of seeking informed consent for radiotherapy.

• Prevention is the main focus of intervention through careful planning techniques.
• Despite careful planning, late radiation damage can occur, as the risk is never negligible when radical doses are being used for a cure.
• If late side effects do occur, it is essential that adequate assessment of the severity and impact on quality of life is recorded.
• It is important to exclude tumour recurrence, especially if the complication occurs within the first 5 years of therapy, and the possibility of second malignancies if it occurs more than 10 years after treatment.
• Symptoms usually form part of a syndrome or cluster of effects: these are best managed by a multidisciplinary team of experts.

CONCLUSION

Late side effects, although rare, can have a substantial impact on patients' functional ability and quality of life. The potential for the occurrence of late effects is a 'Damocles sword' hanging over the person who has received radiotherapy, forming a lifetime risk that does not diminish. To be cured of the cancer but left with a major physical disability iatrogenic to the treatment is the paradox of medicine. However, endeavours to reduce these late effects have occurred through improvements in treatment and recognition of contributing factors. The advent of modern imaging techniques, such as spiral CT and magnetic resonance imaging (MRI), has allowed improved assessment of the tumour extent and its spatial relationship to important adjacent normal tissues or organs. Together with the development of sophisticated radiotherapy treatment planning, delivery and verification systems that provide three-dimensional planning and conformal radiotherapy, these methods have allowed more accurate targeting of the tumour volume and avoidance of normal organs. A further technological advance on conformal radiotherapy techniques is the development of intensity-modulated radiotherapy. The use of these techniques has been applied to several tumour sites with the expected potential of reducing the incidence and severity of late complications. Results and outcomes from these current studies are eagerly awaited. Ongoing work to integrate functional information from positron emission tomography (PET) with the structural information currently available from CT or MRI will provide better assessment of the tumour and guide treatment, as well as potentially allow avoidance of functionally important normal tissues, for example, in cerebral irradiation.

Important steps have been taken to create consensus in the evaluation and recording of radiation-induced complications, such as the Late Effects Normal Tissues/Subjective/Objective/Management/Analytic (LENTSOMA) scale. The onus remains with the medical community to document the frequency of these complications and the factors surrounding them. This will allow for comprehensive assessment of predisposing factors which will lead to a better understanding of the basis of late radiation-induced complications. Mathematical predictive models can be refined to provide a better assessment of late complication probabilities and methods of diminishing late complications can be evaluated, such as tissue radioprotectors, growth factors or pharmacological agents to modulate normal tissue injury. This is a promising area of future research. Many of these agents remain experimental at present, and represent continued challenges for the management of radiotherapy in the future.

REFERENCES

Aristizabel S A, Steinbronn D, Heusinkveld R S 1984 External beam radiotherapy in cancer of the prostate. The University of Arizona experience. Radiotherapy and Oncology 1:309–315

Bhatia S, Robison L L, Oberlin O et al 1996 Breast cancer and other second neoplasms after childhood Hodgkin's disease. New England Journal of Medicine 334:745–751

Boice J D 1988 Carcinogenesis: a synopsis of human experience with external exposure in medicine. Health Physics 55:621–630

Boice J D, Blettner M, Kleinerman R A et al 1987 Radiation dose and leukemia risk in patients treated for cancer of the cervix. Journal of the National Cancer Institute 79:1295–1311

Boivin J F, Hutchison G B, Lubin J H et al 1992 Coronary artery disease mortality in patients treated for Hodgkin's disease. Cancer 69:1241–1247

Border W A, Noble N A 1994 Transforming growth factor beta in tissue fibrosis. New England Journal of Medicine 331:1286–1292

Burger A, Loffler H, Bamberg M et al 1998 Molecular and cellular basis of radiation fibrosis. International Journal of Radiation Biology 73:401–408

Burns R J, Bar-Shlomo B Z, Druck M N et al 1983 Detection of radiation cardiomyopathy by gated radionuclide angiography. American Journal of Medicine 74:297–302

Cassady J R 1995 Clinical radiation nephropathy. International Journal of Radiation Oncology, Biology, Physics 31:1249–1256

Choi K N, Rotman M, Aziz H et al 1991 Locally advanced paranasal sinus and nasopharynx tumors treated with hyperfractionated radiation and concomitant infusion cisplatin. Cancer 67:2748–2752

Cohen E P, Lawton C A, Moulder J E 1995 Bone marrow transplant nephropathy: radiation nephritis revisited. Nephron 70:217–222

Coia L R, Myerson R J, Tepper J E 1995 Late effects of radiation therapy on the gastrointestinal tract. International Journal of Radiation Oncology, Biology, Physics 31:1213–1236

Constine L S, Schwartz R G, Savage D E et al 1997 Cardiac function, perfusion, and morbidity in irradiated long-term survivors of Hodgkin's disease. International Journal of Radiation Oncology, Biology, Physics 39:897–906

Cuzick J, Stewart H, Rutqvist L et al 1994 Cause-specific mortality in long-term survivors of breast cancer who participated in trials of radiotherapy. Journal of Clinical Oncology 12:447–453

Danjoux C E, Catton G E 1979 Delayed complications in colorectal carcinoma treated by combination radiotherapy and 5-fluorouracil: Eastern Cooperative Oncology Group (ECOG) pilot study. International Journal of Radiation Oncology, Biology, Physics 5:311–315

Dearnaley D P, Khoo V S, Norman A R et al 1999 Comparison of radiation side effects of conformal and conventional radiotherapy in prostate cancer: a randomised trial. Lancet 353:267–272

Dion M W, Hussey D H, Doornbos J F et al 1990 Preliminary results of a pilot study of pentoxifylline in the treatment of late radiation soft tissue necrosis. International Journal of Radiation Oncology, Biology, Physics 19:401–407

Emami B, Lyman J, Brown A et al 1991 Tolerance of normal tissue to therapeutic radiation. International Journal of Radiation Oncology, Biology, Physics 21:109–122

Eriksson F, Gagliardi G, Liedberg A et al 2000 Long-term cardiac mortality following radiation therapy for Hodgkin's disease: analysis with the relative seriality model. Radiotherapy and Oncology 55:153–162

Fajardo L F, Berthrong M 1988 Vascular lesions following irradiation. Pathology Annual 23:297–330

Forman J D, Zinreich E, Lee D J et al 1985 Improving the therapeutic ratio of external beam irradiation for carcinoma of the prostate. International Journal of Radiation Oncology, Biology, Physics 11:2073–2080

Fries K M, Sempowski G D, Gaspari A A et al 1995 CD40 expression by human fibroblasts. Clinical Immunology Immunopathology 77:42–51

Ganem G, Saint-Marc-Girardin M F, Kuentz M et al 1988 Venocclusive disease of the liver after allogeneic bone marrow transplantation in man. International Journal of Radiation Oncology, Biology, Physics 14:879–884

Green D M, Gingell R L, Pearce J et al 1987 The effect of mediastinal irradiation on cardiac function of patients treated during childhood and adolescence for Hodgkin's disease. Journal of Clinical Oncology 5:239–245

Hancock S L, Hoppe R T 1996 Long-term complications of treatment and causes of mortality after Hodgkin's disease. Seminars in Radiation Oncology 6:225–242

Hanks G E 1988 External beam irradiation for clinically localised prostate cancer: patterns of care studies in the United States. National Cancer Institute Monographs 7:75–84

Hanks G E, Krall J M, Martz K L et al 1988 The outcome of 313 patients with T1 (UICC) prostate cancer treated with external beam irradiation. International Journal of Radiation Oncology, Biology, Physics 14:243–248

Henk J M, Whitelocke R A F, Warrington A P et al 1993 Radiation dose to the lens and cataract formation. International Journal of Radiation Oncology, Biology, Physics 25:815–820

Hishikawa Y, Kurisu K, Taniguchi M et al 1991 Radiotherapy for carcinoma of the oesophagus in patients aged eighty or older. International Journal of Radiation Oncology, Biology, Physics 20:685–688

Hoopes P J, Gillette E L, Benjamin S A 1985 The pathogenesis of radiation nephropathy in the dog. Radiation Research 104:406–419

Hopewell J W 1986 Mechanism of action of radiation on skin and underlying tissues. Radiation Research 19:39–47

Inskip P D, Stovall M, Flannery J T 1994 Lung cancer risk and radiation dose among women treated for breast cancer. Journal of the National Cancer Institute 86:983–988

Juncos L I, Carrasco-Duenas S, Cornejo J C et al 1993 Long-term enalapril and hydrochlorothiazide in radiation nephritis.Nephron 64(2):249–255

King V, Constine L S, Clark D et al 1996 Symptomatic coronary artery disease after mantle irradiation for Hodgkin's disease. International Journal of Radiation Oncology, Biology, Physics 36:881–889

Kramer S, Gleber R D, Snow J B et al 1987 Combination radiation and surgery in the management of advanced head and neck cancer: final report of study 73-03 of the RTOG. Head and Neck Surgery 10:19–30

Krochak R J, Baker D G 1986 Radiation nephritis. Clinical manifestations and pathophysiologic mechanisms. Urology 27:389–393

Lawrence T S, Ten Haken R K, Kessler M L et al 1992 The use of 3-D dose volume analysis to predict radiation hepatitis. International Journal of Radiation Oncology, Biology, Physics 23:781–788

Lawrence T S, Robertson J M, Anscher M S et al 1995 Hepatic toxicity resulting from cancer treatment. International Journal of Radiation Oncology, Biology, Physics 31:1237–1248

Lawton C A, Won M, Pilepich M V et al 1991 Long-term treatment sequelae following external beam irradiation for adenocarcinoma of the prostate: analysis of RTOG studies 7506 and 7706. International Journal of Radiation Oncology, Biology, Physics 21:935–939

Lewin K, Millis R R 1973 Human radiation hepatitis. A morphologic study with emphasis on the late changes. Archives of Pathology 96:21–26

Moulder J E, Fish B L, Cohen E P 1993 Treatment of radiation nephropathy with ACE inhibitors. International Journal of Radiation Oncology, Biology, Physics 27:93–99

Movsas B, Raffin T A, Epstein A H et al 1997 Pulmonary radiation injury. Chest 111:1061–1076

Parsons J T, Bova F J, Fitzgerald C R et al 1994a Radiation optic neuropathy after megavoltage external-beam irradiation: analysis of time–dose factors. International Journal of Radiation Oncology, Biology, Physics 30:755–763

Parsons J T, Bova F J, Fitzgerald C R et al 1994b Severe dry-eye syndrome following external beam irradiation. International Journal of Radiation Oncology, Biology, Physics 30:775–780

Perrault D J, Levy M, Herman J G et al 1985 Echocardiographic abnormalities following cardiac radiation. Journal of Clinical Oncology 3:546–551

Pilepich M V, Asbell S O, Krall J M et al 1987 Correlation of radiotherapeutic parameters and treatment related morbidity – analysis of RTOG study 77-06. International Journal of Radiation Oncology, Biology, Physics 13:1007–1012

Reike J W, Hafermann M D, Johnson J T et al 1995 Oral pilocarpine for radiation-induced xerostomia: integrated efficacy and safety results from two prospective randomised clinical trials. International Journal of Radiation Oncology, Biology, Physics 31:661–669

Roach M, Gandara D R, Yuo H S et al 1995 Radiation pneumonitis following combined modality therapy for lung cancer: analysis of prognostic factors. Journal of Clinical Oncology 13:2606–2612

Roden D, Bosley T M, Fowble B et al 1990 Delayed radiation injury to the retrobulbar optic nerves and chiasm: clinical syndrome and treatment with hyperbaric oxygen and corticosteroids. Ophthalmology 97:347–351

RTOG-EORTC 1995 LENT SOMA tables: tables of contents. Radiotherapy and Oncology 35:17–60

Rutqvist L E, Lax I, Fornander T et al 1992 Cardiovascular mortality in a randomised trial of adjuvant radiation therapy vs. surgery alone in primary breast cancer. International Journal of Radiation Oncology, Biology, Physics 9:1669–1673

Schilsky R L 1982 Renal and metabolic toxicities of cancer chemotherapy. Seminars in Oncology 9:75–83

Shipley W U, Zietman A L, Hanks G E et al 1994 Treatment related sequelae following external beam radiation for prostate cancer: a review with an update in patients with stages T1 and T2 tumor. Journal of Urology 152:1799–1805

Smit W G J M, Helle P A, van-Putten L J et al 1990 Late radiation damage in prostate cancer patients treated by high dose external beam radiotherapy in relation to rectal dose. International Journal of Radiation Oncology, Biology, Physics 18:23–29

Stewart J R, Fajardo L F, Gillette S M et al 1995 Radiation injury to the heart. International Journal of Radiation Oncology, Biology, Physics 31:1205–1211

Tewfik H H, Buchsbaum H J, Latourette H B et al 1982 Para-aortic lymph node irradiation in carcinoma of the cervix after exploratory laparatomy and biopsy-proven positive aortic nodes. International Journal of Radiation Oncology, Biology, Physics 8:13–18

van-Leeuwen F E, Klokman W J, Hagenbeek A et al 1994 Second cancer risk following Hodgkin's disease: a 20-year follow-up study. Journal of Clinical Oncology 12:312–325

van-Leeuwen F E, Klokman W J, Veer M B et al 2000 Long-term risk of second malignancy in survivors of Hodgkin's disease treated during adolescence or young adulthood. Journal of Clinical Oncology 18:487–497

Werner-Wasik M, Madoc-Jones H 1993 Trental (pentoxifylline) relieves pain from postradiation fibrosis. International Journal of Radiation Oncology, Biology, Physics 25:757–758

Wilson W B, Perez G M, Kleinschmidt-Demasters B K 1987 Sudden onset of blindness in patients treated with oral CCNU and low-dose cranial irradiation. Cancer 59:901–907

Zagars G K, von-Eschenbach A C, Johnson D E et al 1987 Stage C adenocarcinoma of the prostate. An analysis of 551 patients treated with external beam radiation. Cancer 60:1489–1499

20

The future of supportive care in radiotherapy

Mary Wells   Sara Faithfull

INTRODUCTION

In the previous chapters of this book we have identified the physical, psychosocial and organisational context in which radiotherapy takes place and the site-specific issues affecting individuals undergoing treatment. Our emphasis on the experience and impact of radiotherapy at different stages of the cancer trajectory is deliberate. Although the actual delivery of radiotherapy treatment is confined to a relatively short space of time, the impact of that treatment can be far-reaching. Until recently, developments in radiotherapy care have focused on the potential for technical advances in treatment planning and delivery to improve outcomes such as survival, local recurrence and incidence of late effects. To a large extent, the everyday issues affecting patients undergoing radiotherapy have been overlooked, and the supportive care of these patients has been superficial.

The shortage of therapy radiographers, the relatively small number of clinical oncologists in the UK and the general lack of nurses employed in radiotherapy, have hampered the widespread provision of truly supportive care. The environment in which radiotherapy is administered and the sheer volume of patients being treated in most departments, largely prevent the opportunity for individualised support at the time of treatment. Similarly, most conventional on-treatment review clinics offer a brief encounter with a busy clinical oncologist, and are not necessarily conducive to individualised care. Patients' reflections of their experience of radiotherapy indicate that, by and large, their sense of being an individual is somehow lost in the process and delivery of treatment. Recent documents produced by patient groups emphasise the need for radiotherapy services to be more patient-centred (Clinical Oncology Patients' Liaison Group 1999, The National Cancer Alliance 1996).

It is interesting that developments in molecular oncology such as predictive assays (see Ch. 2) are moving us further towards the potential for treatment to be biologically tailored to the individual. Similarly, new radiotherapy techniques, such as conformal and intensity-modulated radiotherapy, also offer a more individualised approach to treatment. It is vital that the quest for an effective treatment approach that is biologically unique is mirrored by the development of a supportive care strategy which meets the needs of the individual person who is undergoing cancer treatment. If we are to change the experience of radiotherapy for individuals, we need investment, reorganisation and creativity. This chapter considers ways in which this might be achieved, and places the concept of supportive care at its centre.

WHAT IS SUPPORTIVE CARE?

Put simply, supportive care is an umbrella term for those aspects of healthcare concerned with the physical, psychosocial and spiritual issues faced by the person with cancer. The provision of supportive care in radiotherapy therefore relies on an understanding of the impact of cancer on the individual, as well as the impact of treatment itself. Our belief is that assessment is fundamental to supportive care, and that effective interventions to support the individual through the physical and psychosocial effects of radiotherapy must be based on that assessment. The previous chapters in this book suggest ways in which assessment and intervention might enhance the support of patients with specific physical and psychosocial concerns.

There are some similarities between the concepts of supportive care and social support, described in the literature as the contact with health carers, family or friends which can influence the stress of illness (Krishnasamy 1996, Wills 1985). Social support needs may be increased for those with cancer, due to the uncertainty and fear experienced during diagnosis and treatment (Courtens et al 1996, Dunkel-Schetter 1984). The support of family, friends and colleagues is seen to be particularly important during radiotherapy (Wengstrom & Haggmark 2001). However, supportive care in radiotherapy not only encompasses the psychosocial support of the patient with cancer, but also incorporates strategies aimed to prevent, alleviate and manage the physical effects of cancer and its treatment.

Without an appreciation of the complexity of support needs, healthcare professionals working in radiotherapy may fail to provide supportive care. The recent national (England and Wales) assessment of cancer care service frameworks and patients' experiences identified limited support and counselling services for patients. Indeed, few patients diagnosed with cancer had access to someone, such as a specialist nurse, who knew about their cancer and could provide the needed support (Commission for Health Improvement, 2001). The report concludes that, although cancer services have undoubtedly improved, there is still much to be achieved. Although better policies and guidelines may provide a template for the support of patients, a more fundamental shift in attitudes is required if care is to be provided in a truly patient-centred way.

Several of the chapters in this book use patients' own words to illustrate the impact of treatment. These narrative accounts provide us with powerful descriptions of the experience and meaning of radiotherapy, and remind us what it feels like to be on the receiving end of care. Such experiences are felt in a context of largely impersonal treatment environments, associated with vivid imagery, as illustrated in Solzhenitsyn's (1968) evocative account of life in a cancer ward, and more recently, in a qualitative study of patients' experiences of radiotherapy (Long 2001):

> *Through the square of skin that had been left clear on his stomach, through the layers of flesh and organs ... poured the harsh X-rays, their trembling vectors of electric and magnetic fields, unimaginable to the human mind*
>
> (Solzhenitsyn 1968, p. 73).

> *I think about the radioactive, like the bombs and everything that go off ... that's what I compare it with ...*
>
> *My father died of cancer many, many years ago ... I have memories of [him] laying on the bed and ... he was burnt on his chest and he looked terrible. That memory stayed with me all these years*
>
> (Long 2001, p. 465).

Several chapters in this book have referred to the fears and misconceptions that exist about radiotherapy, and explained the potential for the context in which care takes place to influence the experience of treatment. In order to develop supportive care into a reality, we must first address the contextual problems which prevent and obscure the provision of support.

THE ORGANISATION OF RADIOTHERAPY CARE

The structure and delivery of radiotherapy services are described in Chapter 1. Increasingly, patients undergoing radiotherapy attend on an outpatient basis, often from some distance away, thus leaving little time to assess, plan and implement supportive care. The demands of technology, the requirement for radiation safety and treatment accuracy and the insidious nature of many radiotherapy symptoms can obscure the support needs of patients on treatment. Services are organised so as to increase the throughput of patients, reduce waiting times and maximise machine time. On-treatment review clinics provide some opportunity to monitor side effects and symptoms as well as check dose and fractionation, but by no means do they enable a holistic assessment of the patient to take place. When treatment ends, discharge communication with primary care may be delayed and lacking in detail (Tanner & Myers 2002), making continuity of care into the community a significant challenge.

Evidence suggests that people feel ill-prepared for treatment and that reduced healthcare contact at the end of radiotherapy may leave those with physical or emotional symptoms feeling unsupported once treatment is complete. Most patients are monitored in conventional follow-up clinics on a monthly basis at most, and the benefits of such follow-up are increasingly being questioned. In the USA, Steinberg & Rose (1996) claim that the provision of hospital-based monitoring is important for two principal reasons: firstly, the early diagnosis of any cancer spread or recurrence, and secondly, the assessment of toxicity. These authors believe that the radiotherapist has a legal responsibility to monitor the effects of treatment and that this information is essential for quality assurance. There is, however, no convincing evidence that routine clinic visits following cancer therapy influence the long-term survival of patients, although they may provide reassurance.

Brada (1995) argues that this feeling of support engendered by clinical visits could be maintained without perpetuating the hospital and cancer physician-centred tradition of follow-up. He suggests that patients might be more accepting of this if they were informed of the lack of value of conventional follow-up, and states:

> If oncological services are to deliver truly patient-centred care, it should be patients themselves who are asked what services they want and what they expect from them. It is likely that the main desire is to be cured. Given the full knowledge that a ritual pilgrimage to the clinic does not provide any better chances of cure, would a patient still want to come? (p. 656)

Controversies about the purpose and value of on-treatment review and follow-up are likely to persist. However, it is clear that patients need support, information and advice during and after radiotherapy, and that toxicity monitoring is crucial. In the UK, alternative methods of achieving this are currently being tested. Recently there has been increasing interest in the potential for nurses and radiographers to review patients on treatment (Campbell et al 2000, Faithfull et al 2001, James et al 1994, Sardell et al 2000). Descriptive studies have shown that review clinic appointments with nurses are significantly more likely to include discussions about side effects, information and advice about treatment and psychosocial interactions than conventional medical appointments (Campbell et al 2000). A recent randomised trial confirms that patients are significantly more satisfied with the support they receive from specialist nurses and that nurse-led care during treatment is cheaper than conventional care, and is more focused on emotional issues and promoting health (Faithfull et al 2001).

The employment of radiographers in follow-up clinics and information/support roles can also make a positive contribution to care (Colyer & Hlahla 1999). Telephone (Collins 2001, Rose et al 1996) and drop-in clinics provide flexible ways of providing support to patients, particularly after treatment has finished, but these have not yet been rigorously evaluated. However, the potential for suitably qualified nurses and radiographers to manage on-treatment review clinics has now been endorsed by the Royal College of Radiologists (1999). Further development of advanced practitioner roles in both professions will provide a structure through which innovative approaches to care can grow (Department of Health 2000a,c).

If nurse- and radiographer-led clinics are to be successful, good communication and clear definition of roles and responsibility must exist. Colyer (1999) states (p. 187) that: 'it has become an article of faith that the quality of health care offered is directly proportional to the effectiveness of the interprofessional team'. Nowhere is this more relevant than in radiotherapy, where nurses, therapy radiographers and clinical oncologists work so closely together. However, the reality is that lack of communication and professional tensions present significant barriers to successful teamwork (Wells 1998). A Delphi survey carried out in Sweden (Wengstrom & Haggmark 1998) revealed that the most difficult nursing problems in relation to working with other professionals were lack of communication, lack of knowledge of their work and competence and lack of respect for or comprehension of each other's work. Given that Swedish nurses are jointly trained in nursing and therapy radiography, it could be assumed that the problems identified in the survey are likely to be felt by *both* professional groups in the UK.

Colyer (1999) suggest that practitioners in cancer care need to be liberated to decide how best to manage care, and that they must advance teamwork by engaging in dialogue at every level, continuing professional development, and devolving and sharing responsibility for clinical care. It is vital that nurses, therapy radiographers and oncologists work together towards a collaborative and coordinated approach to ensure that care is safe, seamless and supportive. Extending the role of nurses and radiographers into areas such as on-treatment review and follow-up requires the operational support and commitment of clinical oncologists as well as the professional development and education of the practitioners involved.

THE CULTURE OF CARE

The deficiencies in teamwork and the organisation of radiotherapy services are not the only constraints to the provision of supportive care. Corner (2001) suggests that there is a gap between 'you' (the health carer or healthcare system) and 'me' (the person in need of treatment). She proposes that the relationship between 'you' and 'me' is compromised by the power and dominance of biomedicine, the boundaries and tensions between professions and the architecture and environment of care settings. In radiotherapy, these obstacles are particularly apparent. The highly technical nature of treatment, the danger associated with radiation and the role conflict existing between different professional groups, contribute to a culture of care which is not always 'patient-friendly'. Patients' experiences demonstrate that the environment of care can be impersonal and alarming, and that although speed and efficiency are welcome, the corollary is that there is little time for any personal discussion about the impact of treatment. As one patient with breast cancer described (www.dipex.org):

> But with radiotherapy you are put in this horrible sort of machine thing. I'd just lie there and you haven't got, you know, you're a bit exposed, and everyone just leaves the room and you're left and there's all these lasers going across you. And it's dark. Yeah, I think I found that really horrible because you just feel so strange. And because you haven't got anybody near you. And no one can sort of sit in there with you and say that it's OK. And it's a strange feeling ... I understand why everyone leaves the room but how can this be good for me if everyone else has to, like, leave the room and go behind a closed door, and I sit here taking all this, these lasers going into my body? And they pull you know, you do feel a bit like a slab of meat because they pull you around and push you. I mean obviously just to get it right and they probably do it all day so it probably drives them mad. But you do feel like a slab of meat eventually, and that's ... yeah they probably don't talk, you know, they don't interact with you in the same way that the chemotherapy nurses did, so I think I found that quite an impersonal experience. I'd say that would probably be the only time when I ever felt that there wasn't much support.

Because of the radiation protection issues, daily contact with radiography staff is inevitably limited to the time immediately before and after treatment. With other patients waiting to be treated, this period of time is unlikely to offer the opportunity for comprehensive support. However, the personal approach of staff at this time can still make a difference. Similarly, the manner and degree of sensitivity shown by nurses and doctors in clinic can either destroy or create an atmosphere conducive to supportive care. The Clinical Oncology Patients' Liaison Group (1999) and National Cancer Alliance report (1996) both emphasise the importance of being treated as a person, and illustrate how much the attitude and approach of healthcare professionals can influence the 'humanity' of the treatment experience. Good communication, continuity of care, privacy, dignity and information are essential components of this humanity. However, these aspects, individually or together, are not enough unless patients feel cared for as people. As Corner (2001) points out, caring environments must change so that they make care of people's 'selves' a priority. In tandem with this, Corner believes that people who use healthcare must be given greater autonomy and assistance to manage their health themselves. She states:

> The challenge is to create a system in which the needs of individuals are addressed in the context of highly sophisticated and technologically advanced biomedicine, and equally sophisticated care-giving practices that sustain people's 'selves' are valued and promoted (p. 59).

THE WAY FORWARD

Turning supportive care into a reality in radiotherapy demands a new way of thinking, a more flexible way of working and a more holistic approach to the needs of patients undergoing treatment. We need to change the culture of care from one that functions for the convenience of the service to one which truly places the patient at its centre. This can only be achieved by looking through patients' eyes, auditing aspects of patients' journeys through the department and eliciting patients' views of services. We need to lobby for more resources for radiotherapy, both locally and nationally. Radiotherapy care has never attracted the funding and attention given to the treatment and care of patients having cytotoxic therapy. It is time to challenge this lack of attention and be proactive about bidding for more resources. In order to provide truly supportive care we need more nurses, more therapy radiographers, more physicists and more oncologists. We need to invest in information technology so as to improve communication and enable patients to access up-to-date information via computers and other media sources. Attention to the physical environment of care is also important. Patients deserve to wait for treatment in comfortable and pleasant surroundings where there is opportunity for privacy as well as interaction. Measures of healthcare quality now take this into account, viewing the patients' endorsement as the hallmark of a good treatment service (Centre for Health Improvement 2001, National Executive 2001).

Nurses, radiographers and oncologists must work together to break down professional boundaries, understand each other's contribution to care and develop complementary supportive care strategies which reflect their areas of particular expertise. Nurses and radiographers are ideally placed to lead the development of pre-treatment support, on-treatment review clinics and follow-up services which address the holistic needs of patients with cancer. Such services must enable comprehensive assessment of the impact of radiotherapy in the context of the patient's life and cancer journey, so that care is not confined to the specific period of time in which radiotherapy treatment is delivered. Assessment of treatment toxicity is a priority, and systematic use of toxicity scores or quality-of-life tools should be the basis for care provision.

Healthcare professionals working with patients undergoing radiotherapy must abandon their somewhat fatalistic approach to acute side effects, and explore ways of preventing and alleviating the discomfort of symptoms. Underlying problems with pain and nutritional difficulties must be addressed in order to prevent further deterioration and promote comfort during treatment. We need to utilise existing evidence for the management of radiation-induced morbidity, and develop benchmarks against which services can be assessed (Ellis 2000). Where there is no evidence, we need to produce creative solutions to the management of symptoms, using the knowledge and experience of patients and members of the multidisciplinary team. We need to create networks with colleagues in other centres to enable collaboration and sharing of practice to take place and research efforts to be streamlined and coordinated.

Research

The lack of an evidence basis for supportive care has been identified in almost every chapter as a barrier to evidence-based practice. To address this deficit, investment is required in both clinical and health evaluation research. The scope for clinical research is enormous, given that relatively few existing studies focus on the experience and effects of treatment from the patient's point of view. There is a need to identify symptoms, physical and psychosocial needs and gaps as well as develop and test interventions designed to meet those needs. In addition, health evaluation research is required, to enable the investigation and evaluation of services and roles aimed at improving standards of care.

One of the problems is that, even where evidence exists, practitioners may be unaware and practice is slow to change. It is important that we identify, collate and disseminate existing research findings through systematic review and guidelines development. However, much of the research literature relating to supportive care in radiotherapy comes from small studies undertaken by nurses for higher degrees, and a great deal of this work lacks statistical power (Faithfull 1996). Despite this drawback, many small qualitative studies provide crucial insights into the experiences and nature of patients' problems, which can then form the basis of intervention research. It is important that intervention studies use well-validated questionnaires and clinical tools which are sensitive to radiation-induced symptoms (Bond & Thomas 1991). If scientific research into the radiobiological response to radiotherapy is able to reveal characteristics that predispose certain individuals to more severe radiation reactions, interventions can be more appropriately targeted to those most at risk. The development of multicentre collaborations is essential, so as to increase substantially the number of patients entering clinical trials.

Undertaking health evaluation research (which aims to evaluate the overall quality of a service) can be a daunting prospect, but many healthcare trusts and universities have experts who can facilitate and assist with the design, implementation and data analysis of such studies. Health evaluation research utilises a whole range of methods – clinical audit, service mapping, needs assessment, patient satisfaction, quality of life and economic evaluation. Adopting a participatory and inclusive approach to research is essential for planning services, encouraging experimentation and evolution of practice (DoH 1992). Clinical staff have a pivotal role to play in the audit and identification of aspects of care which are lacking, and small-scale projects can still influence decision-making by drawing attention to areas of the service which require further development (Robson 2000). As Table 20.1 illustrates, many aspects of practice could be assessed using health evaluation strategies. However, research studies of this nature are inevitably complex and conventional designs are not always appropriate for the purpose. The Medical Research Council has addressed some of the problems of evaluating complex interventions using a framework of theory, modelling, exploration, description, piloting, intervention and evaluation (Medical Research Council 2000). The development and evaluation of supportive care strategies in radiotherapy require a research design that is flexible and dynamic enough to cope with the changing needs of individuals, and the Medical Research Council framework provides the basis for a possible approach.

It is important that new research is both well coordinated and complementary. The expansion of research registers, cancer networks and National Cancer Research Institutes (NCRI) provides a focus for development programmes and contributes much towards this goal (www.doh.gov.uk/research/rd). At a more local level, practitioners must increasingly take responsibility for accessing and disseminating relevant research findings so that their practice is evidence-based. This is by no means straightforward, and they require leadership, support, supervision and

Table 20.1 Health evaluation and research

Type of research	Specific examples in relation to radiotherapy
Mapping patient pathways	Identification of areas of difficulty or delay in the radiotherapy service
	Exploration of transitions in care, e.g. planning and preparation for treatment, on-treatment review, follow-up and continuing care
Needs assessment	Patients requiring palliative radiotherapy
	Care provision for patients from ethnic minorities
	Needs for patients with specific cancers
Systematic review	Management of site-specific and general symptoms
Clinical audit	Waiting times
	Patient-friendly services
	Information resources
	Documentation and assessment
Patient satisfaction	Patients' experiences of treatment
Survey research	Incidence and nature of symptoms/problems in the radiotherapy population, e.g. pain, nutritional difficulties
Qualitative research	The experience and impact of planning, treatment, acute and late side effects and transitions in care
Intervention research	New approaches to the management of toxicity
Economic evaluation	New treatments or models of care delivery
Role/service evaluation	Prescribing practices of clinicians
	Symptom management strategies
	Nurse/radiographer-led clinics

education, as well as an organisational culture that genuinely embraces the concept of clinical governance (Scally & Donaldson 1998).

Education

The lack of an evidence base for supportive care in radiotherapy is certainly influenced by the general lack of knowledge and understanding about radiotherapy, not only amongst patients and their carers, but also amongst many healthcare professionals. One of the reasons for this is that education and training programmes have, historically, placed little emphasis on the supportive aspects of caring for radiotherapy patients, instead concentrating on the technical aspects of radiotherapy or the care of patients receiving apparently more intensive or demanding treatments, such as chemotherapy.

There is a need for investment in the education of healthcare professionals who are in a position to provide supportive care in radiotherapy. Flexible pathways are required, which prepare knowledgeable and skilled practitioners to adapt to the changing needs of radiotherapy patients at different stages of the treatment trajectory and in different care settings. Initiatives are already in place so as to widen the entry base for nurse training and change the style of education offered (DoH 2000a). There is increasing recognition that multiple entry levels allow students with varying academic abilities to enter nursing (DoH 2000a, UK Central Council 1999) and alternative entry routes are currently being considered for radiographers. There is enormous scope for developing common foundation programmes for different groups, whereby healthcare professionals can work alongside each other from an early stage in their careers, thus helping to overcome some of the existing suspicions and barriers between professions. It is also vital that education and service providers work together to develop multiprofessional training opportunities for qualified practitioners which address the complexities of interdisciplinary working as well as the importance of supportive care issues.

These educational initiatives are likely to take many years to come to fruition and, in the meantime, continuous professional development for all practitioners must be seen as a priority. In addition to the core competencies and transferable skills necessary for radiotherapy practice (for example, radiation safety and communication), continuous professional development programmes also need to incorporate the assessment and management of common side effects.

Because funding is limited and workload pressures are intense, many staff are discouraged from undertaking research or developing new initiatives in practice. Much has been written in the past on the theory–practice gap evident in healthcare, and studies have identified that practitioners have difficulty accessing, appreciating and using research evidence in practice. It is now a professional and service requirement that practitioners develop these skills (UKCC 1999), but the organisational support and commitment must also exist so that staff are encouraged to undertake education, initiate changes and evaluate practice. Clinical career pathways, which recognise research as a valid and valuable activity towards changing practice, are also needed (DoH, 2000c,d). The potential for advanced practice roles in nursing and therapy radiography is now being supported at a national level (DoH 2000a) but there is still considerable ambiguity over the precise remit and definition of such roles. None of the new nurse consultant posts in the UK focus on the needs of patients undergoing radiotherapy, and many new senior radiographer roles concentrate on the technical aspects of delivering new therapies rather than the supportive care which is required. Controversy also exists over the educational preparation appropriate to advanced practitioners, although programmes at Masters and Doctoral level are continuously developing so as to meet these needs.

CONCLUSION

The future of supportive care in radiotherapy is a considerable challenge, given ever-increasing patient numbers, continually advancing technology and acute shortages in key staff groups. It is perhaps inevitable that the focus of most radiotherapy services is on the delivery of safe treatment, and that those aspects of care which are seen as optional extras get neglected. The aim of this book is to argue that supportive care is not an optional extra, and that patients' physical and psychosocial needs before, during and after radiotherapy deserve greater attention. We need to build the evidence base, to undertake meaningful research and to invest in education and collaborative practice. In developing guidelines and strategies for supportive care, we must recognise the unique needs of the individual as well as the benefits of a standardised approach to care. The organisation and delivery of radiotherapy care need to be critically examined in order to make services more patient-centred. Recent investment in cancer services (DoH 2000b, Scottish Executive Health Department 2001) presents a unique and timely opportunity for us to reconsider our approach to the care of radiotherapy patients. We need to seize that opportunity and work collaboratively to direct energy and resources towards real improvements in radiotherapy services. Most importantly, we need to listen and respond to the experiences of patients who are undergoing treatment to ensure that supportive care in radiotherapy becomes a reality.

REFERENCES

Bond S, Thomas L 1991 Issues in measuring outcomes of nursing. Journal of Advanced Nursing 16:1492–1502
Brada M 1995 Is there a need to follow-up cancer patients? European Journal of Cancer 31A:655–657
Campbell J, German L, Dodwell D 2000 Radiotherapy outpatient review: a nurse-led clinic. Clinical Oncology 12:104–107
Clinical Oncology Patients' Liaison Group 1999 Making your radiotherapy service more patient-friendly. Board of the Faculty of Clinical Oncology, Royal College of Radiologists, London
Collins D, 2001 Telephone follow-up clinics. Macmillan Voice 17:11–12
Colyer H 1999 Interprofessional teams in cancer care. Radiography 5:187–189
Colyer H, Hlahla T 1999 Information and support radiographers: a critical review of the role and its significance for the provision of cancer services. Journal of Radiotherapy in Practice 1:117–124
Commission for Health Improvement 2001 NHS cancer care in England and Wales. Audit Commission, London
Corner J 2001 Between you and me: closing the gap between people and health care. Nuffield Trust. H M Queen Elizabeth the Queen Mother Fellowship, vol. 9. the Stationery Office, London

Courtens A, Stevens F, Crebolder H et al 1996 Longitudinal study on quality of life and social support in cancer patients: Cancer Nursing 19:162–169

Department of Health 1992 Report of the taskforce on the strategy for research in nursing, midwifery and health visiting. National Health Service, London

Department of Health 2000a Meeting the Challenge: a strategy for the allied health professions. National Health Service, London

Department of Health 2000b The NHS cancer plan. National Health Service, London

Department of Health 2000c The nursing contribution to cancer care. National Health Service, London

Department of Health 2000d Towards a strategy for nursing research and development. National Health Service, London

Dunkel-Schetter C 1984 Social support and cancer: findings based on patient interviews and their implications. Journal of Social Issues 35:120–155

Ellis J 2000 Sharing the evidence: clinical practice benchmarking to improve continously the quality of care. Journal of Advanced Nursing 32:215–225

Faithfull S 1996 How many subjects are needed in a research sample in palliative care? Palliative Medicine 10:259–261

Faithfull S, Corner J, Myer L et al 2001 Evaluation of nurse-led care for men undergoing pelvic radiotherapy. British Journal of Cancer 18:1853–1864

James N, Guerrero D, Brada M 1994 Who should follow up cancer patients? Nurse specialist based outpatient care and the introduction of a phone clinic system. Clinical Oncology 6:283–287

Krishnasamy M 1996 Social support and the patient with cancer; a consideration of the literature. Journal of Advanced Nursing 23:757–762

Long L 2001 Being informed: undergoing radiation therapy. Cancer Nursing 24:463–468

Medical Research Council 2000 A framework for development and evaluation of RCTs for complex interventions to improve health. MRC Health Services and Public Health Research Board, London

National Cancer Alliance 1996 'Patient-centred cancer services'? What patients say. National Cancer Alliance, Oxford

National Executive 2001 Manual of cancer services standards. London, Department of Health

Robson C 2000 Small-scale evaluation. Sage, London

Rose M, Shrader-Bogen C, Korlath G et al 1996 Identifying patient symptoms after radiotherapy using a nurse-managed telephone interview. Oncology Nursing Forum 23:99–102

Royal College of Radiologists 1999 Skills mix in clinical oncology. Royal College of Radiologists, London

Sardell S, Sharpe G, Ashley S et al 2000 Evaluation of a nurse-led telephone clinic in the follow-up of patients with malignant glioma. Clinical Oncology 12:36–41

Scally G, Donaldson L 1998 Clinical governance and the drive for quality improvement in the new NHS in England. British Medical Journal 317:61–65

Scottish Executive Health Department 2001 Cancer in Scotland: Action for change. Scottish Executive Health Department, Edinburgh

Solzhenitsyn A 1968 Cancer ward. Penguin, London

Steinberg M, Rose C 1996 Post-treatment follow-up of radiation oncology patients in a managed care environment. International Journal of Radiation Oncology, Biology, Physics 35:113–116

Tanner G, Myers P 2002 Secondary and primary care communication: impressions of the quality of consultant communication with special regard to cancer patients. Primary Health Care Research and Development 3:23–28

UK Central Council 1999 Fitness for practice. United Kingdom Central Council for Nursing, Midwifery and Health Visiting, London

Wells M 1998 What's so special about radiotherapy nursing? European Journal of Oncology Nursing 2:162–168

Wengstrom Y, Haggmark C 1998 Assessing nursing problems of importance for the development of nursing care in a radiation therapy department. Cancer Nursing 21:50–56

Wengstrom Y, Haggmark C 2001 Coping with radiation therapy. Strategies used by women with breast cancer. Cancer Nursing 24:264–271

Wills T 1985 Supportive functions of interpersonal relationships. In: Cohen S, Syme L (eds.) Social support and health. Academic Press, New York p 61–82

Index

Numbers in bold refer to figures and tables.

G

Gag reflex suppression, topical anaesthetics, 195
Gamma rays, 75
Gargles, 192
Gastric emptying, increasing, 221
Gastrointestinal effects, 79, **115**, **116**, 247–264
  aetiology, 249–252
  areas for further research, 264
  factors influencing occurrence, 252–253
  impact, 254–255
  key clinical points, summary, 263–264
  late complications, 359–362
  management, 255–263
    algorithms, **256**, **257**
    diarrhoea, 259–262
    nausea and vomiting, 255, 256–259
    proctitis, 263
  symptom patterns, 253–254
Gender, and patient information, 44, 45
Gene therapy, 93
General information tapes, 54
General Medical Council, 13, 29
General practitioners (GPs), communication with, 66, 67, 68
Genetic code, 72–73, 77
Genital lymphoedema, 290, 292, 293, 294, 297
Genitourinary side effects, **116**
Gentian violet, 151, 152, **154**, **155**
Gliomas, cranial irradiation effects, 274
Global symptom impact, **103**
Glucose turnover, increased, 205
Glutamine, oral, 194
Glutathione, 92
Glycosaminoglycans, 228
GM-CSF
  mouthwashes, 195
  systemic, 194–195
Gonadotrophin-releasing hormone agonists, 307
Gonads, damage to, 79, 304, 348
  ovarian effects, 305–306
  testicular effects, 306, 348
Gram-negative bacteria, oral mucositis, 195
Granisetron, **258**
Grays (Gy), 75
Grief response, body image changes, 327, 328, 332
Growth factors, 172
Gynaecological cancer
  audit of toxicity data, 99–100
  brachytherapy, 7, 91–92, **121**, 122
  elemental diet study, 259, **261**
  sexual issues, 312–313
  urinary symptoms, **230**, 231
  see also Cervical cancer

H

Habit-based oncology, 31
Haematological side effects, **80**
  radiation morbidity scoring data, **117**
  see also Blood count
Haematospermia, 314
Haematuria, 229, 235, 366
Haemorrhagic cystitis, 365, 366
Hair loss, 325
Hair washing, cranial irradiation, 145, **149**
Hand, small muscle wasting, 271
Head and neck cancer
  breathlessness, **173**, 174
  chemoradiotherapy, 19, 91, 182
  continuous hyperfractionated accelerated radiotherapy (CHART), 9, 106, 184
  dietary advice, **217**, 218
  fatigue, 119, 120
  lymphoedema, 292, 293, 294, 297
  nutritional supplements, 216
  oropharyngeal problems see Oropharyngeal effects
  partial alopecia, 325
  sexual problems, 311
  tumour growth during treatment, 81
  weight loss, 190, 207
Health evaluation research, 378–380
Health Professions Council, 13
Health Technology Board for Scotland (HTBS), 13
Health-related quality of life (HRQOL), 104, 293
Heart
  late complications, 354–357
  side effects, **116**
  tolerance dose, **350**
Heliox administration, 175
Helium laser treatment, 194
Hemibody irradiation, 169
Hepatitis, 362, **363**
Hidden costs, radiotherapy treatment, 65
History, radiotherapy department development, 2
Hoarseness, 185
Hodgkin's disease
  coronary artery disease, 357
  fatigue, 120
  patients' rating of side effects, 50
  pericarditis, 356
  radiation-induced malignancies, 367
Homeopathic preparations, skin reaction management, **149**
Hormone replacement therapy, 305, 306, 308, 312
Horner's syndrome, 272
Hospital Anxiety and Depression (HAD) scale, 49, 106